Management of Back Pain

I will praise you for I am fearfully and wonderfully made;
your works are wonderful, I know that full well.

Psalm 139, 14

For Churchill Livingstone

Publisher: Mike Parkinson
Project Editor: Lowri Daniels
Copy Editor: Nairn Reed
Indexer: Laurence Errington
Production Controller: Debra Barrie
Sales Promotion Executive: Kathy Crawford

Management of Back Pain

Richard W. Porter MD FRCS FRCS(Edin)
Professor of Orthopaedic Surgery, University of Aberdeen,
Aberdeen, UK

SECOND EDITION

CHURCHILL LIVINGSTONE
EDINBURGH LONDON MADRID MELBOURNE NEW YORK AND TOKYO 1993

CHURCHILL LIVINGSTONE
Medical Division of Longman Group UK Limited

Distributed in the United States of America by Churchill
Livingstone Inc., 650 Avenue of the Americas, New York,
N.Y. 10011, and by associated companies, branches and
representatives throughout the world.

First edition 1986
Second edition 1993

ISBN 0-443-04630-1

British Library of Cataloguing in Publication Data
A catalogue record for this book is available from the
British Library.

Library of Congress Cataloging in Publication Data
A catalog record for this book is available from the Library of
Congress.

The
publisher's
policy is to use
**paper manufactured
from sustainable forests**

Produced by Longman Singapore Publishers (Pte) Ltd.
Printed in Singapore.

Contents

SECTION 5
The 'problem back' patient

SECTION 6
Prevention

Contributors

Paul Butt MD FRCR FRCP
Consultant Radiologist, St James University
Hospital, Leeds, UK

John Dove FRCS
Consultant Orthopaedic Surgeon, Stoke on
Trent Spinal Service, Hartshill, Stoke on Trent,
UK

John A. McCulloch MD FRCS(C)
Professor of Orthopaedics, Northeastern Ohio
Universities College of Medicine, Rootstown,
Ohio, USA

John A. N. Shepperd MA FRCS(Edin)
Consultant Orthopaedic Surgeon, Royal East
Sussex Hospital, Hastings, UK

Francis W. Smith MD FRCP(Edin) FFRRCSI
DARD
Consultant in Nuclear Medicine, Aberdeen
Royal Infirmary, Aberdeen, UK

Preface to the Second Edition

This second edition of *Management of Back Pain* is necessary because of the remarkable progress in all disciplines related to the lumbar spine. The basic scientists have expanded our horizons in biomechanics, disc biochemistry, neurophysiology and the pain mechanism, but there is advance on every front like an incoming tide. In the field of imaging we are embarrassed by the wealth of new information. And because these techniques reveal much symptomless pathology, we value new understandings in clinical assessment.

A similar revolution has occurred in therapy, with a plethora of new surgical techniques for the protruding disc, the compromised nerve root and the painful unstable spine. In conservative management we are learning the dangers of enforced bed rest, and functional rehabilitation has come of age. There is hope for the patients in distress with behavioural modification programmes. And manipulative techniques are being favourably reviewed. Inevitably many methods run ahead of our knowledge of the natural history, but progress is remarkable.

This edition remains a monograph but I am indebted to the help from many quarters. John McCulloch with his unique North American experience writes the chapter on MRI. Paul Butt describes the place and scope of radiology, and Frank Smith writes an important chapter on the diagnostic value of nuclear medicine. My friends John Shepperd and John Dove contribute to chapters on surgical techniques, and in the basic sciences Chris Main and Richard Aspden have had their influence.

This book is written from the perspective of a surgeon trying to understand the complexity of lumbar spine disorders. It cannot be comprehensive, but I hope its logical sequence from the basic sciences to clinical investigation, then a description of various back pain syndromes and management methods, will help others who are interested in this fascinating disorder.

Aberdeen, 1993   R.W.P.

Preface to the First Edition

It is not an easy task to write a book about back pain, when one is more aware of our ignorance than our knowledge. Back pain is but a symptom. The possible causes are legion, some of which we find, and some elude us. But the quest lends a fascination that I hope is reflected in these chapters.

The book falls naturally into three sections. We start with the basic sciences, then recognizable back pain syndromes with their management, and finally ways in which back pain may be prevented. 'Management' is a more appropriate word than 'treatment', the latter suggesting therapy that will lead to a cure. With backs this is rarely possible, and even following surgery a cure is relative. Management means sharing with the patients an understanding of the source of pain, and how the natural history of the condition can be used to their advantage, rather than be aggravated by miscalculated daily activity and misplaced therapy. Management is the art of the possible; cures are a little more difficult.

I remember a preacher friend telling me that he always tried to be informative, interesting and inspiring. I hope that you will find these qualities here. Information about backs has exploded in recent years and I pass on in a constructed form what I have learnt from others. Like Paul the apostle, I am a debtor. Backs are interesting when we apply all the available knowledge to unravel the diagnostic riddle of 'what is wrong?', and more

so as we curiously ask: 'what is the mechanism of that patient's behaviour?'.

But we need more. We need a breath of inspiration if our understanding of back pain is to move forward. Some of our steps when tested will be proved wrong, but try we must. The quest has barely started. The history of back pain matches the history of man, and we have only just begun to ask 'Why?'. To think we have made more than the first faltering steps would be presumptuous. Inspiration means freedom to be original, and if there are any new concepts in this book, they are to be tested by experience.

The untimely death of Bill Parke has robbed us of his help in Chapter 8, 'Radiological investigation', but we quote his writings and include his concepts.

No treatise on the subject can be universally acceptable, when the spectrum of opinion is so wide. Neither can it be comprehensive. I have not described in detail surgical technique, nor have I dealt in depth with back pain of inflammatory origin. One can only describe the view from where you are, and mine is an orthopaedic vantage, assisted by my good friend and radiologist, Paul Butt. I hope it will complement the work of other disciplines, stimulate thought, help us move forwards, and ultimately be of value to the patient with the painful back.

Doncaster, 1986   R.W.P.

Acknowledgements

I would like to thank Mrs Irene Wells for her secretarial assistance, and Mr Keith Duguid and members of his photographic department at Aberdeen Royal Infirmary. Thanks, of course, for the tolerance of Christine and the family.

R.W.P.

Introduction

1. Upright man

A book about the management of back pain should really start with a statement about the healthy spine and the harmony of spinal form and function; thus a chapter on 'Upright man', before proceeding to focus on pathology, pain mechanisms and methods to modify disability. Though surrounded by patients with spinal disorders, we are increasingly impressed by the lifetime function of the spine. We question the concept that the spine is a mistake of evolution, struggling to do a good job in the upright posture. Rather, its form seems to match its function.

The one physical attribute making man unique among his vertebrate cousins is his upright stature. Other primates may enjoy the canopy of the tropical forest, sometimes climbing, sometimes semi-upright, but man alone is comfortable and confident with the upright bipedal stance.

The spine has three complementary roles, all taxed by the upright posture. It must be strong and supportive, protect the neurological structures within the vertebral canal and be sufficiently flexible in various postures (Fig. 1.1). To what degree are these three roles compatible with each other, and with the demands of being upright? Is it true that back pain is related to a failure of these roles in the upright stance?

THE STRENGTH OF THE SPINE

Load-bearing

In Chapter 4 we consider the failure of spinal structures, but it is important to be reminded that the spine generally does not fail. Much of the time, and for most people it is successful in its load-bearing characteristics, some of which are quite

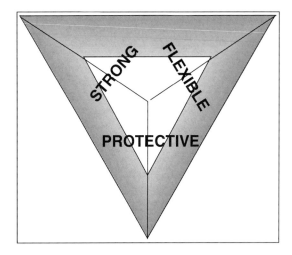

Fig. 1.1 Three complementary functions of the spine.

unique to the human spine. For example, how does the lower lumbar spine accommodate the relatively large loads in the upright posture?

Bone density is related to physical stress, and it would therefore be physiologically possible for the lower lumbar vertebrae to increase in bone density in response to increased load (Fig. 1.2). In practice, however, the density is the same throughout the human spine. In mass per unit volume does not change in relation to load, but rather it matches its increasing load with an increasing cross-sectional area (Fig. 1.3) (Brinckman et al 1989).

Comparative anatomy confirms this principle. Chimpanzees which are semi-upright have larger caudal than cranial vertebrae, but a lesser difference than humans (Fig. 1.4). Quadrupedal sheep have cervical vertebrae as large as those in

3

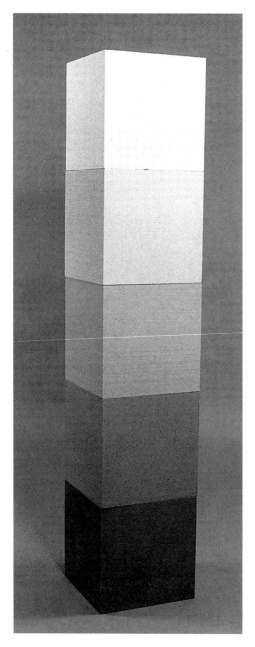

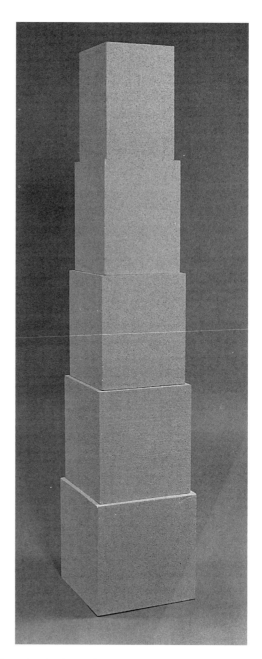

Fig. 1.2   A model of a potentially stable tower system of five cubes of equal size. The cubes of greatest density are at the base, with cubes of lesser density above.

Fig. 1.3   An alternative stable design, with five cubes of equal density, the larger cubes are at the base with an increased cross-sectional area.

the lumbar spine. If human vertebrae had accommodated to load-bearing by increasing density, this would have been compatible with a recent change from quadrupedal to an upright stance, but this is not what we observe. This increase in size of the lumbar spine which matches the increased load-bearing is also preformed. Before the infant stands, the lower lumbar vertebrae are relatively large, ready for the upright posture.

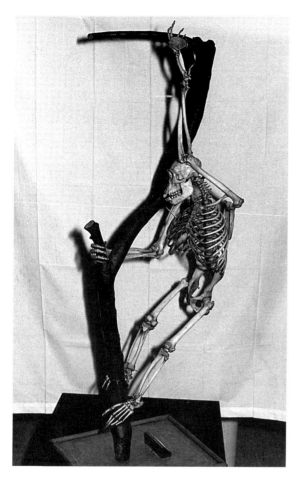

Fig. 1.4 The chimpanzee is semi-upright. The lower lumbar vertebrae are relatively larger than those of the upper spine, but the difference is not as marked as in man. There is no lumbar lordosis, a feature of man's upright stance, and the lower ribs are in close proximity to the pelvic brim.

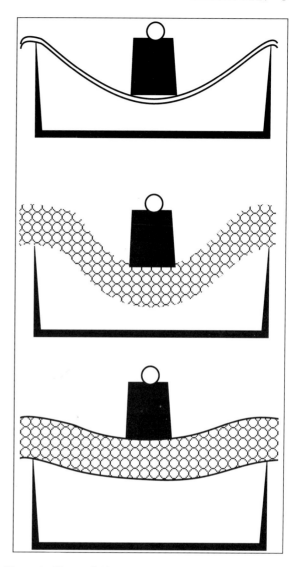

Fig. 1.5 Sheets of thin card on two supports readily deform under load. A block of foam rubber also deforms under load. A sandwich of the same foam rubber between two sheets of card can support a greater load.

VERTEBRAL STRUCTURE

The internal structure of the vertebrae also has useful load-bearing qualities. Figure 1.5 shows a piece of card which might represent a sheet of compact bone. When placed on two supports it readily deforms with a load. Two pieces fare little better. A thick piece of sponge could represent cancellous bone, and this also easily deforms with load. However, when the same test is applied to a composite sandwich of the materials — a sponge between two sheets of card — there is minimal deformation. In the construction industry, this is called 'foam filling'. It is light in weight and strong. It is also the form of many bones, especially the vertebral bodies. Cancellous bone sandwiched between cortical endplates combines lightness of weight and strength.

Lumbar lordosis

The lumbar lordosis is a characteristic of the upright posture. In the past it has been described as an unfortunate necessity, because when man stood erect he had to throw his lumbar spine backwards. But now we find that a lordosis has distinct advantages. The chimpanzee's spine has one long kyphotic curve, but upright man has a secondary lumbar lordotic curve which develops when the infant learns to stand upright. Aspden (1989) was the first to recognize the biomechanical significance of this lordotic curve and suggested that it contributes to the spine's considerable strength. It enables man to lift several times his own body weight when other primates do not even lift the equivalent of body weight. Perhaps they do not try! Biomechanically, however, the lumbar arch has advantages. The principles of the load-bearing characteristics of an arch are described in Chapter 4. Far from being a mistake or a disadvantage, the lumbar lordosis seems to be an integral part of its strength (Fig. 1.6).

We might ask, why does the strength of the spine sometimes fail? Is this not a sign of inherent weakness? The mechanism of osteoporotic fracture is still unresolved, but skeletal failure is not unique to the upright posture. Racehorses and poultry suffer from osteoporotic fractures, and the hunt is on for environmental factors that might affect bone strength in later life. Provided the bone quality and quantity are satisfactory, the gross structure of the spine is not only adequate for a lifetime of load-bearing in the upright posture, but it also enjoys a useful margin of safety.

PROTECTION OF THE NEUROLOGICAL STRUCTURES WITHIN THE VERTEBRAL CANAL

The spine is strong to support the upright human frame but it also has to be protective for the spinal cord and nerve roots. This protection from external trauma is highly efficient, but more complex is its ability to protect the neurological tissues from insult within. Restricted space within the vertebral canal can be a clinical problem when disc or degenerative change or excessive segmental movement compromise the canal. In general, however, the spine is well endowed with a capacious vertebral canal and it enjoys a margin of safety for its neural contents.

In early life the developing neural tissues have an intimate relationship with surrounding bone. Much as hydrocephalus or microcephalus affects the skull size, so the neural contents exert an epigenetic influence on the neural arch. There is

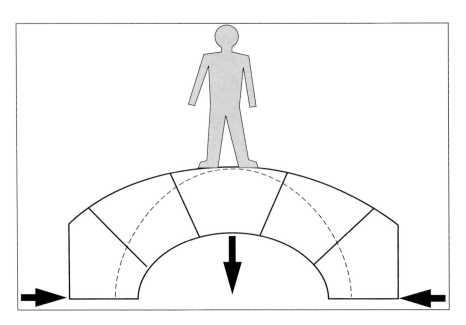

Fig. 1.6   A model of polystyrene blocks shaped into an arch. The system is very strong provided there is satisfactory abutment at each end — the thrust-line stays within the arch.

enough space for comfort and a margin to spare. By 4 years of age the canal's growth is largely complete (Fig. 1.7), and though the vertebral body is still relatively small the canal is mature and is usually adequate. Archaeological measurements show, as expected, a steady reduction in canal size down to the fourth lumbar level. Less nerves in the vertebral canal require less space. The increase in size at L5 (Fig. 1.8) is difficult to explain, but it does confer an advantage at a site where there is an acute lumbosacral angle and sometimes a trefoil shape, and at a site where the spine is prone to develop degenerative change.

Constitutional spinal stenosis which affects a small percentage of the population may have a genetic component, but several studies identify early environmental factors which also might stunt canal growth (Clark et al 1980, Porter & Pavitt 1987) (Chapter 6). Environmental insults before 4 years of age, and particularly in utero, may permanently affect the canal. Never reaching maturity and with little catch-up growth after 4 years of age, it remains stenotic. Given a good start in life, however, the canal is large enough to protect the nerves in health, and it has a margin to spare in disease.

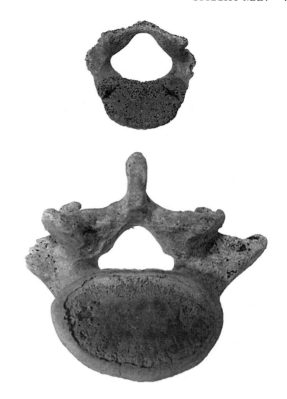

Fig. 1.7 Photographs of a 4-year-old infant's fifth lumbar vertebra above, and an adult fifth lumbar vertebra below. The adult vertebral body is much larger, but the cross-sectional area of the vertebral canal is much the same in the two specimens. (Reproduced with the permission of Doncaster Royal Infirmary.)

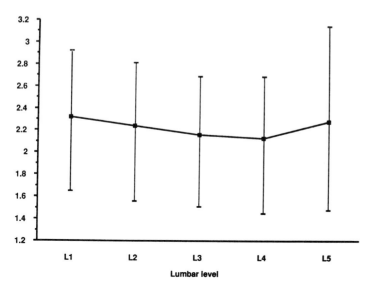

Fig. 1.8 A graph to show the mean cross-sectional area of the vertebral canal and the 10th and 90th percentiles from L1 to L5 from 240 archaeological spines. The canal reduces in area from L1 to L4 and widens again at L5.

FLEXIBILITY

A flexible spine is not essential to upright man, but it makes a big difference. The stiff spine of anky-losing spondylitis is capable of certain function but it is not very efficient. It is the segmental nature of the spine that provides for change of posture and the generation of torque to assist the pelvis and lower limbs when walking. To what degree is flexibility compatible with the spine's other roles of strength and protection, and is this affected by the upright posture?

The role of the intervertebral disc

Segmental failure of an intervertebral disc might be considered the essential key to understanding mechanical back pain, but much of the time the disc is healthy and highly successful in permitting a flexible spine. Although the upright posture increases the stresses on the lumbar discs, there is a small but significant bonus to disc nutrition from being upright. This largest avascular structure of the body receives its nutrition by diffusion. The large interlacing molecules of proteoglycan exert their strong osmotic pressure attracting water into the disc, reaching an equilibrium with the hyd-rostatic pressure which is encouraging water to extrude from the disc (Urban & McMullin 1988) (Fig. 1.9, also Ch. 4). The diurnal changes in posture significantly affect disc volume and aid fluid transport and nutrition. Because a change in axial load also affects the cell biochemistry, there may be a useful cellular compensation for the up-right posture.

The difference between disc degeneration and ageing is unresolved, but disc degeneration is nei-ther an inevitable consequence of being upright nor of being old. Twin studies suggest that the genetic component of disc degeneration is small compared with environmental factors. Smoking is important as is vibration (Frymoyer et al 1983, Deyo & Bass 1989, Boshinzen et al 1992), and there are factors yet to be identified which affect the disc's fluid transport system — at the end-plate, the matrix pathway and the cell membrane.

Structure of the disc

The gross structure of the disc with alternating

Healthy disc

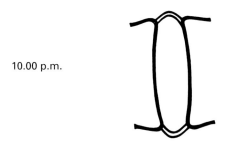

10.00 p.m.

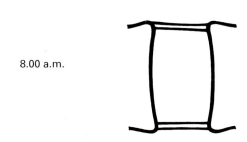

8.00 a.m.

Fig. 1.9   Diagram to show the diurnal change in fluid content of the intervertebral disc. When the hydrostatic pressure is reduced during recumbency, the unopposed osmotic pressure causes fluid to be imbibed.

layers of parallel fibres of collagen in the annulus is also recognized as appropriate for the up-right posture. It produces a strong radial ply effect, withstanding great compression forces (Fig. 1.10). A vertical load to the spine will not damage a healthy disc; the vertebrae will fracture first (Adams & Hutton 1982). The disc morphology is well able to cope with major axial forces applied in the upright posture.

Angular or rotational displacement risks da-mage to the neurological structures, but the angle of fibre orientation of the annulus restrains rotation to about 3° (Hickey & Hukins 1980). Provided the spine is not loaded and the disc is healthy, rotation is easily restrained by the fibres of the annulus. Moreover, a loaded disc benefits from two guardians, the apophyseal joints and the musculoligamentous system.

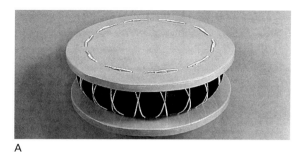

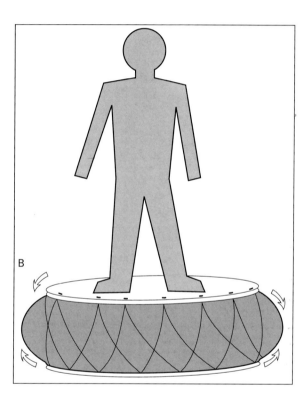

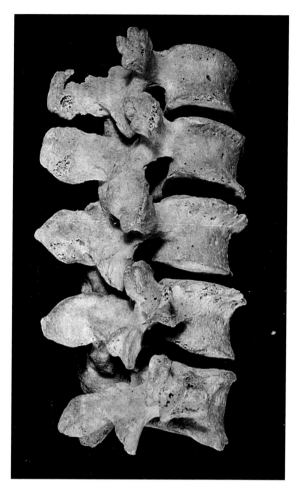

Fig. 1.11   Five Romano-British 3rd century lumbar vertebrae. The sagitally orientated apophyseal joints restrain rotation.

Fig. 1.10   A model of an intervertebral disc, with a football bladder between two wooden plates, supported by oblique strands of rubber (**A**). This system is able to carry considerable loads (**B**).

Apophyseal joints

The sagittal orientation of the lumbar apophyseal joints restrains rotation (Fig. 1.11), more so when the spine is extended. The flexed spine, however, disengages the apophyseal joints, risking dangerous degrees of rotation and injury to the annulus.

The neuromuscular system

In the process of lifting, however, a second guardian — the neuromuscular system — responds to ensure that the lumbar spine remains lordotic and stiff (Fig. 1.12). The diaphragm, the abdominal muscles and the pelvic floor contract, increasing the intra-abdominal pressure. In upright man, the lumbar lordosis uniquely throws the lumbar spine forwards into the abdominal cavity. On three sides it is surrounded by a pneumatic splint. It is impossible to lift a heavy weight without the lumbar spine being stiffened, the apophyseal joints in tight-pack, and the discs protected from rotation — unless, of course, there is a slip, trip or fall, with flexion and torsion before the reflexes can respond.

Closely applied to the spine are the psoas and

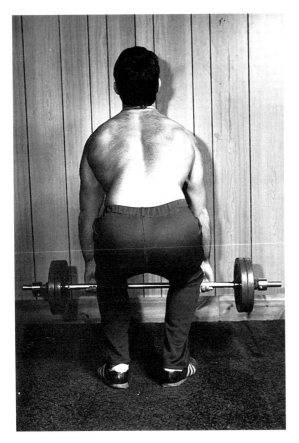

Fig. 1.12 The weight-lifter lifts without flexing the lumbar spine, using mainly the glutei and the quadriceps muscles.

sacrospinalis muscles, wrapped in the envelope of the lumbar fascia which extends laterally to the abdominal muscles and to the latissimus dorsi and glutei. This arrangement confers a double advantage to the spine, making it difficult to flex the spine and lift at the same time, and also stiffening the spinal segments to reinforce the strength of the arch. Upright man when compared with other primates has a more robust abdominal musculoligamentous system. With five lumbar vertebrae and considerable space between the pelvic brim and the lower ribs, he compares favourably with those other primates which have fewer lumbar vertebrae and a lesser space.

The spine's flexibility is not in conflict with strength and protection. Rather, it is compatible with these two roles and with the demands of being upright.

The suggestion that back pain is the result of man's struggle to become upright is no longer tenable. There is an undoubted excellence to the system. Examining the spine is like inspecting pieces of china, each stamped with the maker's mark of excellence. Neither is there evidence of a so-called vestigial structure, that the spine is only half adequate, or that man is only half upright or semi-upright. Furthermore, when spinal pathology does occur (and the spine is no more exempt from pathology than any other system), that pathology, rather than being innate to the system, seems generally to be the result of environmental factors which are potentially preventable; they are not the result of being upright.

REFERENCES

Adams M A, Hutton W C 1982 Prolapsed intervertebral disc. A hyperflexion injury. Spine 7: 184–191

Aspden R M 1989 The spine as an arch: a new mathematical model. Spine 14: 266–274

Boshinzen H C, Bongers P M, Hulshof C T J 1992 Self-reported back pain in fork-lift truck and freight-container drivers exposed to whole body vibration. Spine 17: 59–65

Brinckman P, Biggemann M, Hoilweg D 1989 Prediction of the compressive strength of human lumbar vertebrae. Spine 14: 606–610

Clark G A, Panjabi M M, Wetzel F T 1980 Can infant malnutrition cause adult vertebral stenosis? Spine 8: 99–105

Deyo R A, Bass J E 1989 Lifestyle and low-back pain. The influence of smoking and obesity. Spine 14: 501–506

Frymoyer J W, Pope M H, Clements J H, Wilder D G, MacPhearson B, Ashakaga T 1983 Risk factors in low-back pain. Journal of Bone and Joint Surgery 65-A: 213–218

Hickey D S, Hukins D L W 1980 Relation between the structure of the annulus fibrosus and the function and failure of the intervertebral disc. Spine 5: 106–116

Porter R W, Pavitt M 1987 The vertebral canal, part 1. Nutrition and development. An archaeological study. Spine 12: 901–906

Urban J P G, McMullin J F 1988 Swelling pressure of the lumbar intervertebral discs; influence of age, spinal level, composition and degeneration. Spine 13: 179–187

2. Back pain — a problem — personal, national and clinical

In spite of the spine's excellent form and function, back pain is a national, personal and clinical problem: national because it is experienced by most of the population at some time and is a drain on the nation's resources; personal because it can remain a major unresolved dilemma; and clinical because not only is diagnosis difficult, but methods of treatment are conflicting and often unrewarding.

A PERSONAL PROBLEM

For the patient, back pain is more than an academic manipulation of statistics; it is a personal problem, and it is one of epidemic proportions. It causes half the population to seek help from their general practitioners at some time (Jayson 1981). The incidence of attendance varies from 20 to 37 per 1000 per year (Fry 1974, Lewith & Turner 1982, Drinkall et al 1984), and about one visit in four is a first attendance for back pain. It is the major cause of sickness in early adult life (Fig. 2.1).

Attendance depends not only on the incidence of back pain, but on the ethos of the community (Bremner et al 1968) and the management of health care. We examined over 800 records of 40-year-old men and their wives from four South

Yorkshire practices, over a 20-year period; 50–81% of the men and 26–63% of the women attended at some time with back pain (Table 2.1).

By the time the doctor is approached, the problem is more than the touch of back pain that we can all expect from time to time. It has become unmanageable, interfering with mobility, work, sleep and recreation. The high male incidence, especially in the fifth decade (Wood & McLeish 1974), may not reflect the true perspective. Women, the young and the elderly may be less inclined to seek help. Fin Biering-Sorensen (1982) recorded a high incidence amongst women in advancing years, and there is an increasing incidence in the young (Balagué et al 1988). When children visit hospital with back pain, they often have serious spinal disease (Turner et al 1989).

General practice statistics underestimate the problem. Half the patients treated by registered osteopaths have back pain, and one in three of these have not seen their own doctor (Burton 1978, 1981). Many more suffer without treatment. For all of those, back pain is a problem — because of the severity of the pain, its persistence, its disabling effects, the fear of its origin and apprehension about the future. Too often it is compounded by different practitioners offering various

Table 2.1 Percentage of 40-year-old men and their wives who attended their general practitioner at some time in the previous 20 years with low back pain (n = 855).

	% of men who attended with back pain	% of their wives who attended with back pain	% of men who were heavy manual workers
Practice A	81	54	49
Practice B	65	26	65
Practice C	62	63	18
Practice D	50	39	22

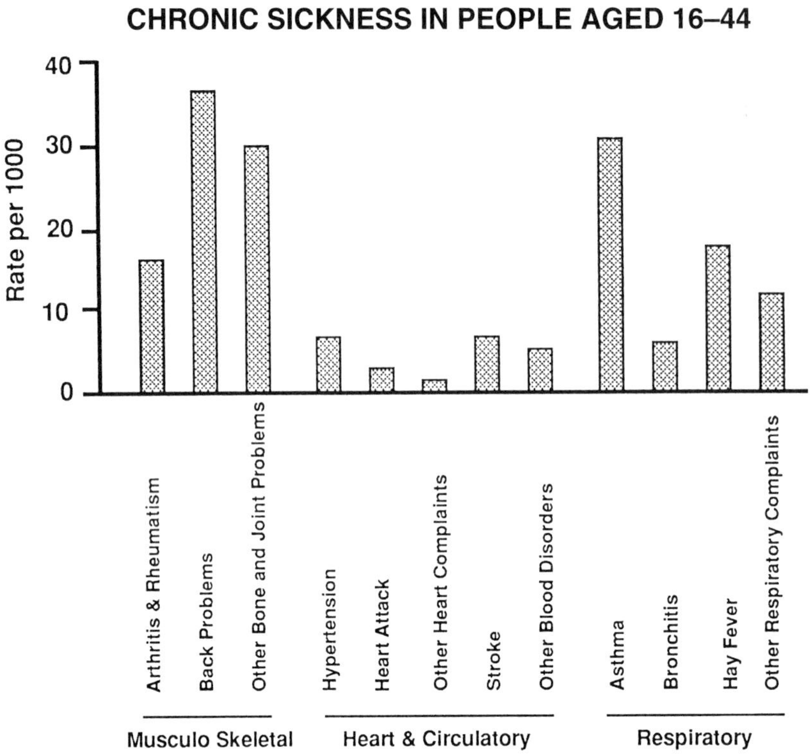

CHRONIC SICKNESS IN PEOPLE AGED 16–44

Fig. 2.1   Back pain had the highest sickness rate in the UK in 1988, when compared with other illnesses. (Source: General Household Survey 1988)

diagnoses, or admitting ignorance by recommending no treatment or contradictory methods. The patient is understandably confused, and for those whose pain does not settle naturally with time, anxiety or depression adds to their dilemma.

Mr GS was a dynamic sales representative who, at the age of 35, was in charge of 15 salesmen serving two counties. Unexpectedly, he found himself in bed with pain in the back and left leg and restricted straight leg raising. He failed to improve over 3 weeks. A lower lumbar disc was speedily excised but recovery was slow; after 3 months, in spite of aching in the back and left leg, he forced himself back to work. For 5 years his employers were satisfied with him, but his wife and two boys suffered — no sex, no sports, no fun; Dad always seemed to be in some sort of pain. He couldn't even walk at a normal pace, and both legs seemed to tighten up after 5 minutes. He would rest and then walk further, but after a heavy day his legs were so restless in bed that he had to sleep in a room of his own. Some experts diagnosed spinal stenosis and he

agreed to have a spinal decompression; now, at 42 years of age, after a second operation he still has very limited walking distance and episodes of back pain that put him to bed from time to time. He stands to lose his job.

Mrs GN is 10 years older than her husband, and at 39 years of age she and her family think she should be able to run her home, engage in an active social life and have energetic holidays. For 3 years, however, she has had a painful back whenever she does heavy work. She has no sex life and she fears for her marriage. Two months ago she spent a week lying on the floor, and all she can remember the orthopaedic surgeon saying to her as she could hardly raise either of her heels from the floor was, 'Never mind dear, we all get back pain and you will have to live with it'.

Mr J McH is 26 years old, plays professional soccer and is the club's best striker. He thought he had a hamstring strain and missed a few games, but when his ankle reflex was affected he was soon in the hands of a surgeon and a prolapsed disc was removed. Now his pain has settled but he has a weak soleus and cannot stand on his toes. The club cannot afford to renew his contract, and with no other work experience he has moved from the glare of the floodlights to the dole queue.

Mrs JD, who is 62 years old, remembers having a couple of bad years with pain in the back and leg in her 20s and has treated her back with respect ever since. For 2 years now she has had periods of severe pain in the right leg from the buttock, thigh and calf to the ankle. The pain is getting worse and now keeps her awake at night. Sometimes she takes 20 analgesics a day. She has had three epidural injections with only temporary relief. She looks strained and nervous, prefers to stand rather than sit when she visits the clinic, and asks if an operation will help her.

Mr HR was a coal-face worker earning good money until his back began to ache after a heavy shift. Within 6 months it became a constant ache, relieved only by lying down. An X-ray showed a spondylolisthesis and he was advised to take a light job in the pit bottom. Even this proved too much until now he is not working at all. Not yet 40 years old, he sits at home whilst his wife goes out to work. He is trying to prove that a fall of coal strained his back and caused his problem, but cannot understand why the doctors say it would have been painful anyway. If he exaggerates a bit, it is only to convince the doctors there is really something wrong with him. They all seem to think he is malingering and no one understands him. Even his wife says it must be 'in his mind'.

These histories are real, and in spite of expert medical help the problems remain.

A NATIONAL PROBLEM

On average, every worker has 3 days off work with back pain each year. Days of certified incapacity have increased threefold in the past 15 years (Fig. 2.2). Viewed from a national perspective the problem is enormous. As many as 35% of patients who visit their general practitioner with back pain may be in sufficient trouble to be referred at some time to hospital (Barker 1977) (Table 2.2). This may be as much as 9% referral in any 1 year (Fig. 2.3). Orthopaedic surgeons and rheumatologists in the UK see 0.4 million patients per year with

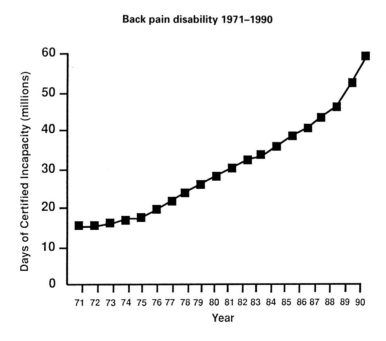

Back pain disability 1971–1990

Fig. 2.2 Days certified incapacity from back pain have increased fourfold in the UK in two decades. (Source: Department of Social Security 1991)

Table 2.2   Use of hospital resources for 40-year-old men (n = 393) who had experienced some low back pain in the previous 20 years, in four general practices.

	% of men with low back pain referred for X-ray	% of men with low back pain referred for orthopaedic opinion
Practice A	44	24
Practice B	23	21
Practice C	33	13
Practice D	37	35

back pain (Jayson 1981). Many of these have been waiting in excess of 3 months for an appointment, with months off work and little prospect of an early return. Their investigations absorb a large proportion of the radiological budget, and their management is an even larger part of the work-load of the physiotherapy and appliance de-partments.

Only a minority of patients will be offered sur-gery, with successes balanced by an equal number of failures. Up to 7500 disc operations are per-formed each year in Britain: 15 per 100 000 of

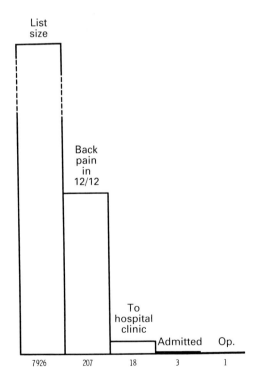

Fig. 2.3   Histogram showing the number of patients attending one general practice in 1 year complaining of back pain, and the number referred to hospital.

the population. There is more enthusiasm for disc surgery in the US, where 69.5 operations per 100 000 are performed each year (Nelson 1983). Waddell (1987) estimated that 300 000 new lam-inectomies were performed each year in the US, and that 15% of these patients will continue to be disabled.

The cost of back pain to the British National Health Service is currently over £350 million per year. Social Security pays out £0.5 billion per year in sickness and invalidity benefits and disablement pensions for back pain. Furthermore, back pain strikes those in their most productive years. The cost to the community in lost output is about £3 billion. The economic cost to the nation is staggering.

Heavy manual workers, who are the main producers of the national wealth, are those most likely to complain of back pain (Fig. 2.4). In the coal-mining industry, 11.9% of certified absences are due to back pain (Afacan 1982); 75% of miners will have some back pain and most of those will be off work with it at some time, whilst 50% of office workers will experience back pain and half of them will need to be off work (Fig. 2.5). Occupational factors are highly important (Riihimaki et al 1989). There is a high incidence of back pain amongst truck drivers (Kelsey 1975); tractor drivers (Allawi 1978, Anderson 1980, Boshinzen et al 1992); helicopter pilots (Fitzgerald & Crotty 1972); bricklayers; nurses in medical, geriatric and orthopaedic wards (Cust et al 1972, Ryden et al 1989); dockworkers (Anderson 1986); coal miners (Lloyd et al 1986); reindeer workers (Videman 1991); and in those parts of an industry where heavy load handling is required (Troup 1968, Chaffin & Park 1973, Frymoyer et al 1983). Measured in economic terms, back pain is probably the largest medical problem awaiting a solution.

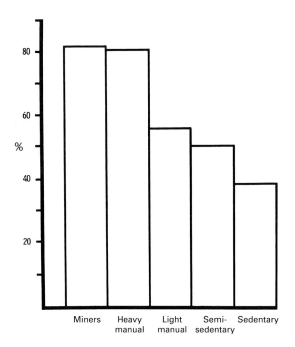

Fig. 2.4 Percentage of 40-year-old men according to occupation who had previously visited their general practitioner with back pain.

A CLINICAL PROBLEM

To the clinician, the problem is pertinent. Faced with a patient asking two questions, 'What is causing the back pain?' and 'Can you put it right?', it is often difficult to give a satisfactory answer to either. In most medical conditions we seek a diagnosis. We listen and question the patient, examine and investigate until we are satisfied we have identified the pathological condition which is responsible for the symptoms. We are content with a pathological diagnosis even if we cannot be too sure how the symptoms are experienced by the patient. When investigating back pain, however, we are frequently uncertain which part of the spinal anatomy is sufficiently deranged to produce pain. Pathology is often symptomless. All too often we cannot find the nociceptive source. We have no diagnosis, and therefore a problem.

Clinicians have described back pain with ambiguous words like 'lumbago', 'fibrositis', 'slipped disc' — as though providing a label was as good as a diagnosis. Other physicians have accepted our ignorance of the pain source, describing undiagnosed back pain as 'non-specific back pain' (Jayson 1984). Our very terminology confirms that all too frequently we have no diagnosis.

If the patient's first question is difficult, the second is no easier. How can you treat a problem when you do not know its cause? It is generally true that when a variety of remedies abound to treat a condition, there is no cure. For back pain this is certainly correct. The methods of treatment

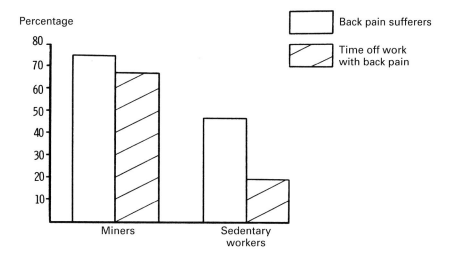

Fig. 2.5 Percentage of coal miners (n = 251) and sedentary workers (n = 198) over 50 years of age who at interview said they had experienced back pain, and who had been off work with back pain.

are legion: from exercise to rest, manipulation to immobilization; drugs by mouth, into muscles, into joints, discs, the spine; needles, endoscopes and knives; micro- and maxi-surgery; relaxation; stimulators; bending the mind and strengthening the faith. When it comes to a scientific appraisal of our efforts to treat back pain, with few exceptions it must be confessed that in the long term, no one method of treatment seems better than doing nothing at all.

These are problems indeed for a clinician in a scientific age, in a consumer-led market fuelled by support industries and in a society where health expectations are high. No diagnosis and no treatment of proven worth. We are left with two choices: nihilism, despair and defeat; or a positive approach of facing up to the difficulties, clearing away the myths, and patiently seeking to answer questions from a base of known facts. The problems are great but so is the reward. Back pain can be one of the most interesting and stimulating fields of medicine: the satisfaction of searching for a diagnosis to find a nociceptive source; the reward of a patient's gratitude that someone is sufficiently interested to try and is prepared to give time to listen and explain; the reward of combining with colleagues in so many disciplines — the bioengineers, biochemists, mathematicians, clinicians and therapists — to answer some of the unsolved questions; and the reward of preventative medicine to reduce the back pain problem for a future generation. We can try.

REFERENCES

Afacan A S 1982 Sickness absence due to back lesions in coal miners. Journal of the Society of Occupational Medicine 32: 26–31

Allawi A 1978 Postmen with driving commitments have higher complaints about LBP than those without. PhD thesis, University of London

Anderson J A D 1980 Back pain and occupation. In: Jayson MIV (ed) The lumbar spine and back pain. Pitman Medical, Tunbridge Wells, p 57–82

Anderson J A D 1986 Epidemiological aspects of back pain. Journal of the Society of Occupational Medicine 36: 90–94

Balagué F, Dutoit G, Waldburger M 1988 Low back pain in school children. An epidemiological study. Scandinavian Journal of Rehabilitation Medicine 20: 175–179

Barker M E 1977 Pain in the back and leg: a general practice survey. Rheumatology and Rehabilitation 16(1): 37–45

Boshinzen H C, Bongers P M, Hulshof C T J 1992 Self-reported back pain in fork-lift, container, tractor drivers exposed to whole body vibration. Spine 17: 59–65

Bremner J M, Lawrence J S, Miall W E 1968 Degenerative joint disease in a Jamaican rural population. Annals of Rheumatic Diseases 27: 326–332

Burton A K 1978 The prior medical contact of osteopath's patients. British Osteopath Journal 11: 19–23

Burton A K 1981 Back pain in osteopathic practice. Rheumatology and Rehabilitation 20: 239–246

Chaffin D B, Park K S 1973 A longitudinal study of low back pain as associated with occupation weight lifting factors. American Industrial Hygiene Association Journal 23: 513–523

Cust G, Pearson J C G, Mair A 1972 The prevalence of low back pain in nurses. International Nursing Review 19: 169–179

Drinkall J N, Porter R W, Hibbert C S, Evans C 1984 The value of ultrasonic measurement of the spinal canal diameter in general practice. British Medical Journal 288: 121–122

Fin Biering-Sorensen 1982 Low back trouble in a general population of 30-, 40-, 50- and 60-year-old men and women. Danish Medical Bulletin 29: 289–299

Fitzgerald J G, Crotty J 1972 The incidence of backache among air crew and ground crew in the Royal Air Force. Flying Personnel Research Committee — Ministry of Defence (Air Force Department) FPRC/1313

Fry J 1974 Common diseases: their nature, incidence and care. MTP Press, London

Frymoyer J W, Pope M H, Clements J H, Wilder D G, MacPhearson B, Ashikaga T 1983 Risk factors in low back pain. Journal of Bone and Joint Surgery 65-A: 213–218

Jayson M I V 1981 Back pain: the facts. Oxford University Press, New York

Jayson M I V 1984 Difficult diagnoses in back pain. British Medical Journal 288: 740–741

Kelsey J L 1975 An epidemiological study of acute herniated lumbar intervertebral discs. Rheumatology and Rehabilitation 14: 144–159

Lewith G T, Turner G M T 1982 Retrospective analysis of the management of acute low back pain. Practitioner 226: 1514–1618

Lloyd M H, Gauld S, Souttar C R 1986 Epidemiological study of back pain in miners and office workers. Spine 11: 136–140

Nelson M 1983 Orthopaedic surgery: proceedings of the international symposium on low back pain and industrial and social disablement. Back Pain Association, p 91

Riihimaki H, Tola S, Videman T, Hanninen K 1989 Low back pain and occupation. Spine 14: 204–209

Ryden L A, Melgaard C A, Bobbitt S, Cohn A, Conway J 1989 Occupational low back injury in a hospital employee population. Spine 14: 315–320

Troup J D G 1968 The function of the lumbar spine. PhD thesis, University of London

Turner P G, Green J H, Galasko C S B 1989 Back pain in childhood. Spine 14: 812–814

Videman T 1991 Back pain in reindeer workers. Presented to the Society for Back Pain Research, London, Nov 8

Waddell G 1987 Failure of disc surgery and repeat surgery. Acta Orthopaedica Belgica 53: 300–342

Wood P H N, McLeish C L 1974 Digest of data on the rheumatic diseases. 5. Morbidity in industry, and rheumatism in general practice. Annals of Rheumatic Diseases 33: 93–105

3. The causes of back pain: aetiology

Back pain is but a symptom and its source may arise in many different structures (Table 3.1). Most people who complain of back pain have a problem with either the spine or associated structures, but back pain can of course be the presenting symptom of pathology in other systems and perhaps we should discuss these first.

BACK PAIN FROM NON-SPINAL CAUSES

Gynaecological pain

Gynaecological causes account for the largest number of patients with back pain when spinal problems are excluded. Pain associated with menstruation is recognized with its periodicity and its constant nature over several hours, and it is unrelated to posture and activity. Uterine prolapse, fibroids, pelvic infection or a retroverted uterus not infrequently produce low back pain which is aggravated by standing and walking and relieved by rest. When there is presumptive evidence of gynaecological pathology, one can usually exclude a spinal cause for the pain if there are no abnormal spinal signs — that is, if there is a good range of lumbar movement and no tenderness. Not infrequently the spine is restricted and tender, and it is difficult to exclude a coexistent spinal problem.

A few patients are referred after pelvic surgery with persistence of their back pain, and it becomes obvious in retrospect that there is also a spinal problem. Mechanical back pain of spinal origin not uncommonly follows pelvic and abdominal hysterectomy. There is no evidence that the lithotomy position is significant in the aetiology of such pain. Some patients are referred with pain after treatment of a pelvic carcinoma in the hope that there is an innocuous mechanical problem. Too frequently the constant nature of the pain suggests a recurrence of the tumour.

Renal pain

It is not usually difficult to distinguish between renal pain and derangement of the upper lumbar spine. The kidney generally produces pain in the loin, an unusual site for spinal pain; it tends to be constant, building up to a peak, gradually settling over several hours and being unaffected by posture and activity. Ureteric pain can radiate to the iliac fossa and groin in the same distribution as a lower thoracic or upper lumbar root lesion, but it tends to be constant for several hours at a time. Frequency and dysuria support the diagnosis, and a full renal investigation is necessary.

Table 3.1 Classification of back pain

1. Non-spinal causes
   a) Gynaecological
   b) Renal
   c) Other retroperitoneal pathologies
   d) Vascular
   e) Peripheral nerve entrapment
   f) Guillain–Barré syndrome
2. Spine and associated structures
   a) Bone (fracture, metastases, primary tumours, blood dyscrasia)
   b) Bone and joints (infective, inflammatory)
   c) Soft tissue pathology
   d) Segmental mechanical derangement
   e) Inflammatory causes.
      i) Neurological symptoms
         disc protrusion
         root entrapment from degenerative change
         neurogenic claudication
      ii) Back and referred pain

occur. Osteoid osteoma and benign osteoblastoma of the vertebrae can present with back pain and a fixed scoliosis, a rare combination in children and adolescents with mechanical derangement only (Freiberger 1960, Kirwan et al 1984). This demands close inspection of the pedicles at the apex of the curve. The most useful and reliable investigations are a technetium bone scan to determine the level of the lesion and a computerized axial tomographic (CAT) scan to identify the precise location of the nidus (Fig. 3.2).

Small osteolytic deposits of multiple myelomatosis can be scattered through many bones causing back pain, and fractures associated with myelomatosis or with leukaemia will produce pain. All too frequently spinal bone tumours are not diagnosed until they produce neurological compression signs. Unremitting pain and an absence of a previous history of back pain, especially in the elderly, should cause one to suspect malignancy. Simple angiomata of the vertebral bodies are usually symptomless and are discovered by chance on routine radiographs. On careful examination they can be recognized in 10% of spines (Finneson 1973), and perhaps should not be considered tumours at all; they do not normally require treatment (Fig. 3.3). Radiotherapy may result in

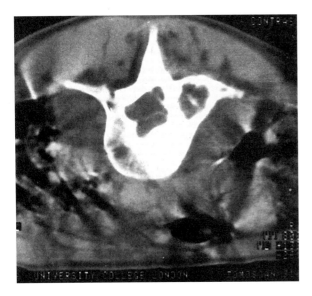

Fig. 3.2   CT of an osteoid osteoma in the pedicle of L3, extending into the body, lamina and transverse process, with a central nidus (by kind permission of Mr E O G Kirwan).

osteoporosis and vertebral collapse (Roaf 1980). Sickle cell disease can cause similar osteolytic vertebrae and back pain (Ozoh et al 1990).

Tumours within the vertebral canal can cause pain with or without neurological signs. Benign tumours may be symptomless and are more common in children (Delamarter et al 1990). Extramedullary tumours such as neurofibromas, angiomas, meningiomas and lipomas (Supik & Broom 1991) may cause compressive lesions of the cauda equina. Neurofibromas can enlarge the intervertebral foramen from bone erosion and cause root pain.

Infection

Spinal sepsis can be divided into three major categories: vertebral osteomyelitis, epidural abscess and discitis.

Vertebral osteomyelitis

Vertebral osteomyelitis is most commonly caused by haematogenous spread of *Staphylococcus aureus*, although a wide range of other bacteria have been isolated including coliforms, pseudomonas, streptococci, brucella and *Mycobacterium tuberculosis*, fungi and anaerobes (Silverhorn & Gillespie 1986). Infection can be introduced during spinal surgery, epidural injections or myelography, or it can spread from adjacent lesions (Digby & Kersley 1979, Farrington et al 1983, Ingram & Redding 1988). It is not easily differentiated from mechanical causes of back pain on clinical grounds alone. An acute pyogenic osteomyelitis of the vertebral body may be superimposed on a pre-existing back problem. Pain is aggravated by activity and relieved by rest. There is frequently a great deal of muscle spasm, more than is usually encountered with an acute disc lesion (Rae et al 1984). However the scoliosis of osteomyelitis and of osteoid osteoma is fixed, whilst the deformity of the patient with disc protrusion is induced by gravity and abolished by lying down. Pyrexia, loss of weight and loss of appetite accompany spinal infection but all too frequently spinal infection is not suspected until a late stage (Flood et al 1983). It may present as abdominal pain, or may be associated with other debilitating illnesses like

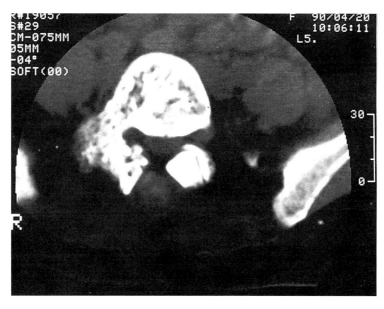

Fig. 3.3 CT scan showing a haemangioma of the body, transverse process and lamina of L5 of a woman who had had part of the lesion excised in childhood. There had been copious bleeding. It was followed by radiotherapy. She had no problems, but developed back pain 40 years later, and the CT scan shows a central foreign body reaction around a swab, posterior to the lamina.

diabetes. It should be considered in the elderly (Thomson et al 1988) and in immunosuppressed patients (Lifeso 1990).

The radiological features of vertebral osteomyelitis are characteristic, with destruction of the end-plate. The disc is soon involved and rapidly destroyed by proteolytic enzymes of the pyogenic organisms with spread to the adjacent vertebrae. Tuberculosis, on the other hand, tends to spread to the next vertebra around the disc under the anterior longitudinal ligament. As in spinal neoplasms, the discs are generally preserved.

In children, haematogenous osteomyelitis is more common in the long bones, and vertebral osteomyelitis is decidedly rare under 9 years of age (Allen et al 1978). The highest incidence is in the third decade, probably because in adults and adolescents the lumbar intraosseous arteries are end arteries, supplying a segment of bone. In children there is an extensive intraosseous arterial anastomosis (Ratcliffe 1982).

Spinal tuberculosis is now fortunately becoming a rare condition. Its previously common involvement of many vertebrae with collapse of the bodies and cold abscess formation is now unusual. The vertebral bodies were commonly affected, often a whole segment of the vertebral column, with progressive destruction of the cancellous bone, vertebral collapse and spread to adjacent vertebrae under the anterior longitudinal ligament. The discs were usually resistant, disappearing at a late stage. Cord involvement was a complication to be feared. Tuberculosis is, however, becoming an occasional disease of the elderly, particularly in men (Horne 1984). Its presentation and features are now much the same as in pyogenic osteomyelitis (Lichtenstein 1975) and it is distinguished only by identification of the causative organism. Sterile granulomatous change can cause late paraparesis.

Discitis

Discitis is an infective inflammatory process involving the paediatric intervertebral disc and adjacent end-plates. The most common organism cultured is *Staph. aureus*. The peak incidence is at 6 years of age and the lumbar spine is most commonly affected. There is a low-grade fever, back pain or abdominal or hip pain, and a refusal to walk or stand. ESR and white cell count are raised. Radiological features of disc space narrowing and irregularities of the end-plate lag behind the clinical symptoms. Technetium-99 bone scanning is the investigation of choice. Spinal rest, with or without immobilization, and antibodies are usually effective treatment.

Epidural abscess

Spinal epidural abscess is encountered rarely, but it should be considered when compressive symptoms are associated with severe pain. There is often a coexisting debilitating disease like diabetes or cirrhosis and a source of infection from spinal surgery, needle investigation or retroperitoneal surgery (Russell et al 1979).

Mr H McC, a 62-year-old farmer and a diabetic for 20 years presented with motor weakness in both legs but with no sensory change. He had a pyelonephritis with an *Escherichia coli* bacteraemia. His white cell count was 17 000 and his ESR 42. X-rays of the lumbar spine suggested an osteomyelitis of the body of the L3 vertebra. A myelogram showed a two-level spinal stenosis (Fig. 3.4) with separation of the dura from the posterior border of L3, suggestive of an epidural abscess. Initially he had classical symptoms of neurogenic claudication on walking only a few paces, but by the time a diagnosis of epidural abscess was made he had recovered dramatically with cefuroxime and then trimethoprim, eventually becoming quite asymptomatic and walking 3 miles. He had no back pain and no spinal tenderness; he had a urinary infection. Radionuclide scanning with 99mTc did not show any increased uptake in the blood pool images nor in the later images (Fig. 3.5).

Causes of back pain from non-spinal pathology and back pain associated with tumour and infection having been described, there remain two broad categories of back pain affecting the spine: inflammatory and mechanical.

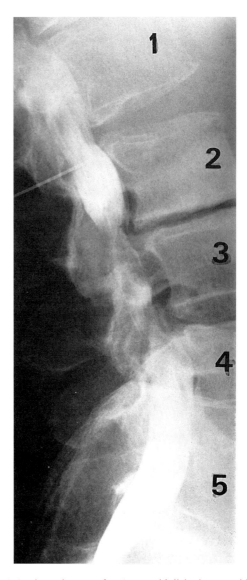

Fig. 3.4 A myelogram of a 62-year-old diabetic man with weakness of his legs. He had a two-level stenosis at L2/3 and L3/4, with a suggestion of a chronic epidural abscess at the posterior border of L3. He had been treated with antibiotics for a urinary tract infection and had made almost full recovery by the time he had the myelogram.

INFLAMMATORY CAUSES OF BACK PAIN

Back pain related to an inflammatory disorder is more common in young men; is worse after rest with early morning stiffness which improves with exercise; tends to be episodic; is referred from the low back to one or other buttock or posterior thigh, but not commonly to both at the same time; and there is often a history of other joint involvement (Calin 1979). There may be a history of urethritis, uveitis, psoriasis or inflammatory bowel disease, and gout is a rare cause of back pain (Das De 1988).

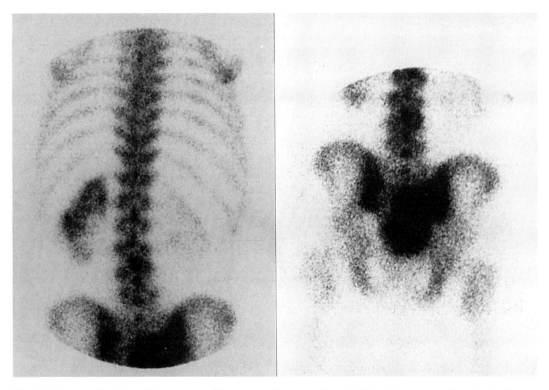

Fig. 3.5 Image of radionuclide scanning of the same patient as in Fig. 3.4. There is no increased uptake in the lumbar spine. The left kidney is poorly functioning, and the right kidney has irregular uptake suggesting pyelonephritis. He has signs also of symphysitis.

Ankylosing spondylitis

In its severe form, ankylosing spondylitis is easily recognized. The spine is stiff, too often in the kyphotic position, with sclerosed sacroiliac joints and a 'bamboo spine' (Fig. 3.6). Involvement of the costovertebral joints restricts chest expansion. In its milder forms the diagnosis depends on a history of an inflammatory type of back pain and a raised ESR. Sacroiliitis may not be manifest radiologically for a year or two after the onset of the illness, and radioscintigraphy with bone-seeking isotopes is more helpful in the early diagnosis (Szanto & Hagenfeldt 1983, Rosenthall & Libsona 1980). Computerized tomographic (CT) imaging is helpful.

Many backache sufferers may have a sub-clinical type of ankylosing spondylitis and the diagnosis is missed for years, if not indefinitely. It is suggested that the condition may affect 2% of the whole population, and the mild form may

occur in the two sexes with equal frequency (Jayson 1981).

There is an increased prevalence of HLA B-27 antigen in ankylosing spondylitis and in up to 40% of patients attending a routine back pain clinic, compared with an incidence of 7–12% in the general population, but this unusually high incidence may be related to the pattern of referral.

Inflammatory changes start in the sacroiliac joints and, if progressive, will gradually spread cranially up the spine involving the apophyseal joints, the vertebral end-plates and ligamentous attachments until the ligaments are ossified. Hips, knees and feet may be affected, and in 15% the disease may start in the peripheral joints. Rarely, the spine will stiffen without much pain. One-third of the patients develop iritis, some ulcer-ative colitis or Crohn's disease, and occasionally aortic valvular disease. (The iritis may affect one eye and then the other, much as the back pain shifts from left to right). In the triad of arthritis,

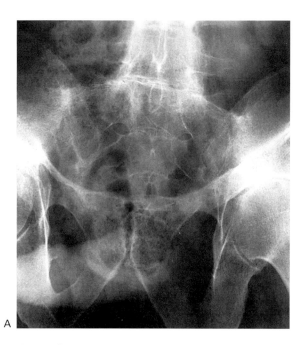

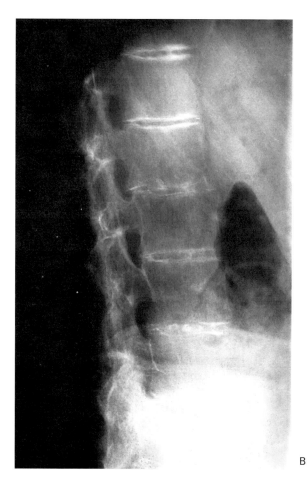

A   B

Fig. 3.6(A)   AP radiograph of a 42-year-old man with an 18-year history of ankylosing spondylitis, showing fusion of the sacroiliac joints and degenerative changes of the hips. **(B)**   Lateral radiograph of the same patient's ankylosed lumbar spine.

uveitis and urethritis (Reiter's disease) 10–30% have associated ankylosing spondylitis.

These patients are most effectively treated by rheumatologists, with care to maintain a good posture and with courses of anti-inflammatory drugs, gold, penicillamine or sulphasalazine and with mobilization regimens.

Sacroiliitis

Sacroiliitis may follow acute salpingitis or prostatitis, and may be responsible for sacroiliac pain and tenderness and morning stiffness. It develops in about one-third of patients with psoriatic arthritis (Benoist 1990). Scintigraphy will be more helpful than radiography in the early diagnosis

although ultimately erosions and sclerosis develop, sometimes with complete fusion of the joint. The ESR does not correlate with the joint activity. There is a high incidence of HLA B-27 antigen. It is worth giving antibiotics when persistent pelvic infection is associated with sacroiliac pain (Szanto & Hagenfeldt 1979, 1983).

It is to be expected that the majority of patients consulting a rheumatologist with back pain will have an inflammatory cause, but this is still only a small proportion of back pain sufferers. The majority of patients with pain in the lower back have had a mechanical disturbance and it is towards an understanding of this problem and its management that we are addressing this book.

REFERENCES

Allen E H, Cosgrave D, Mullard F J C 1978 The radiological changes in infections of the spine and their diagnostic value. Clinical Radiology 29: 31–40

Benoist M 1990 Inflammatory spondyloarthropathies. In: Weinstein J N, Wiesel S W (eds) The lumbar spine. WB Saunders, Philadelphia, p 637–649

Calin A 1979 Back pain: mechanical or inflammatory? American Family Physician 20: 97–100

Das De S 1988 Intervertebral disc involvement in gout: brief report. Journal of Bone and Joint Surgery 70-B: 671

Delamarter R B, Sachs B L, Thompson G H, Bohlman H H, Makley J T, Carter J R 1990 Primary neoplasms of the thoracic and lumbar spine. Clinical Orthopaedics and Related Research 256: 87–100

Digby J M, Kersley J B 1979 Pyogenic non-tuberculous spinal infection. Journal of Bone and Joint Surgery 61-B: 47–55

Farrington M, Eykyn S J, Walker M, Warren R E 1983 Vertebral osteomyelitis due to coccobacilli of the HB group. British Medical Journal 287: 1658–1660

Finneson B E 1973 Low back pain. J B Lippincott, Philadelphia, p 307

Flood B M, Deacon P, Dickson R A 1983 Spinal disease presenting as acute abdominal pain. British Medical Journal 287: 616–617

Freiberger R E 1960 Osteoid osteoclastoma of the spine. A cause of backache and scoliosis in children and young adults. Radiology 75: 232

Galasko C S B 1991 Spinal instability secondary to metastatic cancer. Journal of Bone and Joint Surgery 73-B: 104–108

Horne N W 1984 Problems of tuberculosis in decline. British Medical Journal 288: 1249–1251

Ingram R, Redding P 1988 Salmonella vischow osteomyelitis. Journal of Bone and Joint Surgery 70-B: 440–442

Jayson M I V 1981 Back pain: the facts. Oxford University Press, New York

Jiang G X, Xu W D, Wang A X 1988 Spinal stenosis with meralgia paresthetica. Journal of Bone and Joint Surgery 70-B: 272–273

Kirwan E O'G, Hutton P A N, Pozo J L, Ransford A O 1984 Osteoid osteoma and benign osteoblastoma of the spine: clinical presentation and treatment. Journal of Bone and Joint Surgery 66-B: 21–26

Lichtenstein L 1975 Diseases of bones and joints. CV Mosby, St Louis, p 61

Lifeso R M 1990 Pyogenic spinal sepsis in adults. Spine 15: 265–271

Narakas A O 1990 The role of thoracic outlet syndrome in the double crush syndrome. Annales de Chirurgie de la Main et des Membres Supérieures 9: 331–340

Ozoh J O, Onuigbo M A C, Nwankwo N, Ukabam S O, Umerach B C, Emeruwa C C 1990 'Vanishing' of vertebra in a patient with sickle cell haemaglobinopathy. British Medical Journal 301: 1368–1369

Pryor J P, Castle W M, Dukes D C et al 1983 Do beta-adrenoceptor blocking drugs cause retroperitoneal fibrosis? British Medical Journal 287: 639–641

Rae P S, Waddell C, Venner R W 1984 A simple technique for measuring lumbar spinal flexion. Journal of the Royal College of Surgeons of Edinburgh 29: 281–284

Ratcliffe J F 1982 An evaluation of the intra-osseous arterial anastomoses in the human vertebral body at different ages. A microarteriographic study. Journal of Anatomy 134: 373–382

Roaf R 1980 Spinal deformities, 2nd edn. Pitman Medical, p 65

Rosenthall L, Libsona R 1980 Role of radionuclide imaging in benign bone and joint disease of orthopaedic interest. In: Freeman L M, Weissman H S (eds) Nuclear medicine annual. Raven Press, New York, p 267–301

Russell N A, Vaughan R, Morley T P 1979 Spinal epidural infection. Le Journal Canadien des Sciences Neurologiques 6: 325–328

Saal J A, Dillington M F, Gamburd R S, Fenton G S 1988 The pseudo radicular syndrome. Spine 13: 926–929

Silverhorn K G, Gillespie W J 1986 Pyogenic osteomyelitis: a review of 61 cases. New Zealand Medical Journal 99: 62–65

Supik L F, Broom M J 1991 Epidural lipoma causing a myelographic block in a patient who had sciatica and a lumbo sacral spondylolisthesis. Journal of Bone and Joint Surgery 73-A: 1104–1107

Szanto E, Hagenfeldt K 1979 Sacroiliitis and salpingitis. Quantative 99m Tc pertechnetate in the study of sacroiliitis in women. Scandinavian Journal of Rheumatology 8: 129

Szanto E, Hagenfeldt K 1983 Sacro-iliitis in women. A sequel to acute salpingitis. Scandinavian Journal of Rheumatology 12: 89–92

Thomson D, Bannister P, Murphy P 1988 Vertebral osteomyelitis in the elderly. British Medical Journal 296: 1309–1311

Turek S L 1976 Orthopaedic principles and their applications. Pitman Medical, London

Upton A R M, McComas A J 1973 The double crush in nerve entrapment syndrome. Lancet ii: 359–362

Winer J 1992 Guillain–Barré syndrome revisited. British Medical Journal 304: 65–66

Basic science

4. Structures that fail

If sufficient force is applied to any structure it will deform and fail. The spine is no exception, but the particular structures of the spine which fail depend upon the nature of the applied force, the position of the spine at the time, and the morphological variations. These differ from one individual to another and are age- and sex- related.

THE VERTEBRAE

A vertical compression force tends to cause an anterior wedge fracture of the vertebral bodies, T12, L1 and L2 being most commonly fractured, with decreasing incidence proximally and distally (Young 1973). The compression force necessary to fracture the vertebral bodies is directly related to their mineral content, though it is not necessarily a linear relationship (Ch. 23). Forced flexion of the spine such as that caused by a blow across the shoulders, will also fracture the vertebral bodies, and forced flexion, rotation and shear will sometimes damage the posterior elements and cause neurological injury.

The lumbar articular facets carry 16–40% of the total intervertebral compressive spinal load in the erect posture (Farfan 1973, Adams & Hutton 1980). It would not be surprising if these joints were injured at times of excessive loading.

Fracture of the apophyseal facet may be a more common source of back pain than is generally recognized (Scott 1942, Sims-Williams et al 1978). It may only be demonstrated by computerised tomography and it must be distinguished from an accessory ossicle. We shall make the diagnosis only if it is anticipated in the patient with a short history of sudden pain following a dynamic injury. It will be supported by scintigraphy (Kuusela 1980, Matin 1983).

Microfractures also accompany disruption of the vertebral end-plate by disc herniation and the development of Schmorl's nodes (Hilton 1980), and some degree of skeletal failure results in the 'cod-fish' appearance of demineralized vertebrae (see Ch. 23, Fig. 23.6).

The margin of safety between the strength of vertebrae and the calculated forces they may have to sustain during lifting has long been controversial. In a recent attempt to resolve this, Hutton and Adams (1982) measured the average failure load in young men to be about 10 200 N. They suggested that this was about 23% higher than the forces calculated from the maximum strength of a comparable group in a study by Schultz and Andersson (1981). However, this safety margin is small by engineering standards and, more importantly, the calculations ignored the dynamics of lifting. A more recent study by McGill and Norman (1985) of young men lifting an 18-kg weight (well below maximum lifting capabilities) indicated that, using a static analysis, the lumbar compressive force was about 5200 N but that rose by up to 52% when analyzed dynamically. The values of the vertebral failure loads are not in question, but the forces generated by lifting are calculated from models of the spine and are dependent on the nature of the model being correct.

THE INTERVERTEBRAL DISC

Mechanism of failure

The disc fails as a result of mechanical disruption of the tissues. This may follow or result in biochemical change. Disruption causes a fissure with a variety of configurations. This may extend to form a loose fragment of nucleus pulposus, which can extrude either through a fissure in the annulus or as a Schmorl's node through the vertebral end-plate. The force necessary to produce this failure is dependent upon both individual anatomical variations, and age. For example, a compression force which will produce a wedge fracture in the middle-aged adult will produce vertical extrusion of disc nucleus through the end-plate in an adolescent or young healthy adult.

There is an age-related tendency to disc failure. Disc symptoms (which must post-date failure) present for the first time most frequently in the fourth decade. Either the annulus is more resilient in the young, or there are protective mechanisms resisting failure. There are certainly progressive microscopic and biochemical changes in the nucleus and annulus with age. Urban and Maroudas (1980) have reviewed the chemistry of the intervertebral disc, showing that there is a progressive fall in water content of the nucleus with increased collagen, lower glycosaminoglycans levels, breakdown of the proteoglycans and a fall in the fixed charge density. The nucleus becomes less homogenous with age, more inspissated with loss of its basic hydrostatic properties. Perhaps a fall in annular resilience is balanced by a change in the nucleus making it less vulnerable to prolapse in the elderly, with greatest risk in middle life.

When an annular tear occurs, it generally is posterior, just lateral to the posterior longitudinal ligament (Fig. 4.1) where the non-circular geometry of the disc concentrates stress at the site of maximum convexity (Farfan 1973, Hickey & Hukins 1980). The fissure can develop gradually, from the inner to the outer layers, and if there is a free fragment, with a nuclear herniation. The 15–25 distinct layers of obliquely placed annular fibres (Marchand & Ahmed 1990) are so arranged that each adjacent layer is orientated in an opposite direction, producing a 'radial ply' effect (Fig. 4.2). By this arrangement intact annular fibres will contain the nucleus, even when it is subjected to a vertical compression force that would normally fracture a vertebra. If there is already an annular fissure (either a congenital weakness (Dixon 1973) or from previous trauma), the resilience of the disc is reduced, and the remaining peripheral annular

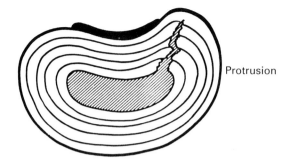

Fig. 4.1 Diagram to show the common site of an annular fissure just lateral to the posterior longitudinal ligament.

fibres can now be disrupted by either a rotational or a vertical compression force.

Opinions differ as to the type of force required to tear the annulus. Hickey and Hukins (1980) suggest that rotation is important whilst Adams and Hutton (1981, 1982) believe that compression of the flexed spine is particularly damaging.

It is probably not axial compression, however, but compression in flexion or torsion that is likely to constitute the first injury to an intact annulus (Hickey & Hukins 1980, Gordon et al 1991). By analogy with behaviour of a tendon, it has been estimated that approximately 4° of torsion will stretch beyond the elastic limit those layers of annular fibres which are orientated against the torsion, and that further torsion or flexion will tear them (Klein et al 1982). Even 4° is probably in excess of the torsion permitted by the

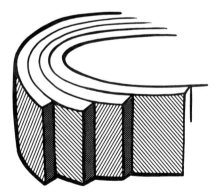

Fig. 4.2 Diagram to show the layers of the annulus having fibres obliquely orientated in alternate directions, producing a radial ply effect.

restraining apophyseal joints at L4/5 and at L5/S1, unless the spine is first flexed to disengage these joints. Rotation of a flexed spine is probably actively resisted by reflex muscle action, but a superadded fall or unexpected strain may overcome that protective reflex and produce sufficient torsion to damage a healthy annulus. This mechanism of disc injury fits both the known facts of the functional anatomy of the spine and also the clinical explanation of the first injury often recounted by patients — a fall or an unexpected strain causing the patient to twist whilst in the stooping position.

Disc resilience

There is some evidence that disc resilience bears a relation to spinal stress in the developing years and early working life (Porter et al 1989). In other anatomical sites, function and form go hand-in-hand, and probably hard work produces a strong annulus. Kelsey (1975) showed that there was a greater incidence of herniated discs in sedentary workers: perhaps 'further education' is responsible for many a weak back and subsequent disc excision. Evans and colleagues (1989) found more degenerate discs in sedentary than in ambulant workers. However, disc degeneration is more common in elite gymnasts than in controls (Sward et al 1991). Our own studies suggest that miners have a lesser incidence of acute disc prolapse and herniation (Porter 1987, 1992), though they are much more prone to the back pain syndromes associated with degenerative change (root entrapment and neurogenic claudication). Cadaveric studies by Videman and colleagues (1990) likewise recorded symmetrical disc degeneration associated with sedentary work, vertebral osteophytosis with heavy work, and least pathology with moderate or mixed physical loads.

Disc nutrition

The lumbar intervertebral discs are the largest avascular structures in the body. Their resistance to injury depends on adequate nutrition, but when is nutrition inadequate? It probably depends on a satisfactory capillary bed in the vertebral body adjacent to the cartilaginous end-plate. Impairment of this capillary bed from bony sclerosis, raised intraosseous venous pressure or the age-related changes in intraosseous arterial anatomy (Ratcliffe 1982) can affect disc nutrition, and may be responsible for some of the progressive biochemical changes in the disc. The epidemiological studies of Frymoyer and his colleagues (1983) and identical twin studies (Battie et al 1991) have shown that back pain is more frequent in smokers and those individuals whose spines are subjected to high frequency vibrations (Pope 1990, Boshuizen et al 1992). They postulate that small changes in the capillary bed from toxic agents or from vibration may significantly affect disc nutrition.

The avascular disc depends on the passage of fluid into the connective tissue matrix for its nutrition. Solutes pass rapidly into the disc by diffusion but large molecules are slow to pass through the fine proteoglycan meshwork. Diurnal changes in fluid volume are considerable and probably aid nutrition (Adams & Hutton 1983). Disc hydration depends upon a balance between the osmotic pressure within the disc and the hydrostatic pressure forcing fluid out of the disc. The volume increases as the hydrostatic pressure is reduced by recumbency, and then the osmotic pressure is largely unopposed. Conversely, the vertical posture increases the hydrostatic pressure, diminishing the fluid volume. Much of the diurnal change in standing height is due to change in the disc's fluid volume. This can amount to 2 cm during the day and it fluctuates fairly quickly with change of posture (Reilly et al 1984, Eklund & Corlett 1984, Adams et al 1990). Postural change and rest between periods of strenuous work affect fluid flow and are probably beneficial to disc nutrition.

One condition which appears to confer an advantage to the resilience of the disc is diabetes. We have observed a low prevalence of diabetes in patients having surgery for disc prolapse (Bremmers et al 1991), and Heliövaara and colleagues (1991) also recorded a low odds ratio for diabetic patients with sciatica and unspecified low back pain. Whether glycosylation of collagen toughens the diabetic annulus, or whether the chondrocytes enjoy a high glucose tolerance is open to speculation.

Disc biochemistry

Collagen

The nature of the collagen molecule and the architectural relationship between molecules determine the structural integrity of the disc. All collagens are constructed in three chains of over 1000 amino acid residues, forming a triple helix. Every third residue is glycine, and the other two are mainly proline and hydroxyproline (Nimni & Harkness 1988). Lysine and hydroxylysine residues are important because they are sites for formation of intermolecular cross-links, giving the fibrils stability (Eyre et al 1984). The fibrils therefore have a high tensile strength and are very inextensible. This changes with age, impairing the mechanical properties.

Twelve different types of collagen have been identified (Mayne & Burgeon 1987) and at least seven of these are found in the disc (Eyre 1989), mainly type I and II.

The gross architectural arrangement of the collagen molecules can be seen with the naked eye. The annulus is constructed as a lamellar structure firmly anchored to the end-plate, whilst the nucleus is an irregular mesh of collagen merging with the annulus but not attached to the end-plate (Inoue & Takeda 1975).

Proteoglycans

These are the other major macromolecules in the disc, formed in chains of carbohydrate bonded to a central core of protein, with a feather-type construction. They exert a fixed charge density to the matrix as a result of a net negative charge, and this controls the distribution of charged solutes and thus the osmotic pressure of the matrix, with implications for cell function (Urban 1990).

A dehydrated disc has densely packed proteoglycan with a small 'pore' size (the space between the molecules), and this reduces fluid diffusion. It will be more detrimental to the flow of macromolecules into the disc, and degraded macromolecules out of the disc. Long periods in the upright posture may therefore impair disc nutrition.

Proteoglycans are probably quickly degraded by enzymes yet undiscovered. Chymopapain will degrade the protein core of proteoglycan, reducing

the fixed charge density and the osmotic pressure. The disc then loses fluid under load.

Matrix synthesis

Little is known about the way in which the cells synthesize the disc matrix, because in vitro the proteoglycan leaches out of the tissue. The turnover of proteoglycan is short in young animals but may be between 2 and 4 years in the adult (Urban et al 1978). Cellular activity may be affected by the pericellular environment, its fluid content, hormones and growth factors. Proteoglycan is synthesized throughout life, but collagen turnover is remarkably slow. The herniated fragment of nucleus is sometimes composed of newly synthesized fibrocartilage (Lipson 1988), and it therefore appears that new collagen can occasionally be laid down. Without restoration of damaged collagen framework, the proteoglycan is no longer anchored and disc function will be permanently impaired.

A free fragment

In vitro a disc protrusion can only be caused experimentally if there is both a fissure of the annulus and a free fragment of the nucleus (Brinkmann et al 1992). As yet, we do not know the mechanism of free fragment formation, whether injury causes a fissure (Fig. 4.3) and alters disc nutrition with the development of further fissure and fragment, or whether altered nutrition affects the disc's biochemistry and then a fissure and fragment are secondary (Fig. 4.4).

Without an annular fissure the loose fragment is contained within the nucleus, but if the annulus is also partially torn, in vivo studies suggest that this combination will cause a protrusion (Fig. 4.5). If a partial tear becomes complete, the loose fragment will extrude or sequestrate (Fig. 4.6). It is theoretically possible for a fissure to so affect disc nutrition that a free fragment develops after a complete annular tear and it then extrudes (Fig. 4.7).

Surgical experience suggests that a free fragment is significant. We examined 104 discectomies. There were 67 patients with free fragments who had sequestrated or extruded or equivocal extruded

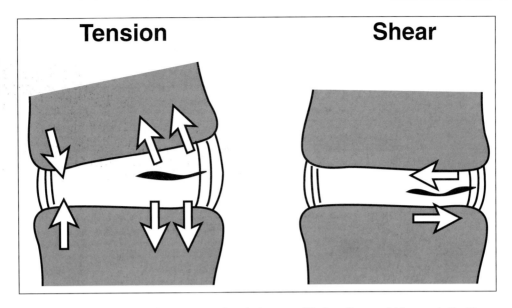

Fig. 4.3 It is possible that injury, acute or chronic, is responsible for a fissure, which secondarily affects disc nutrition, producing a fragment.

free fragments. Of the 37 patients with protrusions and intact outer annulus, 16 had definite loose fragments, though it was not possible to be sure about loose fragments in the remainder (Table 4.1).

The 'motor segment'

It is too easy to think of the disc as an isolated structure and fail to recognize it as part of a 'motor segment' (Lewin et al 1962, Schmorl & Junghams 1971) incorporating the apophyseal joints in a three-joint system. Disruption of a disc must result in disturbed function of the three-joint system, if not at the time of the disc failure then in subsequent years.

Osteophytes result from spinal stress (though they are not necessarily associated with spinal

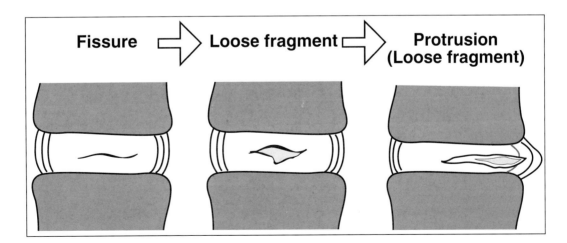

Fig. 4.4 It is equally possible that altered nutrition is responsible for fissure formation with only physiological stress, and a fragment is secondary to this from leaching of the proteoglycan. It will protrude if the fissure then extends to the inner annulus.

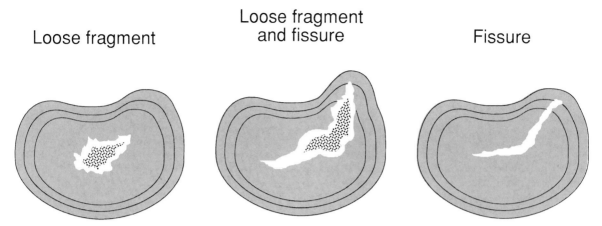

Fig. 4.5   A free fragment without an annular fissure is contained. In the presence of a fissure, the free fragment protrudes. A fissure alone, however, causes no protrusion. This is the experimental observation in vitro (Brinkmann et al 1992), and it agrees with clinical experience.

symptoms). Macnab (1971, 1977) differentiated between claw and traction spurs. Claw type osteophytes develop at the edge of the vertebral body margin around the annulus and sometimes meet and fuse the two vertebrae together (Fig. 4.8). They are commonly seen on the concave side of a scoliosis, and may or may not be associated with disc degeneration. Traction spurs develop a few millimetres from the upper and lower borders of the vertebral bodies (Fig. 4.9) and grow into the attachment of the anterior longitudinal ligament and annular fibres. They are generally accepted as a sign of 'instability' (Harris & Macnab 1954) (Ch. 18), and the majority are associated with disc degeneration (Quinnell & Stockdale 1982). In

practice, there is a spectrum of osteophytes from claw to traction spurs, the classification of a particular osteophyte depending on the particular radiological projection (Macnab 1971). The two particular types may both be related to spinal stress, but from forces in different planes, and may be a sign of protection rather than failure.

If oesteophytes are not an invariable sign of disc failure, nevertheless disc failure is followed by osteophyte formation within a decade, not only by lipping of the anterior or anterolateral margins of the vertebral bodies, but sometimes posteriorly by vertebral bar formation, and generally by osteophytes at the margins of the apophyseal joints (Vernon-Roberts 1980).

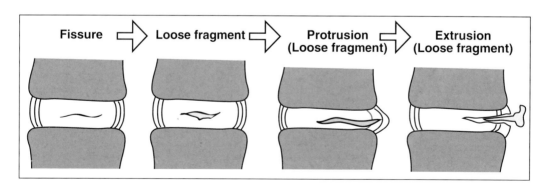

Fig. 4.6   Sequestration could result from a fissure which produces a fragment, then extends to an annular fissure with a protrusion. It can subsequently extrude through a complete tear.

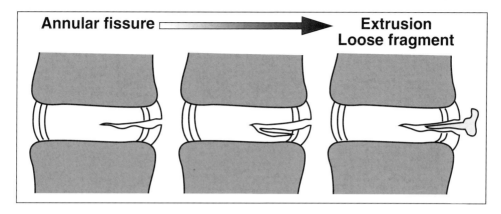

Fig. 4.7   A second method of sequestration could result from a through and through fissure affecting disc nutrition, with a later free fragment forming, and extruding.

SPINAL LIGAMENTS

Isolated disruption of ligaments may occasionally occur as a result of spinal stress but it is a difficult diagnosis to prove, except in the combined bony ligamentous injuries of unstable fracture and fracture dislocation of the spine.

The interspinous and supraspinous ligaments appear to play little part in stabilizing flexion of the spine. Connective tissues can withstand forces directed along the preferred orientation of the collagen fibres, but many papers and anatomy textbooks disagree about the collagen fibre orientation of the interspinous ligament. Confusion began by the inverting of a woodcut for a diagram early this century! The commonly accepted description appears to be that of Heylings (1978, 1980) in which he described the fibres to run posterocranially. However, a study using X-ray diffraction and polarized light microscopy (Aspden et al 1987) showed that the direction of preferred orientation is parallel to the spinous processes with a distribution of fibres about that

Table 4.1   The presence of free fragments in 104 patients who had disc surgery, compared with the operative findings.

Operative findings		Fragment		
	n	Loose	Not loose	Ambivalent
Extrusion or sequestration	(52)	52	0	0
Protrusion	(37)	16	14	7
Equivocal	(15)	15	0	0

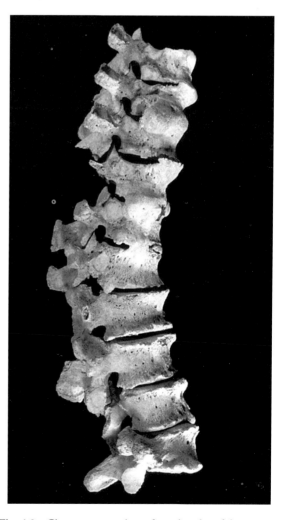

Fig. 4.8   Claw-type osteophytes from the edge of the vertebral bodies, sometimes producing interbody fusion.

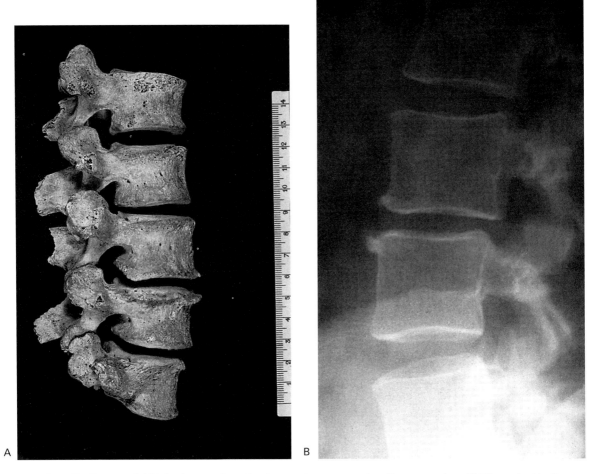

Fig. 4.9(A)   Five Romano-British lumbar vertebrae showing traction spurs on the adjacent margins of L3/4 vertebral bodies.
(B)   Radiograph of a patient with traction spurs at L3/4 level, reduction of the disc space, and signs of rotatory instability
(retrolisthesis and a double posterior shadow of L3).

direction. Flexing the spine did not alter the
direction of preferred orientation but did increase
the width of the distribution. The collagen fibres
of the interspinous ligament pass around the
supraspinous ligament and merge with the
thoracolumbar fascia. Thus, this ligament
appears to have little stabilizing function, but it
does help to anchor the thoracolumbar fascia to
the spine (Tesh et al 1987).

The supraspinous ligament appears to be a
distinctly fatty structure with no single, continuous,
longitudinal collagenous structure. It has a low
stiffness and fails at very low loads. It is suggested
that it provides a protective cushion over the

spinous processes (Hukins et al 1990a).

The complex anatomical arrangement of the
lumbar fascia (Fig. 4.10) provides attachments
between the spinous processes and interspinous
ligaments in the mid-line through the posterior
layer of the fascia, and attachments to the transverse processes through the middle and anterior
layers on the posterior and anterior surfaces of
the quadratus lumborum. These three layers
combine to form attachments laterally to the
three layers of the abdominal muscles, the
latissimus dorsi and the glutei. Thus, together the
layers of the lumbar fascia form a dynamic structure rather than a static rigid mechanism of

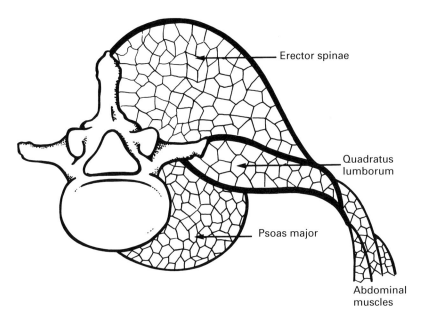

Fig. 4.10   The three layers of the lumbar fascia attached to the spinous and transverse processes of the lumbar vertebrae, which through the abdominal and paraspinal muscles assist stability by stiffening the spine.

stability (Bogduk & Macintosh 1984, Macintosh et al 1986).

There have been two proposals to describe the function of the thoracolumbar fascia, which will increase the extensor moment applied to the spine. The first was a pantograph type of action whereby contraction of the abdominal muscles would pull on the fibres of the thoracolumbar fascia. The fibres were thought to run at about 30° to the spinal axis, and a lateral pull would draw the spinous processes closer together (Gracovetsky et al 1985). The second concept suggested that the thoracolumbar fascia acts like a hydraulic amplifier mechanism in which radial expansion of the contracting back muscles would produce additional tension in the fascia. Both of these hypotheses, however, have been tested and found wanting. The fibre angle was measured to about 70° to the vertical which meant that the pantograph action could only produce a few % of the moment calculated to be produced by the muscles (Macintosh et al 1987); Tesh et al (1987) showed that the hydraulic amplifier mechanism had a 'gain' of only 0.4.

A third concept may be correct. Contraction of the back muscles must generate a radial expansion of those muscles to keep the volume the same. This expansion will be resisted by the fascia and an analysis of this has suggested that the fascia could increase the strength and stiffness of the muscles by about 30% (Aspden 1990, Hukins et al 1990b). Such a mechanism would help to stiffen the spine during a lifting manoeuvre. This hypothesis has yet to be tested but, if correct, then surgical incision of the thoracolumbar fascia should be horizontal and not longitudinal.

Passive stretching of the spinal ligaments provides significant extensor moment during flexion (Gracovetsky et al 1990). It is reasonable to assume, therefore, that damage to the ligamentous complex will predispose the spine to mechanical failure. If the transverse processes can be avulsed by contusion, probably the lumbar fascia can be disrupted by similar forces also. The concept of dynamic ligamentous support is a salutary reminder to the surgeon not to interfere unnecessarily with these structures, either by excision, by promoting scar tissue, or by denervating sections of the muscle.

The pregnancy hormone relaxin has been shown to permit increased spinal mobility in

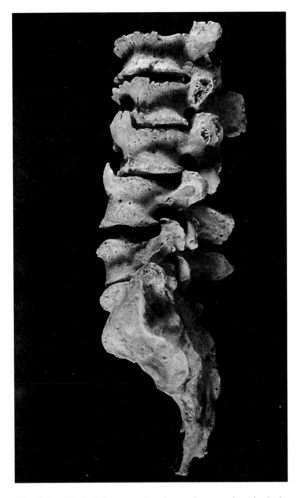

Fig. 5.1 Marked degenerative change in an archaeological Romano-British lumbar spine. Large claw spurs of the vertebral bodies, and osteophytes of the apophyseal joints. Such changes are often seen on radiographs and do not necessarily cause symptoms.

and the toe joints deformed and degenerate without pain.

The apophyseal joints are presumably painful if the capsule is stretched with synovial swelling or by excessive excursion, or if there is increased pressure in the subchondral vessels. Each apophyseal joint has bisegmental innervation (Bogduk & Twomey 1987). Facet joint pathology can cause somatic referred pain, which can be reproduced by pain-provoking injections (see Ch. 14) and relieved by neurolysis. However, degenerative change alone is not necessarily painful. There must be some other factor.

REPAIR

Some structures in the spine can presumably fail and produce pain for a short period, until healing occurs. For example, a compression fracture of a vertebral body often becomes painless after a few weeks. One would expect fractures of apophyseal joints, microfractures, stress fractures and disc extrusion through a vertebral end-plate to produce only temporary pain, unless other structures are affected. Likewise, as at other sites, ligamentous or muscular injuries producing back pain should be self-limiting and not a chronic problem. The majority of patients with back pain, who have a chronic problem, probably have an alternative nociceptive source.

There are probably two major sources of back pain:

1. Segmental pain from;
   a. structures that restrain shear or
   b. structures pain-sensitive to loading
2. Pain-sensitive structures within the vertebral canal.

1. SEGMENTAL PAIN

Structures restraining shear

The thickened capsule and ligaments of an osteo-arthritic hip can cause pain when stretched, and it is not unreasonable to assume that the ligamentous and capsular structures of the spine which restrain shearing forces are likewise a source of pain. They are well endowed with free nerve endings. Injection of hypertonic saline stretching the capsule of the apophyseal joints will produce somatic pain referred to the ipsilateral side of the lower back, the buttock and even into the posterior thigh (McCall et al 1979).

The maximum shearing forces are at L5/S1, but are well resisted by the strong iliolumbar and lumbosacral ligaments, the disc and the coronally orientated apophyseal joint. Lysis of the pars interarticularis negates the effect of the posterior joints, but the other supporting structures are usually still adequate. These are probably a source of pain should they fail. Patients with isthmic spondylolisthesis who attend hospital commonly complain of pain in the back referred into the buttocks and posterior thighs. This would seem to be associated with shearing forces, being worse when standing and shopping, and generally relieved by lying down. A spinal fusion abolishing the effects of shear invariably resolves the problem (Attenborough and Reynolds 1975).

The orientation of the facets at L4/5, the weaker ligaments and the larger disc space mean that shear, though less powerful at this level, is less effectively resisted. This is the commonest site for degenerative spondylolisthesis.

It is reasonable to suggest that structures which restrain shear can be a source of chronic backache when there is segmental failure of the spine (Fig. 5.2). This is developed further in Chapter 7.

Structures which are pain-sensitive to loading

An important question is whether some discs can become pain-sensitive to load rather than movement. The posterior longitudinal ligament has an abundant innervation (Groen et al 1988, Bogduk et al 1981). Nerve fibres have also been reported in the outer third of the annulus (Bogduk et al 1981, Yoshizawa et al 1980, Malinsky 1959). With altered threshold these could respond to load or to movement.

It is worth noting that the peripheral innervation of the disc matches the disc's pressure profile, which in health rises steeply in the outer annulus to a plateau across the remainder of the disc. Perhaps nerves cannot function at such high pressure. Reduced areas of disc pressure occur with degeneration which might permit some innervation. Coppes et al (1990) reported profuse innervation of the longitudinal ligaments, and in two normal discs demonstrated innervation in the outer zone of the annulus. They also observed a few neurofilaments up to the edge of the nucleus pulposus in two degenerate discs. Substance P-related nerves have been found in the discs, and it seems likely that in pathological conditions these fibres can be involved in back pain.

Back pain can accompany discography and chymopapain injections, either from stretching the annulus or from pressure on the end-plate. Painful discography with end-plate disruption suggests that the end-plate can be a nociceptive source (Hsu et al 1988). Pain is associated with bacteriological discitis, and it is therefore possible that some degenerative discs are load-sensitive (Fig. 5.3).

Mrs JR had an uncomplicated excision of a disc protrusion at L5/S1, but had an unexplained pyrexia from the 2nd to the 5th postoperative day. A junior doctor prescribed penicillin tablets for 5 days, without identifying the source of the infection. She continued with severe back pain for 5 weeks and found standing

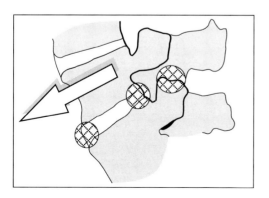

Fig. 5.2 Nociceptive source in structures restraining shear (muscles, ligaments, joint capsule, outer annulus).

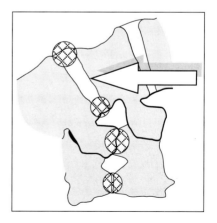

Fig. 5.3 Nociceptive source in structures bearing load (annulus, apophyseal joint, spinous processes).

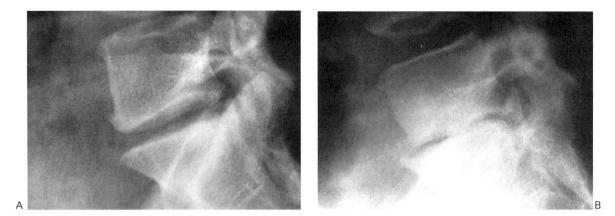

Fig. 5.4   Lateral radiograph of a patient prior to excision of L5/S1 disc protrusion (**A**). She developed severe low back pain that was not recognized as discitis for several weeks. The lateral films 3 months later (**B**) show disc space narrowing and sclerosis of the end-plates.

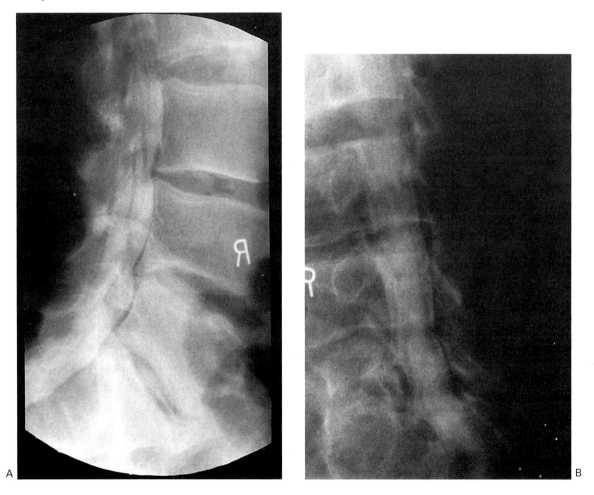

Fig. 5.5   A myelogram of a 54-year-old miner, with back pain radiating round the hips, aggravated by extension.
(**A**)   Lateral view showing a posterior vertebral bar at L4 and a tight dural sac. It is easily understood that extension could produce dural pain. (**B**)   Oblique views of the same patient showing posterior indentation of the dura from the lamina at L5.

and walking very painful. A repeat CT scan failed to identify any remaining disc material compromising the nerve roots, but a scintiscan and later plain radiographs showed evidence of discitis (Fig. 5.4), which became symptom-free over a period of 6 months.

2. PAIN-SENSITIVE STRUCTURES WITHIN THE VERTEBRAL CANAL

The dura

The dura is probably an important source of back pain. Although there are few nerve fibres in the posterior dura, and penetration by needle in the process of radiculography is seldom painful, the anterior dura is richly supplied with nerve fibres and this could be a significant nociceptive source (Cyriax 1978). There is much to support this concept. It can explain the temporary relief obtained by epidural injection of local anaesthetic in the presence of a disc protrusion, why back pain often precedes leg pain in patients with acute disc pathologies, and it might explain the back pain component of the symptoms in spinal stenosis. It can explain the pain and limitation of lumbar extension if there is vertebral displacement and a narrow canal (Fig. 5.5), and when there is a shear strain with a narrow canal, tension on the anterior dura could be a source of pain.

The nerve roots, ganglia and spinal nerve

Anatomy

The true spinal nerve at the lower lumbar levels is only a short segment close to the intervertebral foramen; the greatest part of the length of the nerve in the vertebral canal is composed of ventral and dorsal spinal roots with the dorsal root ganglion and the preganglionic segment (Fig. 5.6). These structures are unquestionably vulnerable to mechanical disturbance within the vertebral canal, the degree depending to some extent on the available space and variable anatomy of the nerve roots and their attachments.

Root excursion is limited by dural fixation and by root attachment at the intervertebral foramen. Proximally the dura is loosely attached by either multiple bands or a solid mid-line septum to the

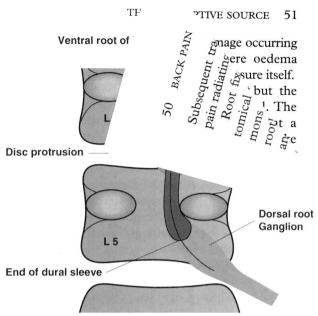

Fig. 5.6 Diagram showing the L5 dorsal and ventral roots, dural sleeve, ganglion and spinal nerve. The L5 roots are vulnerable from a L4/5 disc in the central canal. The dorsal root is more sensitive to ischaemia than the Ventral root, and thus sensory symptoms and signs are more common in disc protrusion than motor signs. The ganglion of L4 may be affected in the root canal.

posterior longitudinal ligament just proximal to the L4/5 and L5/S1 disc and also by more lateral attachments (Spencer et al 1983). The distal attachment of the root to the intervertebral foramen is relatively firm, permitting only slight distal migration of the root when traction is applied to the spinal nerve. The root within the dura is thus partly insulated from the effects of a distal traction force. Spencer and his colleagues described a further ligamentous band from the sheath of the extradural nerve root to the inferior pedicle of the respective foramen. The variable degree of root fixation will affect the extent to which the root is tented over a disc protrusion, and may explain root symptoms in those few patients with a small disc lesion and a spacious canal.

In addition, tension in the attachment of the dura to the posterior longitudinal ligament may produce symptoms similar to those observed by Smyth and Wright (1958), who attached silk threads to the posterior longitudinal ligament and the vertebral periosteum during spinal surgery.

pathology only at spinal level, or is the peripheral nerve itself becoming a nociceptive source by its altered chemistry? Nerve conduction studies suggest that pathological effects of nerve root compression can extend from the original lesion (Watanabe & Tanaka 1990).

Not infrequently a patient who has had previous episodes of disc symptoms with root pain will have a recurrence of symptoms when convalescing from a 'flu-like' illness. This could be a mechanical phenomenon with injury to a disc, bulging from the reduced hydrostatic pressure of a few days' recumbency, and a spine unsupported by weakened muscles. One must question, however, whether the root ganglion could be affected by viraemia if previously bruised from a disc prolapse. Certainly the virus of herpes, latent within spinal ganglia, can be activated periodically (Caplan et al 1977, Warren et al 1978).

There are thus many factors that will affect the response of neural tissue to mechanical injury — the site of the compression; its degree; its duration; its nature, whether soft or bony hard; the diameter of the fibre; and the dynamic factors of root excursion, with irritative, inflammatory (McCarron et al 1987) and biochemical changes. There is much to learn about lumbar root pain, but without doubt the root and ganglion are a significant primary nociceptive source.

Cerebrospinal fluid

The function of the cerebrospinal fluid surrounding the cauda equina is still ill-understood. It buffers the roots and ganglia against physical stress, much as the fetus is protected by liquor. It probably has an insulating effect on nerve conduction, and may be a source of nutrition and remover of nerve metabolites. We do not know what influence a reduced volume of cerebrospinal fluid has on the cauda equina in such syndromes as neurogenic claudication, nor its elimination from the dural sheath of a root compressed by a disc protrusion — 'the cut off sign' commonly seen on radiculography. The absence of cerebrospinal fluid in adhesive arachnoiditis may have symptomatic importance; its influence on nerve function may be highly significant.

The blood supply

Nerve tissue is particularly vulnerable to ischaemia. The function of the ganglia and roots may be adversely affected either by local ischaemia from compression, or by vascular congestion and reduced blood flow. Domminisse (1975) has described the abundant arterial supply to each lumbar nerve root, with the smallest radicular capillaries no larger than 5 μm and the posterior root ganglion having a particularly rich concentration. The supply is abundant presumably because it is necessary, and if it becomes deficient from mechanical compression, scarring or traction, this probably affects nerve function.

The distal cauda equina is supplied segmentally from below by the radicular arteries. If this supply is occluded there is a proximal supply from the spinal arteries at the cord level which provides a rich and adequate anastomosis (Fig. 5.8) (Crock 1981, Crock et al 1986). The concept of a crescenteric watershed of precarious supply in the proximal third of the cauda equina is not correct, but in the presence of an occlusion the roots and ganglia are protected by this rich anastomosis. India ink injected experimentally into the aorta rapidly reaches the radicular arterioles when the proximal or distal supply is impaired (Kobayashi et al 1990).

The physiological relationship between the intraosseous lumbar arterial supply and the radicular arteries has not been established, but it would not be surprising if in certain pathological conditions it became significant. The upper four lumbar arteries are posterior branches of the abdominal aorta arising opposite the bodies of the upper four lumbar vertebrae. A fifth pair usually arises from the iliolumbar artery, but occasionally from the median sacral. These arteries soon divide and run laterally and backwards on the bodies of the lumbar vertebrae, supplying intraosseous branches to the vertebral bodies, then a radicular branch through the intervertebral foramen before further branches supply the muscles of the back and the abdominal wall.

The intraosseous arteries are particularly interesting, showing a marked coiling which increases with age (Fig. 5.9). Ratcliffe (1980, 1981, 1982) described these coils, but their function is and walking very painful. A repeat CT scan failed to identify any remaining disc material compromising the nerve roots, but a scintiscan and later plain radiographs showed evidence of discitis (Fig. 5.4), which became symptom-free over a period of 6 months.

2. PAIN-SENSITIVE STRUCTURES WITHIN THE VERTEBRAL CANAL

The dura

The dura is probably an important source of back pain. Although there are few nerve fibres in the posterior dura, and penetration by needle in the process of radiculography is seldom painful, the anterior dura is richly supplied with nerve fibres and this could be a significant nociceptive source (Cyriax 1978). There is much to support this concept. It can explain the temporary relief obtained by epidural injection of local anaesthetic in the presence of a disc protrusion, why back pain often precedes leg pain in patients with acute disc pathologies, and it might explain the back pain component of the symptoms in spinal stenosis. It can explain the pain and limitation of lumbar extension if there is vertebral displacement and a narrow canal (Fig. 5.5), and when there is a shear strain with a narrow canal, tension on the anterior dura could be a source of pain.

The nerve roots, ganglia and spinal nerve

Anatomy

The true spinal nerve at the lower lumbar levels is only a short segment close to the intervertebral foramen; the greatest part of the length of the nerve in the vertebral canal is composed of ventral and dorsal spinal roots with the dorsal root ganglion and the preganglionic segment (Fig. 5.6). These structures are unquestionably vulnerable to mechanical disturbance within the vertebral canal, the degree depending to some extent on the available space and variable anatomy of the nerve roots and their attachments.

Root excursion is limited by dural fixation and by root attachment at the intervertebral foramen. Proximally the dura is loosely attached by either multiple bands or a solid mid-line septum to the

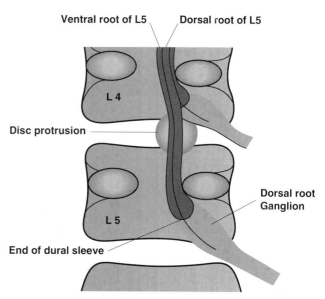

Fig. 5.6 Diagram showing the L5 dorsal and ventral roots, dural sleeve, ganglion and spinal nerve. The L5 roots are vulnerable from a L4/5 disc in the central canal. The dorsal root is more sensitive to ischaemia than the Ventral root, and thus sensory symptoms and signs are more common in disc protrusion than motor signs. The ganglion of L4 may be affected in the root canal.

posterior longitudinal ligament just proximal to the L4/5 and L5/S1 disc and also by more lateral attachments (Spencer et al 1983). The distal attachment of the root to the intervertebral foramen is relatively firm, permitting only slight distal migration of the root when traction is applied to the spinal nerve. The root within the dura is thus partly insulated from the effects of a distal traction force. Spencer and his colleagues described a further ligamentous band from the sheath of the extradural nerve root to the inferior pedicle of the respective foramen. The variable degree of root fixation will affect the extent to which the root is tented over a disc protrusion, and may explain root symptoms in those few patients with a small disc lesion and a spacious canal.

In addition, tension in the attachment of the dura to the posterior longitudinal ligament may produce symptoms similar to those observed by Smyth and Wright (1958), who attached silk threads to the posterior longitudinal ligament and the vertebral periosteum during spinal surgery.

Subsequent traction produced unilateral low back pain radiating into the ipsilateral buttock and thigh.

Root fixation is also variably affected by anatomical anomalies of the roots. Kadish and Simmons (1984) described anastomoses between rootlets, anomalous origins of roots, extradural anastomoses and divisions in 14% of specimens examined, and these will influence root excursion (Okuwaki et al 1991) (Fig. 5.7).

We know little about the function of the sinuvertebral nerve as it returns from the postganglionic segment of the spinal nerve into the root canal. It may at times, with the nerve roots, be a nociceptive source.

The cauda equina within the dura is composed of distinct free-standing nerve rootlets in a cha-

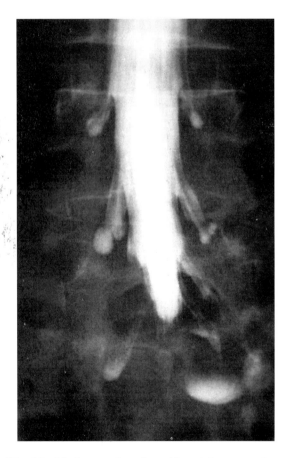

Fig. 5.7 Myelogram of a patient with conjoint roots and cystic expansions of the distal dural sleeves. (Reproduced with the permission of Doncaster Royal Infirmary.)

racteristic anatomical position. The lower sacral and coccygeal roots are located on the dorsal aspect of the sac, and are vulnerable to posterior pressure or surgical injury (Wall et al 1990).

The lumbar root leaves the thecal sac at approximately a 40° angle. The anatomy of its tortuous path has been well described by Amonoo-Kuofi (1991). The S1 root leaves at a more acute angle (Cohen et al 1990). The dorsal root ganglion beneath the pedicles, and one in three have relations of the lateral aspect of the intervertebral disc. The ganglia have an important function and can be impaired by ischaemia. They contain the cell bodies of the dorsal root, which give rise to an axon which bifurcates, a distal process extending to a peripheral receptor and a central process extending to a synapse in the dorsal horn. The cell body will take up amino acids and produce neuronal protein for the axoplasmic transport. It also degrades and restores used protein. It is thus the power-house of the axon transport mechanism, and also the synthesizer of the peptides for nerve transmission at the dorsal horn synapse. Because of this vital function, pathology which affects this dorsal root ganglion is likely to be distinct neurologically from more proximal lesions.

The anatomy of the axons between the cord and the ganglia is also unique, with the cell body of the ganglia at some distance from the synapse in the posterior horn of the cord. Rydevik (1982) has shown that this section of the dorsal root is more sensitive to ischaemia than the ventral root, perhaps explaining why a disc protrusion can produce pain and sensory loss without muscle weakness. The closer the lesion is to the ganglion, the more likely it is to cause permanent damage to the cell in the dorsal root ganglion.

Pathology

There are two distinct types of pathology which affect nerve roots, ganglia and spinal nerves: disc protrusion, and bony or soft tissue degenerative change.

Disc protrusion can be acute or chronic, and in the majority of instances the lesion affects the ventral and/or dorsal roots in the central canal. Occasionally, a lateral disc affects the lumbar root, ganglion or spinal nerve in the root canal.

Bony encroachment into the root canal from the apophyseal joints, from the margins of the vertebral bodies, from thickened ligamentous structures, or perhaps a combination of these with a dynamic component of segmental movement, by contrast, affects the spinal nerves with a different pattern of symptoms. The postganglionic spinal nerve and the ganglion, less commonly the preganglionic nerve and roots, are vulnerable at this level. Occasionally the preganglionic roots may be involved more proximally by the degenerative change of a prominent vertebral bar or the lip of a superior facet in a trefoil central canal, especially in the presence of vertebral displacement or unnatural movement.

The two types of lesion, i.e. the acute disc or the chronic degenerative process, can both affect the roots, ganglia and spinal nerve, but generally at different sites. The chronicity of the lesion, and more particularly the site, may explain the different character of pain and the different signs in patients who have the same root involvement (Leyshon et al 1980).

Pressure on a nerve root from a disc protrusion or in relation to degenerative change often causes pain in the outer buttock, posterolateral thigh, posterolateral calf and outer ankle, with paraesthesia in the big toe or outer foot. Akkerveeken (1989) was not able to find any statistical difference between the pain distribution of L5 or S1 roots, and concluded that the source of the leg pain may be sensors in its nerve root sheath rather than in the root itself. The nociceptive function of the network of the autonomic nerve fibres with many connotations in the nerve roots is not understood (Groen et al 1988), but they may have a protective role. The nerve root adjacent to a disc protrusion is generally swollen (Takata et al 1988).

Experimental compression of a nerve root will produce variable changes related to the degree of pressure. At 30 mmHg intraneural oedema develops affecting nerve function; 50 mmHg affects axoplasmic transport. A high pressure of 200 mmHg, such as could develop from a massive disc prolapse compressing a root against a lamina or adjacent ligamentum flavum, will deform the nerve tissue, the most significant damage occurring at the edge of the compression where oedema affects nerve function more than the pressure itself.

It is possible that not only the root but the peripheral nerve itself becomes pathological. The axonal protein transport may be affected at a spinal level by mechanical disturbance and make the peripheral nerve itself vulnerable to a degree of compression and irritation which would normally be asymptomatic. This would make sense of several clinical observations. A patient with bony entrapment of the nerve root in the root canal not uncommonly states that the root pain is precipitated by sitting on a hard surface, and it is relieved by shifting position. The sciatic nerve in the buttock seems to be sensitive to direct pressure, producing pain from a peripheral source. Likewise some patients with bony entrapment of the root in the root canal have their most severe pain in the outer shin and dorsum of the foot, and digital compression of the common peroneal nerve at the neck of the fibula is acutely tender. Surgical decompression at this level often relieves the discomfort below the knee. The bowstring sign with pain behind the knee when palpating the stretched popliteal nerve, when straight leg raising is limited, is the same phenomenon. Carpal tunnel syndrome has been described as a two-level lesion, one in the hand and the other in the cervical spine (Upton & McComas 1973, Narakas 1990, Wood & Biondi 1990); similarly, meralgia paraesthetica, with spinal stenosis at L3 and associated compression of the lateral cutaneous nerve of the thigh (Jiang et al 1988). There is good evidence that a spinal lesion may produce abnormal axonal chemistry which is subclinical until there is a second pathology in the peripheral nerve itself.

One may also speculate about the source of pain when a patient describes the peripheral spread of sciatic pain, first in the buttock, then in the thigh, and subsequently the calf, ankle and foot. The original pain source was at the spinal level, say from a disc protrusion affecting the nerve root or ganglion, but how significant is the axon transport system of protein at 600 mm per day? Is 'substance P' released from the dorsal root ganglion, increasing the sensitivity of the root to other stimuli (Saal et al 1988)? Is the pathology only at spinal level, or is the peripheral nerve itself becoming a nociceptive source by its altered chemistry? Nerve conduction studies suggest that pathological effects of nerve root compression can extend from the original lesion (Watanabe & Tanaka 1990).

Not infrequently a patient who has had previous episodes of disc symptoms with root pain will have a recurrence of symptoms when convalescing from a 'flu-like' illness. This could be a mechanical phenomenon with injury to a disc, bulging from the reduced hydrostatic pressure of a few days' recumbency, and a spine unsupported by weakened muscles. One must question, however, whether the root ganglion could be affected by viraemia if previously bruised from a disc prolapse. Certainly the virus of herpes, latent within spinal ganglia, can be activated periodically (Caplan et al 1977, Warren et al 1978).

There are thus many factors that will affect the response of neural tissue to mechanical injury — the site of the compression; its degree; its duration; its nature, whether soft or bony hard; the diameter of the fibre; and the dynamic factors of root excursion, with irritative, inflammatory (McCarron et al 1987) and biochemical changes. There is much to learn about lumbar root pain, but without doubt the root and ganglion are a significant primary nociceptive source.

Cerebrospinal fluid

The function of the cerebrospinal fluid surrounding the cauda equina is still ill-understood. It buffers the roots and ganglia against physical stress, much as the fetus is protected by liquor. It probably has an insulating effect on nerve conduction, and may be a source of nutrition and remover of nerve metabolites. We do not know what influence a reduced volume of cerebrospinal fluid has on the cauda equina in such syndromes as neurogenic claudication, nor its elimination from the dural sheath of a root compressed by a disc protrusion — 'the cut off sign' commonly seen on radiculography. The absence of cerebrospinal fluid in adhesive arachnoiditis may have symptomatic importance; its influence on nerve function may be highly significant.

The blood supply

Nerve tissue is particularly vulnerable to ischaemia. The function of the ganglia and roots may be adversely affected either by local ischaemia from compression, or by vascular congestion and reduced blood flow. Domminisse (1975) has described the abundant arterial supply to each lumbar nerve root, with the smallest radicular capillaries no larger than 5 μm and the posterior root ganglion having a particularly rich concentration. The supply is abundant presumably because it is necessary, and if it becomes deficient from mechanical compression, scarring or traction, this probably affects nerve function.

The distal cauda equina is supplied segmentally from below by the radicular arteries. If this supply is occluded there is a proximal supply from the spinal arteries at the cord level which provides a rich and adequate anastomosis (Fig. 5.8) (Crock 1981, Crock et al 1986). The concept of a crescenteric watershed of precarious supply in the proximal third of the cauda equina is not correct, but in the presence of an occlusion the roots and ganglia are protected by this rich anastomosis. India ink injected experimentally into the aorta rapidly reaches the radicular arterioles when the proximal or distal supply is impaired (Kobayashi et al 1990).

The physiological relationship between the intraosseous lumbar arterial supply and the radicular arteries has not been established, but it would not be surprising if in certain pathological conditions it became significant. The upper four lumbar arteries are posterior branches of the abdominal aorta arising opposite the bodies of the upper four lumbar vertebrae. A fifth pair usually arises from the iliolumbar artery, but occasionally from the median sacral. These arteries soon divide and run laterally and backwards on the bodies of the lumbar vertebrae, supplying intraosseous branches to the vertebral bodies, then a radicular branch through the intervertebral foramen before further branches supply the muscles of the back and the abdominal wall.

The intraosseous arteries are particularly interesting, showing a marked coiling which increases with age (Fig. 5.9). Ratcliffe (1980, 1981, 1982) described these coils, but their function is

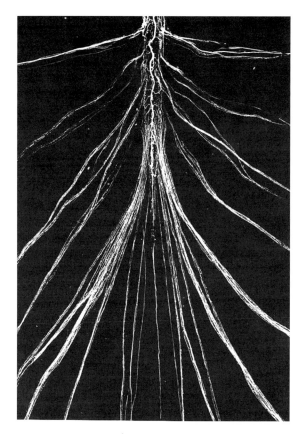

Fig. 5.8 A beautiful dissection of the centripedal arterial supply of the cauda equina, showing an anastomosis at the conus providing for retrograde flow should there be a peripheral block. There is no suggestion of an arc of hypovascularity in the cauda equina. (Reproduced by kind permission of Mr H V Crock.)

not known. It is tempting to suggest that they may produce a resistance to arterial flow, acting as a hydrostatic damp, and if sensitive to autonomic or vasoactive substances, take part in an arterial shunt mechanism diverting blood to the radicular arteries. Intraosseous arterial shunts have been demonstrated in the long bones of rabbits in response to exercise (Pooley et al 1984), and in dogs and mice after the administration of noradrenaline and ATP (McCarthy et al 1984). If the form of these arteries has physiological significance, what is the effect of inserting large interpedicular screws? How does this affect disc nutrition?

Early results of spinal blood flow studies using positron emission tomography (Ashcroft et al 1992) suggest that vertebral blood flow may be an important factor in some types of back pain. In Paget's disease of the spine (Hadjipavlou & Lander 1991) this is also probably significant. The arterial supply to the spinal cord, and presumably the cauda equina, is subject to vasodilatation in response to muscle activity. Blau and Rushworth (1958) described local vasodilatation of the ipsilateral regions of the spinal cord of a mouse whose single hind limb was exercised. Similarly, muscular activity in the pre-paralytic stages of poliomyelitis selectively affects the distribution of the paralysis, probably from vasodilatation of the anterior horn vessels (Buchthal 1949). It would not be unreasonable for the vertebral bodies, which can withstand li-

A

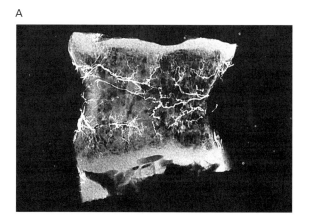

B

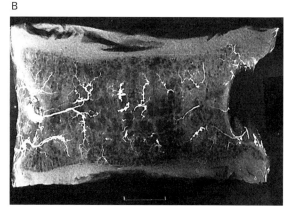

Fig. 5.9(A) and **(B)**   Sagittal sections of the lumbar vertebral bodies showing coiling of the intraosseous branches of the lumbar arteries, the significance of which is unknown (by kind permission of Dr Ratcliffe).

mited ischaemia, to be temporarily deprived of blood, shunting blood to the cauda equina during times of intense muscular activity or during hypovolaemic shock.

The lumbar arteries and their branches must be considered in those cauda equina syndromes which are precipitated by walking. Not infrequently, neurogenic and intermittent claudication coexist (Johansson et al 1982). Atheroma of the abdominal aorta will not only impair flow to the aorta and iliac segments, but will affect lumbar arterial flow. It will be a factor in the root symptoms if space within the vertebral canal is already at a premium and there is incipient root ischaemia.

One of the anomalies of the radiculopathies associated with Paget's disease is that the vertebral canal is not invariably narrow (Herzberg & Bayliss 1980, Ravichandran 1981). A vertebral steal syndrome has been suggested as an explanation of the cauda equina symptoms in Paget's disease, which is sometimes reversible with calcitonin therapy (Walpin & Singer 1979, Douglas et al 1981). The intraosseous branches of the lumbar arteries cannot be neglected when considering cauda equina ischaemia as a pain source.

The complicated venous channels in the extradural compartment of the vertebral canal (Batson's plexus, Batson 1940), freely communicate with the azygous system of veins by the radicular veins. They accompany the nerve roots in the root canal through the intervertebral foramen. These veins are without valves, and thus the pressure within the vertebral canal is increased with raised intra-abdominal pressure. A patient who already has back pain from some lesion within the vertebral canal where limitation of space is a problem, is likely to have an increase in that pain when the venous pressure increases. Coughing, straining and lifting will increase that pressure, and the same mechanism may explain some types of premenstrual back pain.

The venous drainage of the cauda equina is centrifugal, opposite to the arterial flow. The veins of the nerve roots drain peripherally and anastomose with the extradural plexus at the extremity of the dural sleeve (Fig. 5.10). There appears to be a hemi-valve at this site (Suh &

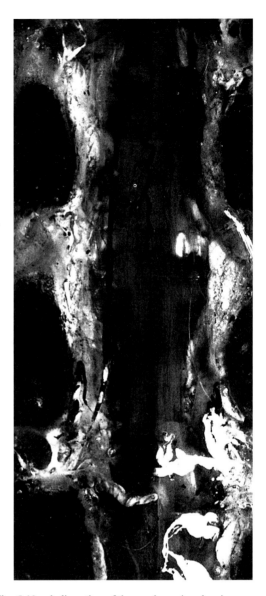

Fig. 5.10   A dissection of the cauda equina showing a centrifugal venous drainage. An attempt to inject barium into the extradural veins to demonstrate the veins of the cauda equina failed because of the hemivalve at the junction of the intradural and extradural veins. Note the small pieces of barium in the radicular vein on the lower left. (By kind permission of Mr H V Crock.)

Alexander 1938), preventing backflow from the valveless extradural plexus into the radicular system of veins. In spite of centrifugal flow, a single level intradural root block may not produce radicular venous hypertension because the

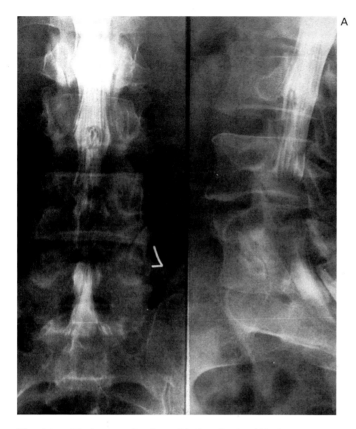

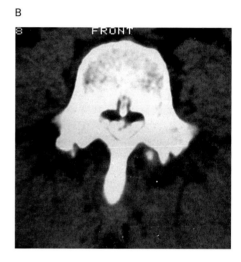

Fig. 5.11 Myelogram of patient with three levels of block at L3/4, 4/5 and L5/S1. The engorged extradural veins produce a circular pattern at L3 and L4 (**A**). These veins are demonstrated in the CT scan (**B**) as the central veins emerge from the back of the body of L3 and encroach onto the tight dura.

radicular veins can reverse flow to the rich anastomosis around the conus of the cord.

Patients with neurogenic claudication often have multiple-level stenosis, and a two-level block at low pressure. The intervening segment of nerve will be affected by venous pooling and a build-up of metabolites. This is probably the mechanism of claudication pain in some patients with spinal stenosis (see page 205).

Patients with neurogenic claudication may also have significant epidural venous engorgement (Fig. 5.11), which can add to the surgical difficulties. Degenerative change in the vertebral bodies with increased interosseous venous pressure may be of some importance in this syndrome. The reduction of osseous venous pressure caused by calcitonin could explain the rapid recovery of impending paraplegia in some patients with Paget's

disease when treated with this drug (Douglas et al 1981), and the same drug's effect on some patients with neurogenic claudication (Porter & Hibbert 1983).

THE SACROILIAC JOINT

The sacroiliac joint is often the first joint of the axial skeleton to be affected by inflammatory disorders. It may produce the first symptom of ankylosing spondylitis, and subclinical forms with intermittent back pain but no abnormal radiological signs may be relatively common in both sexes. Pain and tenderness in the sacroiliac region may follow pelvic infection in women and prostatitis in men, with the appearance of osteitis condensans ilii. The joint is not easily disturbed, however, by mechanical derangement.

The sacroiliac is a large joint of irregular contour, supported by powerful ligaments. It is unusual for it to be a source of pain following a mechanical injury. Its range of movement is the same in symptomatic and asymptomatic joints (Sturesson et al 1989). Sacroiliac over-use may cause pain in military recruits with a positive scintiscan (Chisin et al 1984), but for most patients who complain of pain in the sacroiliac region, a careful assessment of the lumbar spine usually confirms that this is referred from the mid-line. Serious disruption of the sacroiliac joint can accompany pelvic fractures and separation of the pubic symphysis. In those countries where obstructed labour is relieved by symphysiotomy, and in spontaneous disruption of the symphysis, sacroiliac pain can persist for months (Fig. 5.12). Over-enthusiastic removal of donor bone from the posterior ileum will cause long-standing pain and tenderness if the joint is transgressed. However, these instances are rare when considering the total back pain population.

There is no consensus of agreement about the source of pain in most back pain syndromes, but it is not improbable that most patients with a back pain problem of mechanical origin experience pain from two main sources: segmental structures which

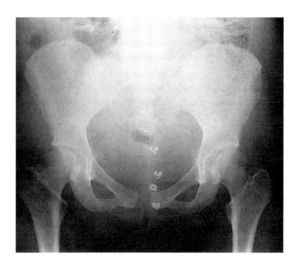

Fig. 5.12 Pelvic X-ray showing spontaneous disruption of the symphysis pubis after obstructed labour. It was relieved by a Caesarian section. The patient experienced back pain and had a waddling gait for several weeks.

restrain shear or are load-sensitive; or tissues within the vertebral canal, especially the dura, ganglia and roots. This at least supports the known facts and provides a working basis for understanding many back pain mechanisms. We shall look at these in detail in the next two chapters.

REFERENCES

Akkerveeken P F 1989 Lateral stenosis of the lumbar spine. Thesis, University of Utrecht

Amonoo-Kuofi H S, El-Badawi M G, Fatani J A, Butt M M 1991 Extra spinal course of the fifth lumbar spinal nerve. Clinical Anatomy 4: 319–326

Ashcroft P, Porter R W, Evans N, Roeda D 1992 Vertebral body and cauda equina blood flow measured by positron emission tomography. Presented to the International Society for the Study of the Lumbar Spine: Chicago, May 1992

Attenborough C G, Reynolds M T 1975 Lumbo-sacral fusion with spring fixation. Journal of Bone and Joint Surgery 57-B: 283–288

Batson O V 1940 The function of the vertebral veins and their role in the spread of metastases. Annals of Surgery 112: 138–149

Blau J N, Rushworth G 1958 Observations of blood vessels of the spinal cord and their response to motor activity. Brain 81: 354–363

Bogduk N, Twomey 1987 Clinical anatomy of the lumbar spine. Churchill Livingstone, Melbourne

Bogduk N, Tynan W, Wilson A S 1981 The nerve supply to the human lumbar intervertebral discs. Journal of Anatomy 132: 39

Buchthal F 1949 Problems of the pathologic physiology of poliomyelitis. American Journal of Medicine 6: 591–597

Caplan L R, Kleeman F J, Berg S 1977 Urinary retention probably secondary to herpes genitalis. New England Journal of Medicine 297(17): 920–921

Chisin R, Milgrom C, Margulies J, Giladi M, Stien M, Kashtan H, Atlan H 1984 Unilateral sacroiliac overuse syndrome in military recruits. British Medical Journal 289: 590–591

Cohen M S, Wall E J, Brown R A, Rydevik B, Garfin S R 1990 Cauda equina anatomy II: extrathecal nerve roots and dorsal root ganglia. Spine 15: 1248–1251

Coppes M H, Marani E, Thomeer R J W M, Ondega M, Geen G J 1990 Innervation of annulus fibrosus in the low back pain. Lancet 336: 189–190

Crock H V 1981 Normal and pathological anatomy of the lumbar spinal nerve roots. Journal of Bone and Joint Surgery 63-B: 487–490

Crock M V, Yamagaishi M, Crock M C 1986 The conus medullaris and cauda equina in man. An atlas of the vascular anatomy. Springer Verlag, Vienna

Cyriax J 1978 Daral pain. Lancet i: 919–921

Domminisse G F 1975 The arteries and veins of the human spinal canal from birth. Churchill Livingstone, Edinburgh

Douglas D L, Duckworth T, Kanis J A, Jefferson A A, Martin T J, Russell R G G 1981 Spinal cord dysfunction in Paget's disease of bone: has medical treatment a vascular basis? Journal of Bone and Joint Surgery 63-B: 495–503

Groen G J, Baljet B J, Drukker J 1988 The innervation of the spinal dura mater: anatomy and clinical implications. Acta Neurochirurgica 92: 39–46

Hadjipavlou A, Lander P 1991 Paget's disease of the spine. Journal of Bone and Joint Surgery 73-A: 1367–1381

Herzberg L, Bayliss E 1980 Spinal cord syndrome due to non-compressible Paget's disease of bone: a spinal artery steal phenomenon reversible with calcitonin. Lancet 2: 13–15

Hsu K, Zucherman J F, Derby R, White A H, Goldthwaite N, Wynne G 1988 Painful lumbar end plate disruptions: a significant discographic finding. Spine 13: 76–79

Jiang G X, Xu W D, Wang A H 1988 Spinal stenosis with meralgia paraesthetica. Journal of Bone and Joint Surgery 70-B: 272–273

Johansson J E, Barrington T W, Ameli M 1982 Combined vascular and neurogenic claudication. Spine 7: 150–158

Kadish L J, Simmons E H 1984 Anomalies of the lumbosacral nerve roots; an anatomical investigation and myelographic study. Journal of Bone and Joint Surgery 66-A: 411–416

Kobayashi S, Yoshizawa H, Hachiya Y, Kurose J 1990 Circulatory dynamics of lumbo sacral spinal nerve roots. Presented to the International Society for the Study of the Lumbar Spine. Boston, June 1990

Leyshon A, Kirwan E O'G, Wynn Parry C B 1980 Is it nerve root pain? Journal of Bone and Joint Surgery 62-B: 119

McCall I W, Park W M, O'Brien J P 1979 Induced pain referred from posterior lumbar elements in normal subjects. Spine 4: 441–446

McCarron R F, Wimpoe M W, Hudkins P G, Laros G S 1987 The inflammatory effect of nucleus pulposus: a possible element of the pathogenesis of low back pain. Spine 12: 760–764

McCarthy I D, Davies R, Hughes S P F 1984 The response of the microcirculation in bone to the administration of noradrenaline and ATP. Presented to the British Orthopaedic Research Society, Stanmore, 1984

McCarthy P W, Carruthers B, Martin D, Petts P 1991 Immunohistochemical demonstration of sensory nerve fibres and endings in lumbar intervertebral discs of the rat. Spine 16: 653–655

Malinsky J 1959 The autogenetic development of nerve terminations in the intervertebral discs of man. Acta Anatomica 38: 96–113

Narakas A O 1990 The role of thoracic outlet syndrome in the double crush syndrome. Annales de Chirurgie de la Main el des Membres Supérieures 5: 331–340

Okuwaki T, Kunogi J, Hasue M 1991 Conjoined nerve roots associated with lumbosacral spine anomalies. Spine 16: 1347–1349

Pooley J, Pooley J E, Stevens J 1984 Evidence for an intraosseous arteriovenous shunt operating in long bones during exercise conditions. Presented to the British Orthopaedics Research Society. Stanmore, 1984

Porter R W, Hibbert C 1983 Calcitonin treatment for neurogenic claudication. Spine 8: 585–592

Ratcliffe J F 1980 The arterial anatomy of the adult human lumbar vertebral body. A microarteriographic study. Journal of Anatomy 131: 57–59

Ratcliffe J F 1981 The arterial anatomy of the developing human dorsal and lumbar vertebral body. A microarteriographic study. Journal of Anatomy 133: 625–638

Ratcliffe J F 1982 An evaluation of the intra-osseous arterial anastomoses in the human vertebral body at different ages. A microarteriographic study. Journal of Anatomy 134: 373–382

Ravichandran G 1981 Spinal cord function in Paget's disease of spine. Paraplegia 19: 7–11

Rydevik R 1982 Pathoanatomy and pathophysiology of nerve root compression. Presented to the International Society for the Study of the Lumbar Spine, Toronto

Saal J A, Dillingham M F, Gambur R S, Fanton G S 1988 The pseudoradicular syndrome. Spine 13: 926–930

Smyth M J, Wright V 1958 Sciatica and the intervertebral disc. Journal of Bone and Joint Surgery 40-A: 1401

Spencer D L, Irwin G S, Miller J A A A 1983 Anatomy and significance of fixation of the lumbo-sacral nerve roots in sciatica. Spine 8: 672–679

Sturesson B, Selvik G, Uden A 1989 Movements of the sacro iliac joints. Spine 14: 162–165

Suh T H, Alexander L 1938 Human spinal cord. Archives of Neurology and Pyschiatry 35: 661–677

Takata K, Inone S, Takahashi K, Ohtsuka Y 1988 Swelling of the cauda equina in patients who have herniation of a lumbar disc. Journal of Bone and Joint Surgery 70-A: 361–368

Upton A R M, McComas A J 1973 The double crush in nerve-entrapment syndromes. Lancet ii: 359–361

Verna-Roberts B 1987 Pathology of intervertebral joints and apophyseal joints. In: Jayson M I V (ed) The lumbar spine and back pain, 3rd edn. Churchill Livingstone, Edinburgh, p 37–55

Wall E J, Cohen M S, Massie J B, Rydevik B, Garfin S T 1990 Cauda equina anatomy 1: intrathecal nerve root organization. Spine 15: 1244–1247

Walpin L A, Singer F R 1979 Paget's disease, reversal of severe paraparesis with calcitonin. Spine 4: 213–219

Warren K G, Brown S M, Wroblewska Z, Gilden D, Koprowski H, Subak-Sharpe J 1978 Isolation of latent herpes from the superior cervical and vagus ganglions of human beings. New England Journal of Medicine May: 1068

Watanabe J, Tanaka H 1990 Identification of the motor nerve fibre potentials in lumbar epidural space and its clinical significance. Spine 15: 1131

Wood V E, Biondi J M 1990 Double crush nerve compression thoracic outlet syndrome. Journal of Bone and Joint Surgery 71-A: 85–87

Wyke B D 1980 The neurology of low back pain. In: Jayson M I V (ed) The lumbar spine and back pain, 2nd edn. Pitman Medical, London, Ch. 11, p 265–339

Yoshizawa H, O'Brien J P, Smith W T et al 1980 The neuropathology of intervertebral disc removed for low back pain. Journal of Pathology 132: 95

6. The significance of the vertebral canal — compromise of its contents and its development

The intervertebral disc has enjoyed an era of popularity since Mixter and Barr described the symptoms of a disc protrusion in 1934. However, the relative importance of the vertebral canal in the symptomatology of back pain has only gradually been appreciated. Sarpyener (1945) documented 10 patients in whom a narrow vertebral canal was responsible for deformity and paralytic problems, and then Verbiest in 1954 described the symptoms of neurogenic claudication resulting from spinal stenosis. The available space in the vertebral canal is now recognized as a significant factor in many back pain syndromes, not only in neurogenic claudication, but also in the root entrapment syndrome, acute and chronic disc lesions, and some of the problems of instability.

ANATOMY

The term 'vertebral canal' refers to a highly complex anatomical space posterior to the vertebral bodies and discs, within the neural arch, which widens and narrows at each vertebral level in both coronal and sagittal planes. There is not only regional variation at each vertebral level, but also considerable individual variation within a population.

The vertebral canal is arbitrarily divided into the central canal and the root canal. At the pedicular level the central canal is bounded laterally by the two pedicles, anteriorly by the posterior surface of the vertebral body, and posteriorly by the cranial aspect of the laminae and the medial aspect of the superior apophyseal joints. Between pedicular levels the central canal has an artificial boundary. It extends from one pedicular level to the next, and contains the cauda equina within the dural envelope (Fig. 6.1).

The root canal is that space lateral to the central canal, in the intervertebral region. Anteriorly it is bounded by the posterior surface of the vertebral body above, the posterolateral aspect of the disc

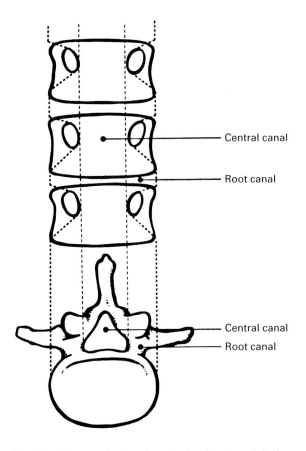

Fig. 6.1 Diagram showing the central and root canals in the coronal and transverse planes.

and the posterior surface of the vertebral body below. Superiorly it is bounded by the pedicle of the vertebra above, and inferiorly by the pedicle of the vertebra below. Its posterior relations are the lateral aspect of the lamina and the superior articulation of the apophyseal joint of the vertebra below. Medially it opens into the central canal, and laterally it ends at the intervertebral foramen. The root canal at L5 is considerably longer than at other levels because of the broad fifth lumbar pedicle.

The lateral recess is that lateral part of the central vertebral canal at the pedicular level, anterior to the medial aspect of the superior apophyseal facet (Schatzker & Pennal 1968). Dome-shaped canals do not have a lateral access, because of the continuous concave posterior surface of this type of canal. Trefoil canals with their 'cocked hat' appearance, however, have a deep lateral recess (Fig. 6.2).

In the sagittal plane the central canal pursues a serpentine course (Fig. 6.3). It is indented posteriorly by the cranial aspect of each lamina, and anteriorly by each intervertebral disc. In the coronal plane, the vertebral canal is narrowest at each pedicular level, widening into each root canal and narrowing again at the next pedicular level.

The general dimensions of the vertebral canal tend to follow a constant pattern from the first to the fifth lumbar levels (Porter et al 1980). In the mid-sagittal plane at the pedicular level, it is generally greatest at L1, reducing to L4 and

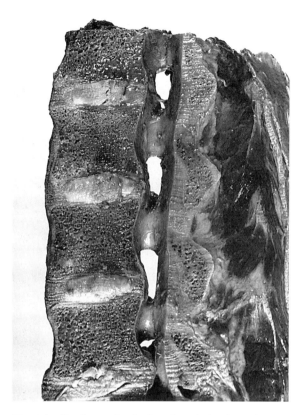

Fig. 6.3 Specimen of sagittal section of a lumbar spine showing the serpentine shape of the central canal, narrowing at each segment level.

increasing again at L5. In the coronal plane, the interpedicular diameter measurements are fairly constant from L1 to L3, widening a little at L4 and then considerably at L5. The total cross-sectional area at the pedicular levels reduces from L1 to L4, and then increases at L5 to an area equal to or even greater than that at L1 (Figs 6.4, 6.5 and 6.6). However, if a canal is trefoil-shaped at L5 its sagittal diameter is then smaller than the sagittal diameter at L4 and its area is also smaller.

There are population differences in the size of the vertebral canal. Spines from the Indian subcontinent are small compared with modern Caucasian spines and with archaeological Anglo-Saxon and Romano-British spines (Porter et al 1980). There is also considerable variation within each population, with approximately 50% increase in the diameters from the 10th to the 90th

Dome shaped   **Trefoil**

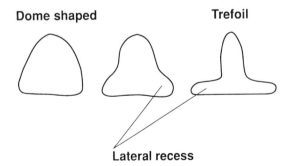

Lateral recess

Fig. 6.2 Diagram to show the variable shape of the central lower lumbar vertebral canal. The dome-shaped canal has no lateral recess, whilst the trefoil-shaped canal has a deep lateral recess.

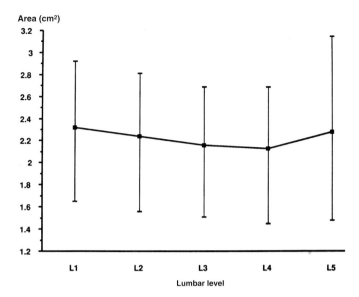

Fig. 6.4 The mean, 10th and 90th percentile measurements of the area of the canal, from three populations of archaeological spines.

percentiles. Eisenstein (1977) noted that women had slightly wider canals than men in the same population. Measuring the mid-sagittal diameter of Caucasoid and Negro spines he found similar absolute measurements with a slight racial difference. The racial variation may have some sig-

nificance when considering the incidence of back pain syndromes.

The range of mid-sagittal and interpedicular diameters is greatest at L5 with more variability in both size and shape of the canal. Eisenstein (1980) described 14% of canals trefoil at L5. The

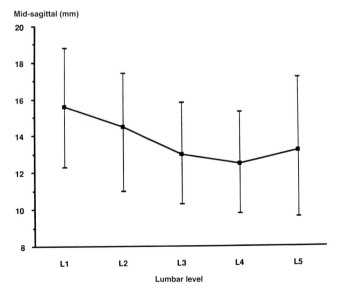

Fig. 6.5 Mid-sagittal measurements from three archaeological populations.

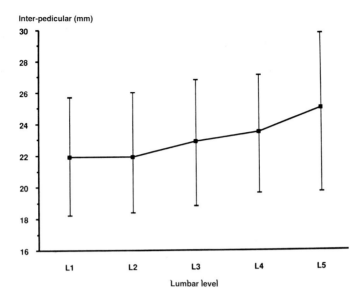

Fig. 6.6 Interpedicular measurements from three archaeological populations.

trefoil configuration is a relative term caused by posterolateral indentation of the neural arch. Two extremes of shape at L5 are shown in Figures 6.7 and 6.8, but in fact no two canals are the same. We measured the trefoil configuration of 240 spines using a photographic method (Figures 5.6, 5.7 and 5.8) and it is apparent that the canal of many spines changes to a trefoil shape from L2 to L5. The change in shape was fairly constant for three archaeological populations.

One would expect the cross-sectional area of the canal to decrease cadually, as there is a gradual reduction in the volume of the neural contents. At first sight, the increased cross-sectional area at L5 (Fig. 6.4) may seem surprising, until we consider the trefoil shape of the canal. A larger cross-sectional area will be advantageous when the surface area of the canal increases, and in addition the lordotic curve, most marked at L5/S1, places some vulnerability on the neural elements unless the cross-sectional area is increased.

Unfortunately, the trefoil-shaped canal is un-healthy if that spine is affected by pathological change. Not only are the L5 nerve roots at risk from encroachment of disc or osteophytes into the lateral recess, but the cross-sectional area of trefoil canals is generally less than that of non-trefoil canals, and the mid-sagittal diameter

is often reduced (Eisenstein 1977, Porter 1980).

SIGNIFICANCE OF CANAL SIZE

An obvious argument against the vertebral canal being a significant factor in the pathogenesis of back pain is that, although the canal does vary in size and shape from one individual to another, this variation is probably adequate for each subject. In other words, the neural contents may be greater with a large canal, but less in a small canal. The lordotic curve and the range of movement for one individual may also be reflected in the canal's dimensions and be satisfactory for that person.

The neural contents undoubtedly influence the dimensions of the vertebral canal to some degree (Rothman 1972), much as the brain determines epigenetically the size of the skull in hydro-cephalus and microcephalus (Lindborgh 1972). In the spine, however, this is not the only factor. There must be other influences at work, both genetic and environmental, because clinical observations show great variation in the propor-tion of intradural to extradural space. We know from CT scans and surgical experience that many patients with back pain have a canal with a small mid-sagittal diameter, a trefoil shape and a tightly

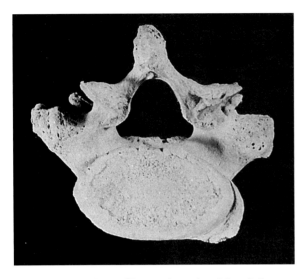

Fig. 6.7   A specimen of L5 vertebrae viewed from below with a large dome-shaped vertebral canal.

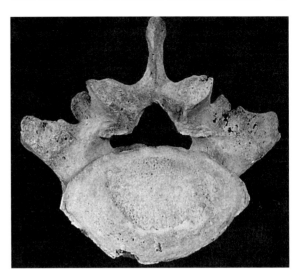

Fig. 6.8   A contrasting L5 vertebra with a shallow trefoil-shaped canal and a deep lateral recess.

packed cauda equina. In fact, the canal will often determine the pattern of symptoms from any particular pathology.

Sarpyener (1945), Schlesinger and Taveras (1953), Verbiest (1954), Van Gelderen (1958), the Epsteins (1962), Ehni (1969), Salibi (1976) and many others have described how spinal pathology in the presence of a small vertebral canal can produce a variety of back pain syndromes. Edwards and La Rocca (1985) showed that 71% of patients with back pain and degenerative change had diameters below the mean. Kornberg and Rechtine (1985) demonstrated an inverse relationship between the vertebral canal size and the morbidity of disc protrusion. Forsberg and Walloe (1982) reported that patients who made a poor recovery from disc surgery had canals that were narrower than those patients who recovered uneventfully. It is the sagittal diameter rather than the inter-pedicular diameter that is critical, the exception being in achondroplasia, in which a narrow inter-pedicular diameter can cause stenotic symptoms (Epstein & Malis 1955, Nelson 1970).

The argument that the canal size is insignificant because it matches the size of the contents and is adequate for the individual runs contrary to anatomical and clinical observations. There is a degree of mismatch, and subjects with limited extradural space are vulnerable to a variety of back pain syndromes when there is added pathology.

A disc protrusion into a restricted space can produce more troublesome symptoms than a protrusion into a wider canal. The trefoil shape places the nerve root at considerable risk in the presence of a posterolateral protrusion. However, a far-lateral disc protruding into the root canal quickly involves the root irrespective of the central canal's size.

Similarly, the variable space in the root canal is a significant factor in the development of root entrapment syndrome from lateral canal stenosis. The root can be spared when degenerative change develops in a wide root canal, but be at risk when similar pathology occurs in a small canal (Fig. 6.9).

In the presence of segmental instability, the neural contents may not be compromised by dynamic changes when the canal is of adequate size, but stenotic symptoms can arise with segmental deformation if the canal is small (Farfan & Gracovetsky 1984, Penning 1992). The vertebral canal size is undoubtedly a risk factor in many back pain syndromes (Fig. 6.10).

THE SOFT TISSUE COMPONENT OF THE VERTEBRAL CANAL

The cauda equina and nerve roots are generally compromised at the intersegmental region of the

parison between the size of the vertebral canal and the length of skeletal long bones showed a useful correlation between the length of the femur and the interpedicular diameter; a tall subject had a large transverse diameter of the vertebral body with widely spaced pedicles (Porter & Hibbert 1981). There were few useful correlations between the mid-sagittal diameter of the canal and other bony measurements. The anteroposterior and lateral diameters of the skull had a weak correlation with the mid-sagittal diameter of the canal, but it seems that this clinically important diameter is largely independent of other skeletal growth. Perhaps this is not surprising when much of the long bone growth occurs in childhood and adolescence, whilst the sagittal diameter of the vertebral canal is already mature by 4 years of age. There is a weak correlation between the size of the clavicle and the sagittal diameter of the lumbar canal (Porter 1980), interesting when one recollects that the clavicle is the first bone to ossify.

Clark and co-workers (1985) suggested that the size of the vertebral canal may be affected by factors that impair early childhood development. They examined two archaeological populations and found that a malnourished population tended to have shallow vertebral canals. Another study of two archaeological populations (Porter & Pavitt 1987) compared the canal size with four physiological stress indicators (cribra orbitalia, porotic hyperostosis, dental hypoplasia and Harris lines). Dental hypoplasia correlated with a small mid-sagittal diameter at L1, L3 and L5, a small area at L5, and a more trefoil canal at L4 and L5. There was supportive evidence that an adverse environment in early life is associated with a shallow vertebral canal. No doubt genetic factors have some influence on the size of the canal, but an adverse early environment is probably also important in impairing its growth. The correct model is probably a consideration of early events operating on a genetic background (Joffe 1992).

The trefoil canal

The trefoil shape occurs in approximately 15% of canals at L5; it is less common at L4 and rare at

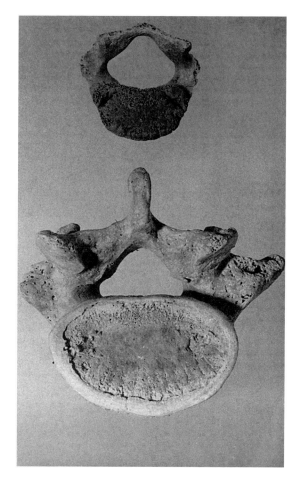

Fig. 6.11 Photographs showing comparisons between the size of the vertebral bodies and the vertebral canals in a 4-year-old child and in an adult.

more proximal levels (Porter et al 1980). It is clinically significant, not only because the L5 root is at risk in the shallow lateral recess, but also because trefoil-shaped canals tend to have small mid-sagittal diameters.

The differential growth of the canal's mid-sagittal and interpedicular diameters makes possible a hypothesis about the trefoil development. The mid-sagittal diameter matures first before 4 years of age, and probably much of this diameter is established in utero. The interpedicular diameter, however, marches to a different tune and continues to mature throughout childhood. Impaired early neuro-osseous development can result in an infant having a small mid-sagittal diameter, and in the absence of spinal catch-up growth that subject will be left with a permanently shallow canal. After infancy, however, an improved environment may allow for adequate growth in stature, resulting in a tall individual with broad vertebral bodies, wide pedicles and a wide interpedicular diameter of the canal. The sagittal diameter remains small but the interpedicular diameter broadens out to a trefoil shape.

Malcomb (1981) has suggested that because body tissues are crystalline in structure, it is to be expected that their growth would resemble that of crystals and liquid crystals. Crystal spirals are logarithmic, as in the spiral growth commonly found in sea shells, and the shape of the human ribs fits well into a hexagonal logarithmic spiral. Spirals may occur of opposite sense and when conjoined produce a variety of forms, and re-entrant angles may be a source of self-perpetuating growth steps. He suggests that the complicated shape of the vertebrae may be explained in terms of crystal growth; it may yet account for some of the variations in form.

There is an interrelationship between different levels of the vertebral canal with regard to morphology. Measurements from over 1600 specimens showed that the cross-sectional area of the lumbar vertebral canal correlates fairly well with that of the cervical spine ($r = 0.65$, $p < 0.001$), at least for the upper and mid-lumbar levels (Table 6.1), and the interpedicular diameters at the mid-cervical and mid-lumbar levels also show a useful correlation (Table 6.2). It is interesting that the mid-sagittal diameters correlate only between the cervical and lower lumbar levels ($r = 0.54$ between C3 and L5, $p < 0.001$) (Table 6.3), levels of both cervical and lumbar regions which are likely to develop pathological change (Rothman 1972, Porter et al 1983, Jacobs et al 1990).

The canal and its contents

If the growth of the neural arch is affected epigenetically by the neural contents (Fig. 6.12), how is it possible to develop a disparity between the canal's size and its contents? A mismatch can be explained by the differential growth of the cord and canal.

In utero, when the conus is in the sacral canal, the epigenetic influence of the spinal cord on the surrounding structures probably causes the size of the cord and the canal to be related. Impaired nutrition and impaired neuro-osseous development will result in a small vertebral canal matched at that time to small contents. In early life, as the conus rises to L2, improved nutrition may arrive too late to benefit the sagittal diameter of the canal, but with improved stature, longer limbs, good muscles and larger peripheral nerves, the cauda equina will also become relatively large yet housed in a shallow vertebral canal left behind by an ascending cord (Fig. 6.13) — a clinically dangerous situation if that canal becomes pathologically compromised.

Spina bifida occulta

The neural tube develops in a craniocaudal manner and is usually complete at the 26th day of gestation. Failure of closure results in spina bifida overta, and failure of closure of the neural arch, in spina bifida occulta. Spina bifida occulta is not an affection of a single segment, even when there is deficiency of only one neural arch; rather, there are subtle changes in the more proximal vertebrae. The mid-sagittal diameter of the vertebral canal in the vertebrae more proximal to the bifid segment is wider than in unaffected skeletons in the same population (Sand 1970, Porter et al 1991). A delay in closure of the neural arch influences at least the two more proximal vertebrae, leaving the canals wider than those of unaffected skeletons. This is a clinical bonus in the syndromes where space is important (Table 6.4).

Spina bifida occulta and overta appear to be related conditions. The parents of children with open spina bifida are four times more likely to

Table 6.1   Correlations between cross-sectional area of lumbar and cervical canals from over 1600 archaeological specimens. Significance of $p = 0.001$ is marked 'x'. The best correlations were between L1 and C3, and L2 and C2.

	C2	C3	C4	C5	C6	C7
L1	x	x[†]	x	x	x	x
L2	x[*]	x	x	x	x	x
L3		x	x	x		x
L4	x	x	x	x		x
L5						x

[*] $r = 0.64$; [†] $r = 0.65$.

Table 6.2 Correlations between interpedicular diameters of lumbar and cervical canals, the best being between L3 and L4 with C3 and C4. Significance of $p = 0.001$ is marked 'x'.

	C1	C2	C3	C4	C5	C6	C7
L1		x	x	x	x	x	x
L2	x	x	x	x	x	x	x
L3	x	x	x†	x‡	x	x	x
L4		x	x★	x‡	x	x	
L5					x		x

★ $r = 0.41$; † $r = 0.42$; ‡ $r = 0.43$.

have the occult lesion than are other members of the population (Lorber & Levic 1967). Neural tube defects are probably related to periconceptional vitamin deficiency (Laurence et al 1981). If at one time vitamin deficiency is related to the development of the occult lesion with a wider canal proximally, and then in another situation impaired nutrition and development can result in a spinal stenosis, there must be two opposite interacting environmental factors.

Spondylolisthesis

Vertebral displacement in isthmic spondylolisthesis widens the sagittal diameter of the vertebral canal, as the floating lamina is left behind and the vertebral body displaces forwards; the pars becomes elongated and the canal dome-shaped. The trefoil configuration is unusual in the presence of spondylolisthesis. Because the canal is so wide, it is unusual to find an isthmic spondylolisthesis in patients with a symptomatic disc protrusion or with neurogenic claudication (Porter & Hibbert 1984). The L4/5 disc is not uncommonly pathological above an isthmic defect at L5, but the large vertebral canal protects the cauda equina.

Table 6.3 Correlations between mid-sagittal diameters of lumbar and cervical vertebral canals, the best being between L5 and C3 and C7. Significance of $p = 0.001$ is marked 'x'.

	C2	C3	C4	C5	C6	C7
L1						
L2	x					x
L3	x	x	x		x	x
L4	x		x		x	
L5	x	x†	x	x	x	x★

★ $r = 0.31$; † $r = 0.54$

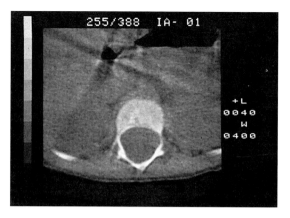

Fig. 6.12 A CT scan of a child with an intradural tumour showing marked expansion of the vertebral canal from the epigenetic influence of the neural tissues.

Vertebrae with unilateral spondylolisthesis occur at about one-quarter of the incidence of bilateral spondylolysis. The asymmetry of the canal in these unilaterally affected vertebrae provides some understanding of the changes observed in the bilateral condition, and of the effect of mechanical forces on the plasticity of the growing canal. There is elongation of the pars, horizontal orientation of the lamina, and asymmetry of the inferior apophyseal joints and the posterior elements in vertebrae with unilateral spondylolysis. The combination of these effects produces a rotation of the spinous process away from the side of the lesion, and the inferior facet joint on the side of the defect is placed more dorsally than the superior facet. This produces a unilaterally capacious vertebral canal (Porter & Park 1982) (Ch. 20).

Table 6.4 The incidence of spina bifida occulta in consecutive patients attending with different back pain syndromes, compared with the incidence in patients with osteoarthritis (OA) of the hip in the same population. The incidence is low in the patients with root pain, and high in those with back pain alone.

	Incidence of spina bifida occulta	(%)
Protruded intervertebral disc	9/142	(6.3)
Root entrapment	3/55	(5.4)
Neurogenic claudication	2/62	(3.2)
Low back pain (undefined)	51/270	(19.0)
Low back pain (instability criteria)	41/86	(47.7)
OA hip	8/70	(11.4)

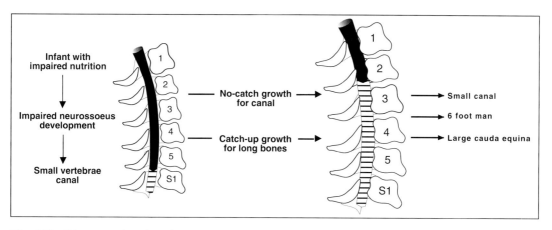

Fig. 6.13 Diagram to show how the ascending cord can leave behind a lower lumbar canal matching the size of the cord. With catch-up growth, the large cauda equina is disproportionately large, in a canal which remains small.

If unrestrained shearing forces can alter the shape of a vertebral canal in subjects with unilateral spondylolysis, what might be the effect of other mechanical forces on the vertebral canal? If a pliable triangular tube is bent it will develop a trefoil configuration, which could be a factor in some spines becoming trefoil with the development of the secondary curve of lumbar lordosis. This might explain why the trefoil shape is uncommon in small children.

Neuro-osseous development and the immune system

Clark and colleagues (1985) suggested that infantile malnutrition may not only impair the development of the vertebral canal, but also may affect the simultaneously developing immune and central nervous systems. It this hypothesis is correct, one might expect the small adult vertebral canal, being a marker of deficient early development, also to be associated with poor function of the adult immune and central nervous systems. The growth curves of the thymus, the central nervous system (Hack et al 1991), the cardiovascular system (Barker et al 1990) and the liver (Barker et al 1992) are similar to that of the neuro-osseous development, and they are similarly affected by an adverse early environment. A small canal is often associated with poor health status.

A relationship exists between the size of the vertebral canal and the thymus hormone thymosin-

α_1 (Clark et al 1988). This is compatible with the observations that adults with spinal stenosis attended their doctors with infections in childhood and in adulthood more frequently than did subjects with wider canals (Porter et al 1987). There is a relationship between bone mineral content and the sagittal diameter of the vertebral canal (Porter et al 1989b). There is also some evidence that the academic performance of children with wider vertebral canals at 16 years of age is better than that of their peers with smaller canals (Figs 6.14 and 6.15); whether this is a reflection of the socioeconomic status or their early neurological development is not established. A Swedish population with back pain had been less successful in a childhood intelligence test and had a shorter education than non-back pain sufferers, but this was not compared with the canal size (Bogenudd & Nilssen 1988).

There is growing evidence that subjects with spinal stenosis are at risk of being disadvantaged, not only in developing back pain when the canal is compromised but also in their general health, academic and socioeconomic status (Table 6.5). A search for factors which affect spinal development is likely to have wider significance than the epidemiology of back pain. Possible culprits are smoking, alcohol, toxins, infections (both bacterial and viral) and placental insufficiency (Tanner 1989). Impaired growth is suspected at birth by a discrepancy between placental and birth weight,

Below 10th percentile

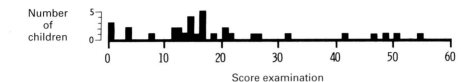

Fig. 6.14 The GCE examination score for 16-year-old children (n = 33) whose canals were below the 10th percentile for a population of 331 children previously measured by ultrasound at 13 years of age.

rather than birth weight alone (Barker et al 1992). Growth abnormalities are most likely to occur during the rapid growth phase from the 8th to the 16th intrauterine week, when the crown–rump length increases from 5 to 15 cm (Thompson 1942). Specific insults to the sensitive fetal enzyme systems at this stage are likely to be more significant than maternal malnutrition, to which the fetus is remarkably resistant (Ounstead & Ounstead 1973).

The vertebral canal is not only a factor that cannot be ignored when attempting to understand the mechanism of a patient's back pain and the high incidence of back pain within a population, but it has far-reaching medical, social and economic consequences.

Table 6.5 Mechanism and implications of spinal stenosis; the small size of the fetus results from infection, toxins , drugs, smoking or alcohol use in the mother, or placental insufficiency; an improved environment after birth with selective catch-up growth results in a tall adult.

Small fetus	Tall adult
Small musculoskeletal system	large musculoskeletal system; large limbs, muscles, nerves, large cauda equina
Impaired neuro-osseous development	large vertebral bodies, wide pedicles wide interpedicular diameter of vertebral canal permanently small sagittal diameter of the vertebral canal trefoil-shaped vertebral canal because of wide pedicles disproportion between lumbar canal and its contents permanently impaired neurological system?
Poorly developed immune system Possibly socioeconomically disadvantaged	permanently impaired immune system? compounding of socioeconomic disadvantage

Above 90th percentile

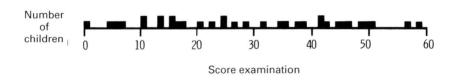

Fig. 6.15 The GCE examination score for 16-year-old children (n = 34) whose canals were above the 90th percentile at 13 years of age ($p = 0.01$) (Porter et al 1987).

REFERENCES

Adams M A, Dolan P, Hutton W C, Porter R W 1990 Diurnal changes in spinal mechanics and their clinical significance. Journal of Bone and Joint Surgery 72-B: 266–270

Barker D J P, Bull A R, Osmond C, Simmonds S J 1990 Fetal and placental size and risk of hypertension in adult life. British Medical Journal 301: 259–262

Barker D J P, Meade T W, Fall C D H, Osmon C, Phillips K, Sterling Y 1992 Relation of fetal and infant growth to plasma fibrinogen and factor VII concentrations in adult life. British Medical Journal 304: 148–152

Bogenudd H, Nilssen B 1988 Back pain in middle life; occupational workload and psychologic factors in an epidemiological survey. Spine 13: 58–60

Clark F A, Pnjabi M M, Wetzel F T 1985 Can infant malnutrition cause adult vertebral stenosis? Spine 10: 165–170

Clark G A, Hall N R, Aldwin C M, Harris J M, Borkan G A, Srinivasan M 1988 Measures of poor early growth are correlated with lower adult levels of thymosin. Journal of Human Biology, 60(4): 436–451

Edwards W C, La Rocca S H 1985 The developmental segmental sagittal diameter in combined cervical and lumbar spondylolisthesis. Spine 10: 42–49

Ehni G 1969 Significance of the small lumbar spinal canal. Cauda equina compression syndromes due to spondylosis. Journal of Neurosurgery 31: 490–494

Eisenstein S 1977 Morphometry and pathological anatomy of the lumbar spine in South African Negroes and Caucasoids with specific reference to spinal stenosis. Journal of Bone and Joint Surgery 59-B: 173–180

Eisenstein S 1980 The trefoil configuration of the lumbar vertebral canal. Journal of Bone and Joint Surgery 62-B: 73–77

Epstein J A, Malis L I 1955 Compression of spinal cord and cauda equina in achondroplastic dwarfs. Neurology 5: 875–881

Epstein J A, Epstein B S, Levine I 1962 Nerve root compression associated with narrowing of the lumbar spinal canal. Journal of Neurology, Neurosurgery and Psychiatry 25: 165–176

Farfan H F, Gracovetsky S 1984 The nature of instability. Spine 9: 714–719

Forsberg L, Walloe A 1982 Ultrasound in sciatica. Acta Orthopedica Scandinavica 53: 393–395

Hack M, Breslan N, Weissman B, Aram D, Klein N, Borawski E 1991 Effect of very low birth weight and subnormal head size on cognitive abilities at school age. New England Journal of Medicine 325: 231–237

Jacobs B, Ghelman B, Marchiello P 1990 Co-existence of cervical and lumbar disc disease. Spine 15: 1261–1264

Joffe M 1992 Influence of early life on later health. British Medical Journal 304: 1509

Kadish L J, Simmons E H 1984 Anomalies of the lumbosacral nerve roots: an anatomical investigation and myelographic study. Journal of Bone and Joint Surgery 66-B: 411–416

Kornberg M, Rechtine G R 1985 Quantitative assessment of the fifth lumbar spinal canal by computed tomography in symptomatic L4/L5 disc disease. Spine 10: 328–330

Laurence K M, James N, Miller M H, Tennant G B, Campbell H 1981 Double-blind randomised controlled trial of folate treatment before conception to prevent recurrence of neural tube defects. British Medical Journal 282: 1509–1511

Lindborgh J V 1972 The role of genetic and local environmental factors in the control of postnatal craniofacial morphogenesis. Acta Morphologica Neerlando–Scandinavica 10: 37–47

Lorber J, Levic K 1967 Spina bifida cystica. Incidence of spina bifida occulta in parents and controls. Archives of Diseases in Childhood 42: 171–173

Malcomb J E 1981 Crystalline structure of the vertebral column–thoracic region. Journal of Anatomy 133: 148–150

Mixter W J, Barr J S 1934 Rupture of the intervertebral disc with involvement of the spinal canal. New England Journal of Medicine 211: 210–215

Miyamoto S, Takaoka K, Yoenenobu K, Ono K 1992 Ossification of the ligamentum flavum induced by bone morphogenic protein. Journal of Bone and Joint Surgery 74-B: 279–283

Nelson M A 1970 Orthopaedic aspects of the chondrodystrophies. Annals of the Royal College of Surgeons of England 47: 185–210

Ounstead M, Ounstead C 1973 On foetal growth rate. Clinics in Developmental Medicine 46: 9

Penning L 1992 Functional pathology of lumbar spinal stenosis. Clinical Biomechanics 7: 3–17

Porter R W 1980 Measurement of the lumbar spinal canal by diagnostic ultrasound. MD Thesis, University of Edinburgh

Porter R W, Hibbert C 1981 Relationship between the spinal canal and other skeletal measurements in a Romano-British population. Annals of the Royal College of Surgeons of England 63: 437

Porter R W, Hibbert C W 1984 Symptoms associated with lysis of the pars interarticularis. Spine 9: 755–758

Porter R W, Oakshott G H L 1988 Familial aspects of disc protrusion. Journal of Orthopaedic Rheumatology 1: 173–178

Porter R W, Park W 1982 Unilateral spondylolisthesis. Journal of Bone and Joint Surgery 64-B: 344–348

Porter R W, Pavitt D 1987 The vertebral canal: nutrition and development, an archaeological study. Spine 12: 901–906

Porter R W, Hibbert C, Evans C 1983 Relationship between the cervical and lumbar spinal canal. Annals of the Royal College of Surgeons of England 65: 334

Porter R W, Hibbert C, Wellman P 1980 Backache and the lumbar spinal canal. Spine 5: 99–105

Porter R W, Drinkall J N, Porter D E, Thorp L 1987 The vertebral canal part 2: health and academic status. Spine 12: 907–911

Porter R W, Adams M A, Hutton W L 1989a Physical activity and the strength of the spine. Spine 14: 201–203

Porter R W, Roy A, Johnson K, Bavington M 1989b Osteoporosis and the constitutionally small vertebral canal. Journal of Anatomy 2: 120

Porter R W, Powers R, Pavitt D 1991 Vertebral changes proximal to spina bifida occulta. Physical Medicine and Rehabilitation 1: 97–100

Rothman N R 1972 The patho-physiology of disc degeneration. Clinical neurosurgery. Proceedings of the Congress of Neurological Surgeons 1972

Salibi B S 1976 Neurogenic claudication and stenosis of the lumbar spinal canal. Surgical Neurology 5: 269–272

Sand P G 1970 The human lumbo-sacral vertebral column: an osteometric study. Thesis University of Oslo

Sarpyener M A 1945 Congenital stricture of the spinal canal. Journal of Bone and Joint Surgery 27: 70–79

Schatzker J, Pennal G F 1968 Spinal stenosis, a cause of cauda equina compression. Journal of Bone and Joint Surgery 50-B: 606–618

Schlesinger E B, Taveras J M 1953 Factors in the prediction of cauda equina syndromes in lumbar discs. Transactions of the American Neurological Association 78: 263

Spencer D L, Irwin G W, Miller J A A 1983 Anatomy and significance of fixation of the lumbo-sacral roots in sciatica. Spine 8: 672–679

Tanner J M 1989 Foetus into man, 2nd edn. Castlemead Publications, Ware, p 46

Thompson D'A W 1942 Maximum velocity of growth at fourth month intra-uterine life. Growth and form, 2nd edn. Cambridge University Press, London

Tomita K, Kawahara N, Baba H, Kikuchi Y, Nishimura H 1990 Circumspinal decompression for thoracic myelopathy due to combined ossification of the posterior longitudinal ligament and ligamentum flavum. Spine 15: 1114–1120

Van Gelderen V 1958 Ein Orthotisches (lordotisches) kauda

Verbiest H 1954 A radicular syndrome from developmental narrowing of the lumbar vertebral canal. Journal of Bone and Joint Surgery 36-B: 230–237

7. Structures that restrain shear — and their failure

A second major source of back pain is the failure of structures to restrain shear. The spine moves as one intact unit, flexing, extending and rotating as a flexible rod, but it is a segmental system and displacement can occur if the shear forces are not adequately restrained. In the upright posture the disc space between L3 and L4 is horizontal (Farfan 1973), but the intervertebral segments L4/5 and especially L5/S1 are subject to sagittal shearing forces. Shear is generated through the disc when the direction of thrust is not perpendicular to the vertebra. The direction of thrust is affected by both gravity and the anatomy of muscle attachments (McGill & Norman 1987). Small variations in muscle force can change the direction of shear and, when not restrained, account for displacement in any of the three planes of rotation. However, shear forces are normally restrained by the apophyseal joints, by the intact disc, by paraspinal muscles and ligaments and by the abdominal pressure. In normal conditions this is adequate to prevent segmental displacement.

THE STRUCTURES

The apophyseal joints

The apophyseal joints are orientated towards the sagittal plane in the upper lumbar spine and more coronally at the lower lumbar levels. The mean measurements for 119 skeletons are shown in Table 7.1. The angle of inclination is difficult to measure because the joints are curved in the two planes, and in the transverse plane they tend to form the arc of a circle. In the upper lumbar spine, the sagittal orientation restrains rotation but permits flexion and extension. There is less need to

Table 7.1 Mean measurement of the superior lumbar facet angle of 119 skeletons.

	Facet angle in the coronal plane (degrees)	
	Mean	SD
L1	66.5	13.3
L2	61.3	6.8
L3	54.4	10.0
L4	41.5	10.8
L5	38.8	7.4

restrain forward shear in the upper lumbar spine, except in positions of flexion. The coronal orientation of the joints in the lower lumbar spine is, however, a powerful restraint to shear (Farfan 1978), and at L5 the torque is also buttressed by the broad pedicles of L5. The inclination of these lower joints does not prevent rotation as effectively as at upper lumbar levels. The restraint to shear is at the expense of rotation, significant perhaps in disc pathology.

It has been suggested that asymmetrical orientation of the apophyseal joints may be a prelude to disc degeneration (Farfan 1973, Cyron & Hutton 1980), though this was not supported in the study of Hagg and Wallner (1990). In our series, 28% had asymmetry between the L5 facets of more than 5° (Table 7.2). Asymmetry may be the initiating factor in some patients developing rotational instability.

We correlated facet tropism with asymmetry of the vertebral canal, and with rotation of the canal in respect to the vertebral body, but found no useful correlation in 119 skeletons. Nor did degenerative change measured by the size of the vertebral body osteophytes correlate with either the degree of asymmetry of the facet joints or the angle of the joint at that level (McGlen et al

Table 7.2 Percentage of vertebrae with facet asymmetry greater than 5°, and the mean difference between these facet angles (n = 119).

	Vertebrae with more than 5° asymmetrical facets (%)	Mean difference for these facet angles (degrees)
L1	21	10.4
L2	26	9.0
L3	34	10.4
L4	32	9.8
L5	28	10.1

1983). If asymmetry does predispose an individual to rotational displacement, then it is either not necessarily associated with degenerative change, or it is so infrequent an occurrence that it was not detected in this series of specimens.

The most frequent site for degenerative spondylolisthesis is at L4/5 where the shearing forces are not adequately restrained by the apophyseal joints. Microfractures and remodelling occur in the subchondral bone of the joints. The vertebra slowly displaces forwards with gradual bony deformity, loss of disc integrity and stretching of the ligaments. The causative factors and their related importance are uncertain. Possibly osteoporosis is significant as well as the sagittal orientation of the joints and disruption of the disc. There is no evidence that joint laxity is significant.

An intact neural arch is essential for the apophyseal joints to effectively restrain shear. However, the fact that spondylolysis can be present with no vertebral displacement suggests that spinal structures other than the neural arch play a significant part in resisting shear forces.

Soft tissue integrity

The apophyseal joint capsules; the anterior and posterior longitudinal ligaments; the supraspinous, interspinous and intertransverse ligaments; the lumbar fascia with muscle attachments; and the strong lumbosacral ligament between the fifth lumbar transverse process and the sacrum are, in combination, efficient restrainers of shear. The paraspinal muscles within the envelopes of the three layers of the lumbar fascia and the psoas muscle anteriorly provide a splint to support the spine, reinforced by intra-abdominal pressure (Tesh et al 1987). It is probable that this musculoligamentous complex prevents further forward displacement occurring in lytic spondy-

lolisthesis, after the cessation of growth. In spite of bilateral pars defects at L5, there is little further displacement even though the forces of shear remain. It probably is prevented by the soft tissue restraint, especially by the lumbosacral ligament and an intact disc.

Ligamentous laxity that accompanies pregnancy in the last trimester (Calguneri et al 1982) increases the risk of injury from the increasing shear forces. Many women date their first onset of chronic back pain to pregnancy (Svensson et al 1990, Ostgaard & Andersson 1992).

Shear is particularly resisted by an intact intervertebral disc. The biochemical anomalies recorded in the lumbosacral disc in spondylolisthesis and in the thoracic discs of scoliosis may be a response to restrained shear, rather than a primary cause. The gross anatomy of the annulus, with layers of oblique fibres of collagen, restrains shear as effectively as it resists rotation, but a degenerate nucleus with loss of disc height and a horizontal fissure is invariably associated with excessive or erratic motion.

FAILURE TO RESTRAIN SHEAR

The symptoms

Fatigue

Can soft tissues which attempt to restrain shear forces become so fatigued that they are a pain source? There are clinical situations in which this is a logical explanation of the pain mechanism. In isthmic spondylolysis, for example, there is an increased shear force as a result of a defective neural arch. Many of these patients frequently experience pain in the back and around the pelvis when standing, compatible with soft tissue fatigue. It is eased by lying down, and can be cured by a spinal fusion.

Momentary pain

When shear is inadequately restrained, can excessive or erratic segmental movement produce a sudden nociceptive insult responsible for momentary microsubluxation pain? Such a mechanism would be compatible with sudden back pain when twisting or rising from the stooped position described by some patients with degenerative spondylolisthesis. Furthermore, segmental pathology can cause under-damping of spinal motion, with jerky erratic movement, an overshoot and the feeling of spinal weakness and insecurity.

The signs

Jerky movement

Failure of restraint of shear forces will produce excessive or erratic segmental motion. Gertzbein et al (1985) have demonstrated this in cadaveric motion segments. In addition, Hukins (1990) has used simple concepts of dynamics to illustrate how jerky movement might occur. Figure 18.3 shows how an under-damped system displays the jerky behaviour characteristic of segmental instability. Ideally a system is 'critically damped', moving to the desired position without overshooting. In an 'over-damped' system, the desired position may never be attained; in an 'under-damped' system, however, movement is jerky.

Climbing up the legs

This sign when rising from the stooped posture is an attempt to reinforce an under-damped segment or segments. Under-damping could occur in isthmic spondylolysis, with impaired energy dissipation of the intervertebral joint. Degenerative discs with inadequate fluid hydration also result in an under-damped spine (Maroudas 1980, Hukins 1990). With these types of inadequate restraint, jerky movement is to be expected. Even with a healthy disc and normal bony anatomy, under-damping and erratic movement can occur from weak ligaments or inadequate neuromuscular control of one or several segments. Conversely, muscle or ligamentous hypertrophy can compensate for a deficient neural arch or degenerative disc, ensuring the spine remains stable. Similarly, a patient who rises from the stooped position by 'climbing up the legs' recruits extra support to maintain stability.

We may try to relate symptoms and signs to the biomechanics of segmental failure, but at the present time we are unsure how often and why unrestrained shear causes symptoms, and why at times it is painless. There is no reason why erratic or excessive movement should invariably produce pain, but many segmental nociceptive structures will be affected by unrestrained shear and it is probably a common source of back pain. This will be discussed further in Chapter 18.

REFERENCES

Calguneri M, Bird H A, Wright V 1982 Changes in joint laxity occurring during pregnancy. Annals of the Rheumatic Diseases 41: 126–128

Cyron R M, Hutton W C 1980 Articular trophism and stability of the lumbar spine. Spine 5: 168–172

Farfan H F 1973 The mechanical disorders of the lower back. Lea and Febiger, Philadelphia

Farfan H F 1978 The biomechanical advantage of lordosis and hip extension for upright man as compared with other anthropoids. Spine 3: 336

Gertzbein S D, Seligman J, Holtby R, Chan K H, Kapasouri A, Tile M, Cruickshank B 1985 Centrode patterns and segmental instability in degenerative disease. Spine 10: 256–261

Hagg O, Wallner A 1990 Facet joint asymmetry and protrusion of the intervertebral disc. Spine 15: 356–359

Hukins D 1990 Clinical signs and dynamics of segmental instability in back pain: descriptions of symptoms. In: Fairbank E A, Pynsent P B (eds) Back pain: classification of syndromes. Manchester University Press, Manchester 139–144

McGill S M, Norman R W 1987 Effects of anatomically detailed erector spinae model on L4/L5 disc compression and shear. Journal of Biomechanics 20: 591–660

McGlen B, Hibbert C, Evans C, Porter R W 1983 The lumbar apophyseal joints in an archaeological collection. Annals of Royal College of Surgeons of England 65: 198

Maroudas A 1980 Physical chemistry of articular cartilage and intervertebral disc. In: Sokaloff L (ed) The joints and synovial fluid. Academic Press, York, vol 2, p 248–293

Ostgaard H C, Andersson G B J 1992 Post partum low back pain. Spine 17: 53–55

Svensson H, Andersson G B J, Hegstal A, Janssen P 1990 The relationship of low back pain to pregnancy and gynaecological factors. Spine 15: 371–375

Tesh K M, Shaw-Dunn J, Evans J H 1987 The abdominal muscles and vertebral stability. Spine 12: 501–508

8. Pain perception and behaviour

Any stimulus above a certain threshold can become a nociceptive source, but it is considerably modified by the nociceptive system before it becomes perceived as pain. The same nociceptive source will produce different pain perception in different subjects and perhaps by changing thresholds, in the same subject at different times. This is apparent in many situations. Two patients having identical operations will estimate their pain perception very differently, and have variable post-operative analgesic requirements. In fact, the same patient having sequential bilateral procedures will frequently comment that for some unexplained reason one operation was more painful than the other. Two individuals with apparently identical fractures will assess their pain very differently, one experiencing little discomfort, and the other feeling intense pain with no obvious explanation from the nociceptive source. The nervous system between the receptors and the higher centres has considerable potential to modify pain in the so-called 'nociceptive system', so that pain perception is not directly proportional to the stimulus (Bonica 1990).

THE NOCICEPTIVE SOURCE

There are probably two types of nociceptive source, the first from a specific group of primary afferent neurons — the nociceptors — which are activated at a high threshold. They respond maximally to intense potentially damaging stimuli and result in the flexion withdrawal reflex, an autonomic response, and the sensation of pain; this is protective.

The second nociceptive source is the plexiform nerve endings in the joint capsule or free nerve endings in ligaments and tendons. They are triggered by a low intensity or innocuous stimulus from tissue injury, inflammation or nerve damage, with an alteration in the transduction sensitivity and with abnormal membrane excitability. There is a mismatch between the stimulus and the response (Woolf 1989, 1990).

The peripheral nociceptive stimulus is considerably modified by central changes.

THE POSTERIOR HORN

The posterior horn cell does not simply receive a sensory stimulus from the peripheral afferent fibre and pass it to higher centres in an unmodified form. In the posterior horn of the spinal cord there are probably side-circuits which can excite or prolong the activity of the original impulse, with secondary circuits able to inhibit transmission of the impulse. Substance 'P', neurotensin, oxytocin, encephalins and other peptides have been identified in many of the intermediary cells of the posterior horn of the spinal cord: substances which have an ability to modify the impulse received by sensory afferents from the nociceptive source.

The function of substance P is unclear, but in patients with chronic back pain it has been found to be decreased in the cerebrospinal fluid, the saliva and plasma (Almay et al 1988) when compared with healthy volunteers (Parris et al 1990). The impulse modification explains the reduction in pain perception by such activities as rubbing the skin over a painful site or applying local heat to a painful area, and it explains the benefits of massage, vibration and transcutaneous nerve stimulation. These all stimulate mechanoreceptors which could produce an inhibitory effect on pain at the posterior horn level. These observations in practice are supported by neurophysiological studies (Wall 1979) and, although the pathways have not been identified, the theory has stood the test of time. The activity of the nociceptive complex in the posterior horn is probably modified by a control mechanism from higher centres, as descending inhibitory pathways under central control may modulate conduction of nerve impulses in the posterior horn mechanism over many segments (Dickenson & Le Bars 1987).

The apparent analgesia in war casualties, quite specific to the area of trauma, can be explained by local endorphin and encephalin secretion causing posterior horn inhibition. Nociceptive and other sensory modalities from other parts of the body are retained. This is probably a horn inhibition, but it may be under mid-brain control.

THE MID-BRAIN

Modification of pain was first recognized by animal experimentation when stimulation of the periaqueductal grey matter made the animal unresponsive to a peripheral nociceptive stimulus. Subsequently, it was observed that the injection of radioactive labelled morphine was identified at precisely the same area of the mid-brain. The identification of encephalin and other morphine-like substances, the endorphins, manufactured in the periaqueductal grey matter and released by electrical stimulation at this site, suggests a mid-brain system of pain inhibition (Kosierlitz et al 1977, Terenius & Wahlstrom 1979). Nalorphine blocks the effects of morphine by being so similar to the morphine molecule that it can become attached in the mid-brain to the specific morphine receptor. The peripheral nociceptive stimulus is then consciously perceived.

There exists a complex mid-brain system of pain modification before it is experienced as an abnormal unpleasant sensation. The control of this mid-brain system of nociception has yet to be resolved, but a central control does explain the apparent absence of pain experienced by casualties in war, boxers, athletes enduring ischaemic pain, and a large percentage of the population arriving at the dentist's surgery. Certainly they have a no-

ciceptive source, but they have modified perception, at least temporarily.

PAIN ENHANCEMENT

We are aware, therefore, of the possibility of a nociceptive source with no pain perception, and can perhaps explain its mechanism. When dealing with some patients suffering from severe back pain, we ask whether it is possible to have pain perception with no continuing nociceptive source. Experiments under hypnosis would suggest that it is, when pain can be genuinely experienced from an imaginary source. At least 35% of amputees suffer from phantom pain (Feinstein et al 1954), though the stump is usually healthy and there is no obvious source. Melzack and Wall (1965) explained spontaneous pain of causalgia and neuralgia in terms of a summation mechanism. The pain experience is not a 'one to one' relationship with the stimulus. We now appreciate that current back pain may reflect more the history of the previous input to the spinal cord than the afferent signals at any one moment (Woolf 1990).

BEHAVIOURAL ASPECTS OF PAIN

When pain is perceived at a conscious level, it has three recognizable components, described by the Hilgards (1975) as sensory pain, suffering and mental anguish. Sensory pain is simply the appreciation and localization of a painful sensory stimulus. The suffering component involves the frontal cortex. When fibres from the thalamus to the frontal cortex are transected by orbito-frontal leucotomy, the subject is still aware of the sensory stimulus of pain but the suffering element is largely removed. He is no longer 'in pain'. The 'mental anguish' component of pain is associated with anxiety and a complexity of emotions, with a resultant pattern of pain behaviour (Gibson 1982). It is this objective response of the patient to the original source — the pain behaviour — that the clinician observes. This psychological component is uniquely individual. That is, the same pain experience can be expected to produce a very different individual behavioural response.

An individual's response to pain will depend on inherited characteristics, previous environmental experience, and the present situation — not least the meaning ascribed to the sensation and an intellectual assessment of the probable outcome of different response strategies. The psychological traits of phobia, anxiety, depression, obsession, hysteria or a tendency to somatize may be influenced by genetic characteristics, and certainly by the imprinting of life's early experiences in infancy and childhood. A child who finds illness rewarding by receiving parental attention and being able to escape the demands of school, may look for benefits from pain in later life. A more disciplined childhood, with demands for a 'stiff upper lip', can produce a stoical attitude to pain. Different ethnic groups have contrasting behavioural responses to back pain, when the anatomical and pathological variations seem relatively insignificant (Bremner et al 1968, Eisenstein 1977, Glass 1979). Many fears and anxieties in adult life are projections from childhood. A child's observation of his parents' attitude to pain will influence his behaviour. The sins of the father are visited on his children to the third and fourth generation.

The immediate environmental situation also will influence the behaviour to pain: the response of the spouse, family, friends and colleagues at work (Battie et al 1989, Magnusson et al 1990). Behaviour will be affected by the rewards of attention or lack of it from doctors and therapists, by financial benefits and the opportunity to avoid unpleasant work. It does not seem to be affected by social class (Larson & Marcer 1984).

Therefore it is as important to ask, 'What kind of patient has back pain?' as 'What kind of back pain has the patient?'. The influence of many known and unknown factors on the patient's basic psychological character will produce a variable response. The obsessional individual may have little time to dwell on pain, and may neglect the conscious pain experience. If, on the other hand, an anxiety state is superimposed on the obsessional character, the pain may become exaggerated and new symptoms added. Depression or phobia may cause abnormal pain behaviour, or prolong its course.

A readiness to somatize in adverse circumstances may cause a patient to seek medical help for pain which others manage alone (Wolfkind &

Forrest 1972, Waddell 1987). We carried out an epidemiological study of the incidence of attendances for back pain in four general practices, examining the records of over 400 men and their wives over 40 years of age and covering an average period of 20 years. The mean attendance rate for conditions other than back pain was significantly higher for both men and women who attended with back pain than for those individuals who never attended with back pain (Table 8.1). Becker and Karch (1979) similarly observed that patients complaining of low back pain are a group who present their symptoms to doctors more readily than other individuals.

We noted in this series that the role of the spouse is highly important in pain behaviour. Husbands and wives tended to polarize, those men and women who were high attenders with back pain having a spouse who was a low attender (Table 8.2).

ASSESSMENT OF PAIN BEHAVIOUR

A clinician treating patients with back pain eventually develops an intuitive sense about pain behaviour. The manner in which the patient enters the consulting room, the way he walks, sits, talks and his facial expression all give a hint of appropriate or inappropriate behaviour, which is supplemented by the examination (Waddell et al 1980, Main & Parker 1989, Main et al 1992). Most patients fall into the middle ground of what would be considered an acceptable response to pain. A few have an exaggerated response, more so if the history is long. These we can identify but we are less skilled at recognizing the stoic.

Table 8.1 Comparison between mean attendances for conditions other than back pain, in 403 men with and without back pain.

	Mean attendances/year for non-back pain conditions	
	Men with back pain ($n = 255$) (SD)	Men without back pain ($n = 148$) (SD)
Mining practice A	5.57 (3.98)	3.22 (2.47)
Mining practice B	6.01 (7.67)	3.65 (2.71)
Town practice A	3.34 (2.45)	2.22 (1.87)
Town practice B	2.57 (1.85)	1.74 (2.08)

Table 8.2 Comparative mean general practice attendance rate per year for all conditions for wives of 40-year-old miners who had an above average attendance rate for all conditions, and for wives of miners with a below average attendance rate, over a 20-year period (n = 96).

	Wives attendance rate/year for all conditions
Wives of miners with above average attendance rate (mean 6.01 visits/year)	2.97
Wives of miners with below average attendance rate (mean 2.53 visits/year)	4.08

We can identify the exaggerating patient who has a small or non-existent nociceptive source (page 96). This does not mean that there was not originally some mechanical failure of the spine, a genuine nociceptive source and a pain experience. With the passage of time the organic cause can cease, but the experience remains. We are not dealing with malingering. Symptoms persist even when they seem to have no gainful value, and when litigation has been settled.

Recognizing inappropriate behaviour warns the clinician that he is faced not only with a complex diagnostic problem, but one difficult to manage. Sophisticated investigations may be counterproductive, and invasive methods of treatment positively harmful. We recognize a problem but find it difficult to modify and change it (Ch. 29).

Attempting to identify the source of back pain, by observing a patient's pain behaviour, can in no way be compared to identifying a fault in a machine. Modification at posterior horn, midbrain and cortical level is to such a degree that it is a wonder that a nociceptive source can be discovered at all. Fortunately, in spite of the fascinating complexity of the nociceptive system and the factors that influence the patient's behaviour, the majority of patients respond to their pain in a rational, appropriate manner. What they experience is in proportion to the organic lesion, and their behaviour is not exaggerated. It is upon this premise that we attempt to make a reasonable diagnosis of the cause of the pain.

REFERENCES

Almay B G L, Johansson F, Vonknossing B 1988 Substance P in CSF of patients with chronic pain syndromes. Pain 33: 3–9

Becker L A, Karch F 1979 Low back pain in family practice: a case control study. The Journal of Family Practice 9: 579–582

Battie M C, Bigos S J, Fisher L D et al 1989 A prospective study of the role of cardiovascular risk factors and fitness in industrial back pain complaints. Spine 14: 141–147

Bonica J J 1990 Management of pain, 2nd edn. Lea & Febiger, Philadelphia

Bremner J M, Lawrence J S, Miall W E 1968 Degenerative joint disease in a Jamaican rural population. Annals of the Rheumatic Diseases 27: 327–332

Dickenson A H, Le Bars D 1987 Supraspinal morphines and descending inhibitors acting on the dorsal horn of the rat. Journal of Physiology 384: 81–107

Eisenstein S 1977 Morphometry and pathological anatomy of the lumbar spine in South African negroes and caucasoids with specific reference to spinal stenosis. Journal of Bone and Joint Surgery 59-B: 173–180

Feinstein B, Luce J C, Langton J N K 1954 The influence of phantom limbs. In: Wilson P, Klopsteg P (eds) Human limbs and their substitutes. McGraw-Hill, New York

Gibson H B 1982 Pain and its conquest. Peter Owen, London

Glass J B 1979 Acute lumbar strain. Clinical signs and prognosis. Practitioner 222: 821–825

Hilgard E R, Hilgard J R 1975 Hypnosis in the relief of pain. W Kaufmann, Los Altos, California, p 29

Kosierlitz H W, Hughes J, Law J H, Waterfield J A 1977 Encephalins, endorphines and opiate receptors. Neurosciences Symposium. Society for Neuroscience, vol 2, p 291–307

Larson A G, Marcer D 1984 The who and why of pain: analysis by social class. British Medical Journal 288: 883–886

Magnusson N, Granqvist M, Jenson R 1990 The loads on the lumbar spine during work at an assembly line. The risks for fatigue injuries of vertebral bodies. Spine 15: 774–779

Main C J, Parker H 1989 The evaluation and outcome of pain management programmes for chronic low back pain. In: Roland M, Jenner J R (eds) Back pain. New approaches. Manchester University Press

Main C J, Wood P L R, Hollis S, Spanswick C C, Waddell G 1992 The distress and risk assessment method. Spine 17: 42–52

Melzack R, Wall P D 1965 Pain mechanisms: a new theory. Science 150: 331

Parris W C V, Kambam J R, Naukam R J, Sastry B V R 1990 Immunoreactive Substance P is decreased in saliva of patients with chronic back pain syndromes. Anaesthesia Analgesia 70: 63–67

Terenius L, Wahlstrom A 1979 Endorphines and clinical pain. An overview. Advances in Experimental Medicine and Biology 116: 261–277

Waddell G 1987 Understanding the patient with back pain. In: Jayson M I V (ed) The lumbar spine and back pain, 3rd edn. Churchill Livingstone, Edinburgh

Waddell G, McCulloch J A, Kummell E, Venner R M 1980 Non-organic physical signs in low back pain. Spine 5: 117–125

Wall P D 1979 Modulations of pain by non-painful events. In: Bonica J J, Albe-Fessar D (eds) Advances in pain

research and therapy. Raven Press, New York

Wolfkind S N, Forrest A J 1972 Low back pain: a psychosomatic investigation. Postgraduate Medical Journal 48: 76–79

Woolf C J 1989 Recent advances in the pathophysiology of acute pain. British Journal of Anaesthesia 63: 139–146

Woolf C J 1990 The contribution of both peripheral and central nervous systems to the pain that follows peripheral nerve injury. In: Samii M (ed) Peripheral nerve lesions. Springer Verlag, Heidelberg, p 51–58

Clinical assessment and investigation of back pain

9. The consultation

The clinician's heart should be gladdened, not saddened, by the patient with backache. It is a symptom with so many possible causes in the soma and psyche that it should challenge our detective skills. Besides the thrill of the chase, it is a condition that will probably get better in spite of us.

There is a danger of becoming too academic, too absorbed by the problem with neglect of the patient. If he feels like a 'case', an interesting condition, a 'statistic in our research programme', we have neglected our primary purpose. We should remind ourselves why the patient seeks a consultation: it is to satisfy the patient, not the doctor. Unless the patient leaves us with a sense of fulfilment, we have failed. However, patients with back pain can be difficult to please, especially when the condition becomes chronic. The general practitioner is reluctant to refer them, and the specialist is often unable to help them. Explanations of the pain mechanism can fall on deaf ears and many hospital patients are dissatisfied with the information they receive (Roland et al 1991). They want an answer to two questions: 'What is wrong?', and 'Can you put it right?'. The whole consultation should encompass these two questions.

But academic we must be. We need to listen, observe, record and learn from this patient's experience in order to unravel the mysteries of back pain. We cannot escape trying to satisfy the doctor because back pain becomes such a fascinating study. From our understanding of this patient, we can help a patient yet to come; the consultation involves more than helping the patient before us, important as that is. Back pain has qualities that are probably unique in medicine. Here is a quest to find the elusive cause of a complex problem and influence it. We may not be too confident about treating the patient before us but with every piece of information, every correct observation recorded, assimilated and correctly interpreted, we should gradually improve our understanding and management. Patient care and research are not only mutually compatible, they are both essential and complementary.

The consultation begins as the patient enters the room. It is good psychology to rise and invite the patient to sit down — and to sit within a few feet, not on the other side of the desk. A smooth flow of conversation is possible if a secretary can unobtrusively record an accurate history without the need to stop for dictation. The patient should be given plenty of time (Wright et al 1982).

THE HISTORY

Past history

Generally the patient wants to begin with the recent history, but it helps to direct him to the first episode of back pain perhaps many years before. Not only is this important in appreciating the present problem, but the patient is often pleasantly surprised that someone is at last prepared to listen to the whole story. At what age did he first experience back pain? Did there appear to be a causative episode? We need to know if there was an injury, what was the mechanism, was litigation involved, and what were the subsequent symptoms. We want to know the distribution of pain at that time, if the symptoms affected the back only or the leg, what treatment was offered, and how long it took to recover. In this history there is generally a clue to the pathology responsible for the first episode of back pain which is relevant to the present problem.

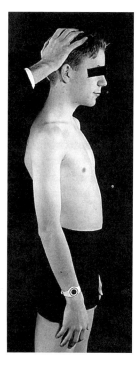

Fig. 9.2 If axial loading produces pain in the lower back, this is inappropriate.

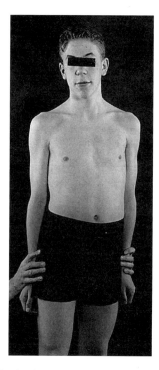

Fig. 9.3 Low back pain when the pelvis is rotated without the spine, is inappropriate.

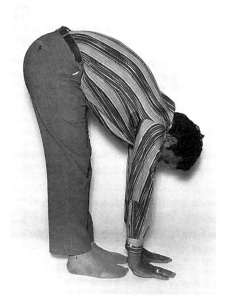

Fig. 9.4 Flexing forwards to reach to the floor with straight knees is a combined test of straight leg raising and lumbar flexion. Patients with back pain can rarely put their hands on the floor, unless they have a spondylolisthesis.

those with isthmic or degenerative spondylolisthesis may easily place the flat of the hands on the floor, in spite of considerable back pain (Fig. 9.4). And as the patient bends forwards, is there evidence of rotary movement? This dynamic trunk list may only be apparent in forward flexion, and is suggestive of disc protrusion.

Mobility of the spine is usefully measured with a tape measure (Fig. 9.5), measuring skin distraction. Three marks are made on the skin with the patient sitting in an upright position: a mark over L4, one 100 mm above and one 50 mm below L4. The patient, sitting on the edge of a chair with the legs apart, then bends over with the trunk, and the arms are dropped fully between the knees. The mean value of this modified Schober's test is 6.5 mm, depending on age (Moll & Wright 1971, Scott 1983). It can be measured by a flexicurve (Burton 1986, Tillotson & Burton 1991) or more rapidly and accurately with a goniometer (Loebl 1967, Reynolds 1975, Salisbury & Porter 1987) or kyphometer (Fig. 9.6).

Observe how the patient stands up again. Is the movement accomplished smoothly or with an

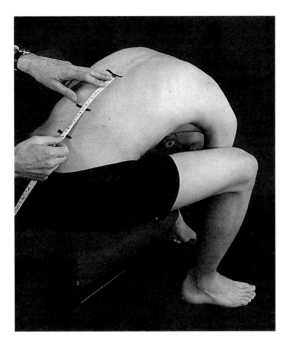

Fig. 9.5 The changing distance between two defined points measured with a tape measure provides an objective record of spinal sagittal mobility.

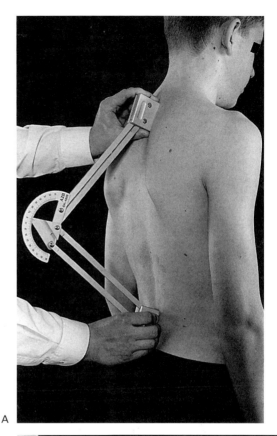

A

extension catch? The catch is a jerky hesitancy half-way through the process of standing up from the stooped position, and is a sign of spinal instability. Another instability sign (though sometimes seen in other back pain syndromes and in distressed patients) is the necessity to use the hands to support the trunk by 'climbing up the legs'.

Ask the patient to lean backwards, supporting the shoulders. An assessment of extension is highly subjective, but one gets an impression of loss of extension, to a third or two-thirds of the normal range. Some patients, in whom space in the vertebral canal is at a premium, have a flexion deformity and cannot even stand upright. They adopt a 'simian' stance (Simkin 1982), standing with the hips and knees slightly flexed. They may temporarily force a more normal stance but will relapse again when distracted.

Lateral flexion is usually good in patients with lumbar pain of mechanical origin, and is equal on both sides unless there is a list. Is it painful? Does it produce contralateral pain? The patient with

B

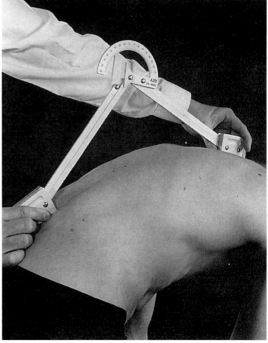

Fig. 9.6 A kyphometer can be used to measure spinal range, recording the difference between two postures, (**A**) and (**B**).

gross restriction of lateral flexion has other spinal or paraspinal pathology, or perhaps a non-organic lesion.

Assessment of the spine prone

Sacrospinalis hypertrophy is difficult to quantitate, but it sometimes accompanies instability, and is more easily detected with the patient prone (Fig. 9.7).

The spinous processes are identified by palpation. A list associated with a disc lesion will have corrected, but not a structural scoliosis. Firm pressure on the spinous processes will reveal the level of the nociceptive source. An L4/5 disc can be very tender over L4 and L5 spinous processes and an L5/S1 disc over L5. A patient who fractured the body of L2 a year ago and who is now tender over L5 probably has lower lumbar pathology sustained at the same time and still a source of pain. One suspects upper lumbar pathology with lower lumbar pain if L1 or L2 is tender; the pain source is then more likely to be in the upper lumbar spine with pain referred to the lower lumbar region. Root pain can occasionally be reproduced by maintaining pressure on a spinous process, called by the French a 'doorbell sign'.

Sacroiliac tenderness is not uncommon. Many patients have pain in the region of the sacroiliac joints and, to convince the clinician of its site, may admit to some tenderness. When specifically asked, 'I know this is where you feel the pain, but I want to know if it is tender', they generally confess the tenderness is over the lower lumbar spinous processes and not over the sacroiliac joints. Sacroiliac tenderness suggests an inflammatory lesion either of these joints, or of the soft tissues of the posterior pelvis.

Sacral tenderness should be regarded with suspicion. It is either a sinister sign of bony metastases or a sign of an exaggerated response. Coccygeal tenderness is compatible with a recent history of trauma, but if long-standing it is probably inappropriate. At this stage, gently squeeze the skin over the site of lumbar tenderness. If unduly painful, it is an inappropriate sign. Sensation over the sacrum, buttocks and posterior thighs is assessed with the patient prone. Saddle anaesthesia has serious implications. Hyperaesthesia is common, but we do not know its significance.

The femoral stretch test is best elicited with the patient prone. Flexing the knee alone will cause tension of the L2 and L3 roots, and may be sufficient to produce back pain. It will be increased by extending the hip. Pain arising in the hips is not influenced by flexing the knee alone. If lying prone is too painful, the tension signs can be elicited with the patient on the side.

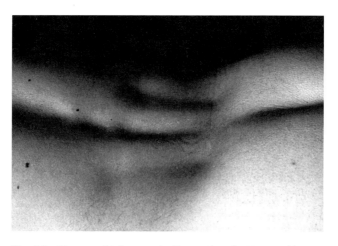

Fig. 9.7 Hypertrophied sacrospinalis muscles of a 48-year-old man, relaxed and lying prone. He had back pain associated with a degenerative spondylolisthesis.

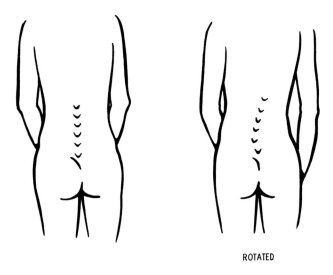

ROTATED

Fig. 9.8   Diagram to show that the floating segment of L5 will remain in line with S1 as the spine is rotated.

In the prone position, it is also possible to identify the floating segment of an isthmic spondylolisthesis. As the lumbar spine is rotated, the spinous process of a floating segment will fail to move. There is sequential lateral movement in an intact spine (Fig. 9.8).

Lower limbs supine

Look at the lower limbs. Is there asymmetry of girth or length to be objectively measured? It is difficult to detect less than 5 mm of leg length discrepancy with a tape measure (Friberg et al 1988), and the association between mild leg length inequality and back pain is questionable (Soukka et al 1991). Is there atrophy of the quadriceps or extensor digitorum brevis?

There is no universal agreement about the correct way to perform the straight leg raising test. One method is to support the heel in the cupped hand of the examiner and, having explained the method to the patient, gently lift the heel from the couch with the knee still extended. The opposite hand rests on the pelvis to limit pelvic rotation (Edgar & Park 1974), though some pelvic rotation will always accompany straight leg raising (Bohannon 1990). The patient's head should be resting on one pillow and the arms relaxed by the sides. The elevation can stop when the patient complains of pain; the angle is assessed and he is asked about the site of that pain. However, although a little uncomfortable for the patient, better repeatability is obtained by lifting the leg to the maximum permitted level. Using a goniometer with this technique (Fig. 9.9), we obtained repeatability within 2° (Porter & Trailescu 1990).

A repeat of the straight leg raising test after an hour of strict recumbency can help distinguish a disc protrusion from a sequestration (Porter & Trailescu 1990). There will be no change in straight leg raising if the disc is incompetent with a complete annular tear. However, changes in the tension of a protrusion can reduce straight leg raising by as much as 30° after a period of recumbency (page 175).

Crossed leg pain, or well leg pain is pathognomonic of a disc herniation. Lifting the asymptomatic leg produces pain in the opposite buttock or thigh. It suggests a poor prognosis for conservative management (Khuffash & Porter 1989).

Modifications of the straight leg raising test can be helpful. At maximum straight leg raising, the foot is dorsiflexed to see if tension on the posterior

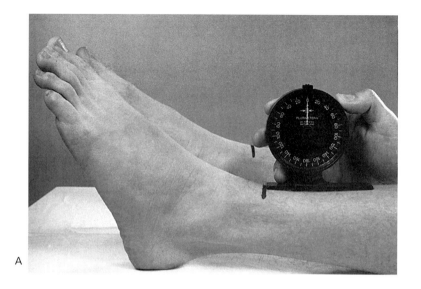

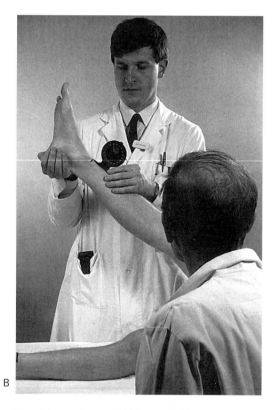

Fig. 9.9   A precision goniometer (**A**) is essential for accurate measurement of straight leg raising. The repeatability is good, when recording the angle at the maximum permitted level (**B**). (Reproduced with the permission of Doncaster Royal Infirmary.)

tibial nerve increases the sensation of pain (Bragaad's test). In the same position, the limb is externally rotated, relaxing the sacral plexus, and then internally rotated, increasing root tension; the experience of pain (Breig & Troup 1979) is recorded. At the limit of straight leg raising, the knee is first flexed and then extended, and the tibial nerve compressed with the examining fingers of one hand, the 'bow string test'. The Lasègue test elicits pain in the leg or back, when at the limit of straight leg raising the knee is slightly flexed, the hip further flexed, and the knee then extended. These tension signs are generally present when a lower lumbar or sacral root is involved in the pathological process of pain. They are marked with acute root involvement from a disc protrusion, but mild or absent with nerve root irritation from long-standing degenerative change.

Many patients are aware of the straight leg raising test and for many reasons, conscious or unconscious, will influence its result. The examiner learns to suspect voluntary resistance and can confirm this by combining the various stretch tests. He can flex the knee and record the range of hip flexion. If with the flexed knee the hip is limited in flexion, there is either hip pathology, or an exaggeration (though low back pain can at times

be so severe that even flexing the hip aggravates the pain). Suspicions of exaggeration are confirmed if on the pretext of examining the back, the patient is asked to sit up and lean forwards on the couch, and with extended knees he can reach well forwards to the feet. The 'flip test' is similarly useful; when the knee of the seated patient is extended, he will 'flip over' backwards if straight leg raising is genuinely limited (Fig. 9.10).

The Burn's test expects a patient to be able to kneel on a bench with knees and hips fully flexed, and place the fingers on the floor. Failure to do so is inappropriate and is said to correlate with hysteria in the MMPI (Evanski et al 1979).

An inflammatory lesion of the sacroiliac joint is painful if the hip is flexed to 90° and then forcibly adducted. This pain is, however, also experienced when there are positive root tension signs, and when there is an inflammatory lesion of the soft tissues of the posterior pelvis. Distraction of the pelvis and compression on the anterior superior iliac spines also aggravates sacroiliac pain.

Internal rotation and resisted abduction of the flexed hip are said to be painful in the piriformis syndrome, when the sciatic nerve is compressed deep and inferior to the piriformis muscle.

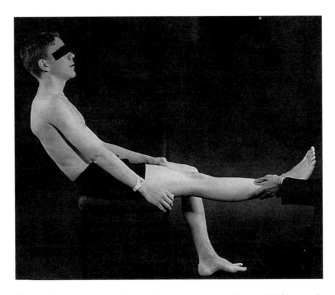

Fig. 9.10 A patient with genuine root tension signs will 'flip over' backwards when seated and the affected leg is lifted.

The knee and ankle reflexes should be symmetrical. Equal diminution is not significant, but asymmetrical reduction helps to identify an affected root. The knee reflex is usually subserved by the L3, L4 and L5 roots, and the ankle reflex by the L5 and S1 roots. An ankle reflex which is normal or slightly depressed in the supine position may be more depressed or absent if examined with the patient prone or sitting (Postacchini & Perugia 1992).

The motor power of selected muscles is recorded — extensor hallucis longus (L5 or S1), peronei (S1), quadriceps (L4 and 5) — but with the variability of muscle innervation, it is unwise to rely on muscle wasting or reflex change to identify the spinal nerve of the lesion. Wasting of the quadriceps can be measured, and the extensor digitorum brevis is a useful little muscle; its wasting can be observed and palpated in some S1 root lesions. Weakness of the extensor hallucis longus is not uncommon, but when other muscles are affected there is either serious pathology or exaggeration. Weakness without wasting is highly suspect.

The sensation is recorded using a sharp pin. Numbness of the big toe (L5) or of the outer foot (S1) are encountered most frequently. A non-dermatomal sensory reduction may be an inappropriate sign, but it is highly subjective for both patient and doctor.

An extensor plantar reflex identifies an upper motor neuron lesion. This is not very reproducible (Maher et al 1992), and clinical decisions should not be made on a single sign. Upgoing toes should be supported by brisk reflexes or clonus. Ataxia may have been suspected from the patient's gait, and confirmed by abnormal position sense of the big toe. If there is hesitancy, impaired proprioception will be supported by a tuning fork vibration test, and by asking the patient to run the heel of one foot down the opposite shin.

Palpate the dorsalis pedis and anterior tibial arteries and, if absent, check the femoral arteries in the groin. Is there a femoral bruit? Impaired peripheral circulation may explain the source of claudication pain or it may coexist with spinal pathology. One absent pulse may be irrelevant.

The examination is not complete without being sure that the hip and knee are not responsible for lower limb pain. Palpation of the abdomen is also mandatory, as an abdominal mass may explain the cause of pain.

We have mentioned many signs that would suggest an exaggerated response. Strange postures, abnormal gait, almost falling, resisted or jerky movements which change during the period of consultation, widespread and variable weakness with no muscle wasting, sweating, collapsing and grasping movements, and closed eyes whilst being examined (Gray et al 1988) are inappropriate signs (Waddell et al 1980, 1984) (Fig. 9.11). Further signs are:

- Pain in the lumbar region when the head is compressed vertically; axial loading
- Pain when the pelvis is rotated on the lower limbs whilst the patient is standing; simulated rotation

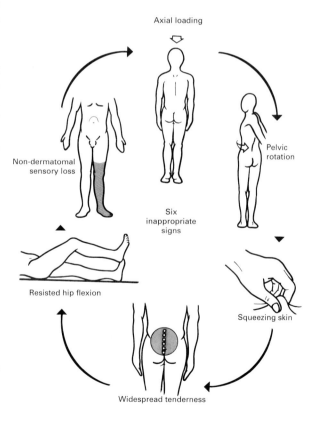

Fig. 9.11 Diagrammatic representation of six inappropriate signs.

- Widespread tenderness
- Pain when the skin of the back is lightly squeezed
- Straight leg raising resisted voluntarily but improved with distraction
- Non-dermatomal sensory reduction.

Their presence does not indicate the absence of an organic lesion, but unfortunately they make the identification of that lesion more difficult and its response to treatment disappointing. They are an exhibition of distress.

The history has provided the clinician with an understanding of the patient's problem subjectively perceived, with its apparent dimensions in time, severity, and disability. The examination points to the diagnosis and helps to distinguish how much of the problem has an organic element.

THE DISCUSSION

From the patient's position, this is the crux of the consultation. He wants to know if we have reached any conclusions about the cause of back pain, if any further tests are necessary, and what is needed to put things right. We probably err on the side of not talking enough to our patients. They want information; we should not withhold it. The first consultation is the best opportunity to explain the probable mechanism of the pain, and mismanagement at this stage will compound problems which can be difficult to resolve.

The only investigation that is required for many patients with back pain is a plain radiograph, and if this has been performed previously it allows the consultation to be completed at one sitting. If we have reached a presumptive diagnosis, it should be explained in simple terms with a description of any necessary confirmatory tests. Discussion of methods of treatment or management and a word about prognosis allays the patient's anxiety, and he should now leave the consulting room in a lighter frame of mind.

INVESTIGATIONS

Investigations supplement but are no substitute for a good history and examination. No single investigation will identify the source of back pain. We need to know the scope of each investigation, its indications, limitations and risks.

No assessment of a spine is complete without radiographs. There has been debate about their value, and in isolation they are positively unhelpful (Halpin et al 1991). The patient is exposed to unjustified radiation. A report of radiographs describing perhaps degenerative changes or a spondylolisthesis is irrelevant if divorced from the history and examination. In combination, however, they add valuable information and also provide a rational approach to diagnosis and management (Ch. 10). Magnetic resonance imaging (MRI) as a first-line investigation, though it spares the patient irradiation, is an unjustified luxury.

Haematological and biochemical investigations will be required if we suspect an inflammatory lesion or intraosseous pathology. It is not cost-effective to screen every patient, nor indeed is it necessary. A raised erythrocyte sedimentation rate (ESR) will support an inflammatory disorder, but it can be raised from many other unrelated conditions. A high ESR may be associated with bony pathology and if this is suspected there is need for other blood tests: acid and alkaline phosphatase, serum proteins and a differential white cell count. It may be necessary to examine the bone marrow and test the urine for Bence-Jones protein. Skeletal demineralization requires estimation of serum calcium, phosphorus and alkaline phosphatase, and sometimes bone biopsy to diagnose osteomalacia and metabolic bone disease.

Only a few patients need further investigation. These are generally patients whose back is causing severe disability and surgery is being considered.

Ultrasound Doppler scan is of particular value in the claudicant patient to ensure the patency of the peripheral arteries. It will give an objective and quantitative record which will be useful with the doubtful peripheral pulse, especially in the obese.

Ultrasound measurement of the vertebral canal can add a further dimension to the diagnostic quest. It is not an investigation that has gained widespread acceptance, and will probably not be generally used until improved imaging offers better results.

Nerve conduction tests will support a diagnosis of peripheral nerve entrapment of the common peroneal nerve at the neck of the fibula, and of the posterior tibial nerve in tarsal tunnel syndrome. Unilateral delayed conduction and/or reduced latency are helpful signs.

Electromyographic studies will confirm the presence of impaired nerve function 5 weeks from the onset of symptoms, or after a change of symptoms (Wilbourn 1992). Selective muscle degeneration can be identified and can suggest the nerve root responsible, but the root cannot be identified with complete confidence because of anomalies of nerve supply to individual muscles (Merriam et al 1982). Electrical studies are useful in the patient who has exaggerated signs, and yet there is a possibility of genuine root pathology. Negative electromyographic findings do not exclude genuine symptoms, but positive results confirm significant root damage.

Thermography, being non-invasive, is an attractive investigation if it can be confidently interpreted, but its assessment to date has been disappointing (So et al 1989, Hoffman et al 1991).

Spinal scintigraphy helps to diagnose facet fracture, stress fracture of the pars and acute disruption of an existing pars defect. It is of more value than radiography in the early diagnosis of

sacroiliitis and of spinal tumour or infection (see Ch. 12).

MRI is the investigation of choice when surgery is a serious possibility, and there are times when it should be supported with computerized tomography (CT) or radiculography. These will tell us where to operate and how rather than when. New imaging has improved spinal assessment, expanding the horizons of the clinician. It offers information about the hidden areas of the spine, the vertebral canal, its size and shape, the degree and extent of stenosis, and soft tissue involvement and the state of the disc.

The expansion of investigative techniques, however, can be counter-productive if they outstrip our skill in taking the patient's history and performing a good examination. These are paramount, and any gross pathology we may identify by sophisticated investigation has little value unless it corresponds to the patient's symptomatology. In addition, we should pause to question what is to be gained by exposing our patients to high-powered technology, when our therapeutic skills have not kept pace with these investigations. Investigation is of value only if it affects the patient's management, and can never be a substitute for a good history and examination.

REFERENCES

Bohannon R W 1990 Letter to editor. Spine 15: 985
Breig A, Troup J D G 1979 Biomechanical considerations in the straight leg raising test. Spine 4: 242–250
Burton A K 1986 Regional lumbar sagittal mobility: measurement by flexicurves. Clinical Biomechanics 1: 20–26
Edgar M A, Park W M 1974 Induced pain patterns on passive straight leg raising in lower lumbar disc protrusion. Journal of Bone and Joint Surgery 56B: 658–666
Evanski P M, Carver D, Nehemkis A, Waugh T R 1979 The Burn's test in low back pain. Clinical Orthopaedics and Related Research 140: 42–44
Friberg O, Nurminen M, Korhonen K, Soininen E, Mänttäri T 1988 Accuracy and precision of clinical estimations of leg length inequalities: comparisons of clinical and radiological measurements. International Disability Studies 10(2): 49–53
Gardner A D, Pursell L M, Murty K, Smith D G 1986 The management of the clinical problem of spinal pain with the assistance of a micro-computer. In: Hukins D W L, Mulholland R C (eds) Back pain. Manchester University Press, p 23–41
Gray D W R, Dixon J M, Collins J 1988 The closed eye sign: an aid to diagnosing non-specific abdominal pain. British

Medical Journal 297: 837
Greenough C G T, Fraser R D 1992 Assessment of outcome in patients with lower back pain. Spine 17: 36–41
Gunzburg R, Fraser R D, Fraser G A 1990 Lumbar intervertebral disc prolapse in teenage twins. Journal of Bone and Joint Surgery 72(5): 914–916
Halpin S F S, Yeoman L, Dundas D D 1991 Radiographic examination of the lumbar spine in a community hospital: an audit of current practice. British Medical Journal 303: 813–815
Hoffman R M, Kent D L, Deyo R A 1991 Diagnostic accuracy and clinical utility of thermography for lumbar radiculopathy. Spine 16: 623–627
Khuffash B, Porter R W 1989 Cross leg pain and trunk list. Spine 14: 602–603
Kirwan E O G, Hutton P A N, Pozo J L, Ransford A O 1984 Osteoid osteoma and benign osteoblastoma of the spine: clinical presentation and treatment. Journal of Bone and Joint Surgery 66-B: 21–26
Leavitt F, Garron D C, D'Angelo C M, McNeill T W 1979 Low back pain in patients with or without demonstrable organic disease. Pain 6: 191–200
Loebl W Y 1967 Measurement of spinal posture and range of spinal movement. Annals of Physical Medicine 9:103–110

McCombe P F, Fairbank J C J, Cockersole B C, Pynsent P B 1989 Reproducibility of physical signs in low back pain. Spine 14: 908–918

Maher J, Reilley M, Daly L, Hutchinson M 1992 Planter power: reproducibility of the plantar response. British Medical Journal 302: 482

Merriam W F, Smith N J, Mulholland R C 1982 Lumbar spinal stenosis. British Medical Journal 285: 515

Moll J M H, Wright V 1971 Normal range of spinal mobility: an objective clinical study. Annals of Rheumatology 30: 381–386

Nelson M A, Allen P, Clamp S E, de Dombal F T 1979 Reliability and reproducibility of clinical findings in low back pain. Spine 4: 97–101

Porter R W, Miller C 1986 Back pain and trunk list. Spine 11: 596–600

Porter R W, Oakshott G H L 1988 Familial aspects of disc protrusion. Journal of Orthopaedic Rheumatology 1: 173–178

Porter R W, Trailescu I F 1990 Diurnal changes in straight leg raising. Spine 15: 103–106

Postacchini F, Perugia D 1992 Changes in the ankle reflex related to posture. Journal of Bone and Joint Surgery 74-B: 155

Remak E 1881 Deutsche Medizinische Wochenschrift 257

Reynolds P M G 1975 Measurement of spinal mobility: a comparison of three methods. Rheumatology and Rehabilitation 14: 180–185

Roland M O, Porter R W, Matthews J G, Redden J F, Simonds G W, Bewley B 1991 Improving care: a study of orthopaedic outpatient referrals. British Medical Journal 302: 1124–1128

Salisbury P J, Porter R W 1987 Measurement of lumbar sagittal mobility: a comparison of methods. Spine 12: 190–193

Scott J H S 1983 Clinical examination, 6th edn. Churchill Livingstone, Edinburgh

Simkin P A 1982 Simian stance: a sign of spinal stenosis. Lancet 2: 652–653

So Y T, Arminoff M J, Olney R K 1989 The role of thermography in the evaluation of lumbosacral radiculopathy. Neurology 39: 1154–1158

Soukka A, Alaranta H, Tallneth K, Heliövaara 1991 Leg length inequality in people of working life. Spine 16: 429–431

Tillotson K M, Burton A K 1991 Non-invasive measurement of lumbar sagittal mobility. Spine 16:29–33

Varlotta G P, Brown M D, Kelsey J L, Gedden A L 1991 Familial predisposition for herniation of a lumbar disc in patients who are less than twenty one years old. Journal of Bone and Joint Surgery 73-A: 124–128

Waddell G 1982 An approach to backache. British Journal of Hospital Medicine, September

Waddell G, McCulloch J A, Kummell E, Venner R M 1980 Nonorganic physical signs in low back pain. Spine 5: 117–125

Waddell G, Main C J, Morris E W, Di Paola M, Gray I C M 1984 Chronic low back pain. Psychological distress and illness behaviour. Spine 9: 209–213

Wilbourn A J 1992 The electromyographic examination. In: Rothman R H, Simeone F A (eds) The Spine, 3rd edn. W B Saunders, Philadelphia, p 155–172

Wright V, Hopkins R, Burton K 1982 How long should we talk to patients? A study in doctor patient communication. Annals of the Rheumatic Diseases 41: 250–252

10. Radiological investigation of patients with back pain

P. Butt

Radiographs can never diagnose low back pain. Most patients who have symptomatic back pain have had pre-existing spinal pathology; much pathology is symptomless and therefore the radiological findings alone cannot provide the clinical diagnosis; they only partially influence management. Informed clinical judgement is the prerequisite for adequate and accurate radiological investigation. Radiological imaging is tailored to the patient, after it has been decided whether the patient is suffering from mechanical or non-mechanical back pain.

NON-MECHANICAL BACK PAIN

This represents but a small group of the patients with low back pain who are referred for X-ray. Although they are only 5% of the total, patients with non-mechanical back pain provide a much greater percentage of the disastrous misdiagnoses.

Traditionally, the first radiological investigation of a patient with non-mechanical back pain is the standard X-ray. False-negatives are common, but metastatic disease with bone sclerosis or destruction, and infection with cortical loss of the endplate or anterior body, may show on a standard X-ray. Absence does not exclude the pathology. Ideally, bone scintigraphy is the first investigation of the patient with non-mechanical back pain and it should always be considered if the plain films are non-contributory. It will save many a misdiagnosis and its value cannot be overemphasized.

High definition computerized tomographic (CT) scanning may be necessary but it cannot be performed for the whole spine. Preinvestigation localization of the area of interest is important and this can be done either with scintigraphy or clinically from specific root signs, localized tenderness and girdle pain. Magnetic resonance imaging (MRI) can cover a greater range than CT scanning and it is more sensitive than bone scintigraphy.

MECHANICAL BACK PAIN

This accounts for the majority (95%) of patients with low back pain referred for radiological investigation. Most of these will get better with rest, reassurance and medication and they need no X-ray examination (Nachemson 1983). This is not to save money nor to spare the radiological department work, but rather because investigation may well demonstrate symptomless pathology. Many symptomless patients have pathological lesions such as disc protrusion, degeneration or spinal stenosis, all of which could be treated surgically (Wilberger & Pang 1983, Wiesel et al 1984, Bell et al 1984, Booth et al 1984, Rothman et al 1986, Stewart et al 1987).

Most patients with an acute episode of back pain recover spontaneously, but if as a result of some inappropriately ordered radiological examination they are diagnosed as having significant pathology which is really symptomless, the clinician is then under considerable pressure to alter his management. Many patients have followed this path to unnecessary surgery. Nothing untoward will happen to the patient with mechanical back pain who waits for 2 months for his first X-ray provided there are none of the standard accepted criteria for urgent surgery.

What are we looking for with plain films?

We all recognize that patients can have severe degenerative disc disease radiologically with no symptoms at all, and that patients can have no radiological evidence of degenerative disc disease and yet suffer incapacitating back pain; therefore, usually we are not looking for degenerative disc disease. There are exceptions, particularly the young patient with an isolated, grossly degenerative disc above L4, whose spine is otherwise pristine.

The reason for plain radiographs in the patient with mechanical back pain is to identify those other conditions which mimic mechanical back pain sufficiently frequently that they are a cause of mismanagement: ankylosing spondylitis, spondylolysis and metastasis at the base of the pedicle. All three can present with back pain, nerve root irritation and nerve root signs, and lead to inappropriate surgery. We have a patient who had two laminectomies and two fusions before ankylosing spondylitis was recognized.

Ankylosing spondylitis

The bamboo spine of the fused spondylitic is well known, but it is the early stage or the less severe form that mimics mechanical back pain. The majority of patients, and women in particular, with symptomatic ankylosing spondylitis do not progress to solid fusion. For this reason, women present at back pain clinics with ankylosing spondylitis more commonly than men, having been misdiagnosed as mechanical back pain. The plain films of the lumbar spine must include adequate views of the sacroiliac joints, and also demonstrate the thoracolumbar junction. Sacroiliitis can be difficult to diagnose on plain films, and CT scanning is the technique of choice (Fig. 10.1a). Sacroiliitis alone is not ankylosing spondylitis; it is necessary to demonstrate Romanus lesions of the spine (Fig. 10.1b), most commonly seen at the thoracolumbar junction, but at an early stage they involve L5. Although unilateral sacroiliitis can be recognized by increased scintigraphic activity, most authorities find that bone scintigraphy is not useful in demonstrating bilateral sacroiliitis.

Spondylolysis

Although spondylolisthesis is not difficult to appreciate, it is not always easy to determine if the displacement is due to a lysis or degeneration. A lateral film may be needed to demonstrate whether the spinous process of the displaced body has moved with the body (degenerative) or stayed behind (lytic).

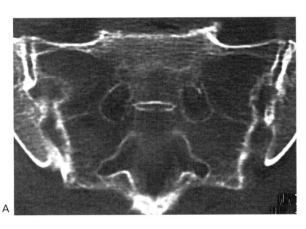

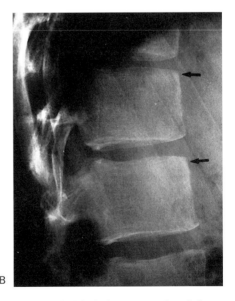

Fig. 10.1(A) CT scanning (here with the gantry parallel to the main axis of the SI joint) is the best way to show inflammatory sacroiliitis. **(B)** The Romanus lesion which describes erosion of the vertebral corners and sclerosis deep to the erosion must be demonstrated to diagnose inflammatory spondylitis. Sacroiliitis alone is not enough. (Reproduced with the permission of St James's University Hospital, Leeds.)

Oblique, lateral or inclined frontal films may be necessary to demonstrate a spondylolysis, but occasionally it is not seen on any of these; 60° oblique tomography (Fig. 10.2) can demonstrate lysis not visible on standard projections. CT scanning has become the method of choice to demonstrate the spondylolysis and there should be no false negatives if the gantry is perpendicular to the table top rather than parallel to the disc space. Gantry angles parallel to the disc space are frequently parallel to the lysis, and the lysis will not then be visible. Reversing the gantry angle shows the posterior elements to better advantage, and this is the best method to demonstrate the lysis (Fig. 10.3).

A positive scintigram (Fig. 10.4) is not necessarily diagnostic of a lysis as there are other causes of increased scintigraphic activity. It has been suggested that a lysis which is not scintigraphically active is not symptomatic (Pennel et al 1985), but this needs confirmation.

Pain-provoking injections attempt to reproduce the patient's symptoms but are of doubtful value.

The lysis invariably communicates with the facet joints above and below, making the origin of the pain uncertain. Communication with the facet joint on the other side may occur via the extradural space, and therefore therapeutic response to injection of a lysis is of somewhat doubtful significance.

Pedicle metastasis

Normally patients with metastatic disease do not present with mechanical pain, but if the metastasis is at the base of the pedicle close to the existing nerve root, the patient may present with back pain and sciatica, made worse by exercise. An X-ray study that does not show the pedicles is incomplete. The pedicles of L5 are not seen on standard frontal films, and therefore the routine radiographic examination of the patient with mechanical back pain should include a frontal supine film of L5, obtained at a cephalic angulation of 20°. This film is also ideal for imaging the sacroiliac joints.

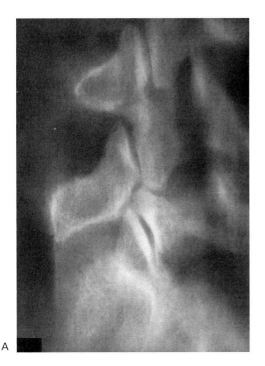
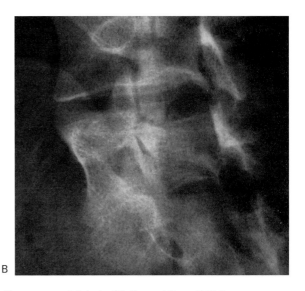

Fig. 10.2(A)   Standard oblique films are not always enough to diagnose spondylolysis. **(B)** Steep oblique (60°) linear tomography is a useful way of demonstrating the lysis. (Fig. 10.2(B) reproduced with the permission of St James's University Hospital, Leeds.)

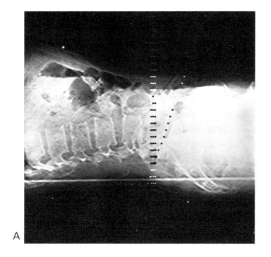

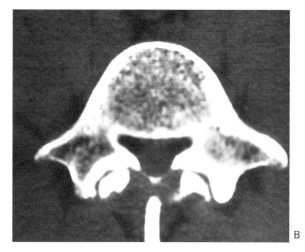

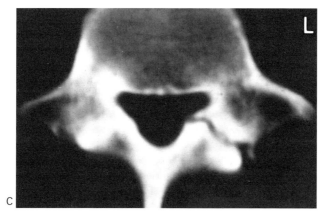

Fig. 10.3(A) The two standard ways of obtaining CT films of the lumbar spine are with the gantry perpendicular to the table or with it parallel to the disc spaces. Gantry angles parallel to the disc space **(B)** may not show a spondylolysis which is shown if the gantry is perpendicular to the table top **(C)**.

What of the majority of patients who do not have one of the above three?

Once again the answer is not radiological but clinical. If the patients do not fulfil the criteria for surgery, then no further radiological studies should be performed. Otherwise, many asymptomatic pathologies will be demonstrated, half of which will be on the same side as the pain and these will put pressure on the clinician to make an inappropriate diagnosis. Radiological criteria must not be used to decide whether patients should have surgery. The X-ray examination may say where, but can never say on whom or when. Just because an examination has no complications (CT) or no danger (MRI), does not mean that the indications for its use should be any less strict than for more invasive techniques (myelography).

What examination should be performed next?

The answer to that question depends on what type of surgery is planned.

Discectomy

Objective nerve root tension signs in a patient who has failed to respond to conservative management are generally the accepted indications for discectomy, be it chemical, percutaneous, micro- or macrosurgical.

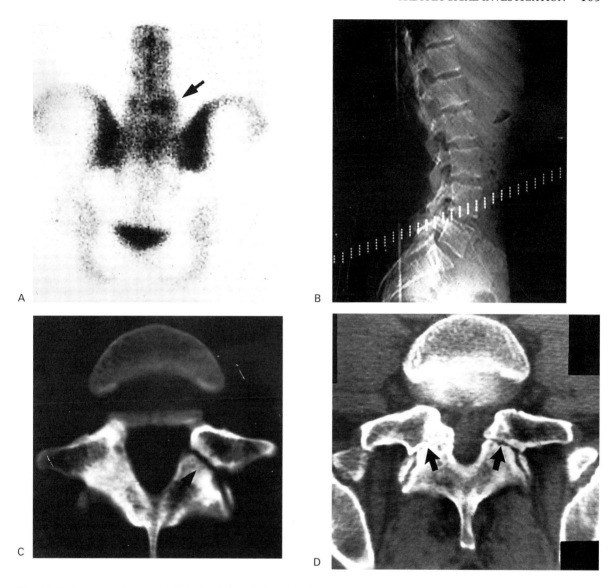

Fig. 10.4 Symptomatic spondylolysis should be scintigraphically active (**A**). CT examination with the gantry angle at maximum reverse tilt (**B**) is the best method of showing the unilateral spondylolysis (**C**) in the patient with the active scintigram or (**D**) in a patient with a bilateral lysis. (Reproduced with the permission of St James's University Hospital, Leeds.)

It is generally agreed that CT scanning should be the first radiological investigation of the pre-surgical discectomy patient. The vast majority of discs, be they lateral, central, foraminal or anterior, will be accurately demonstrated by CT scanning. Scanners are available, safe and involve no greater radiation dose than myelography. There are no false-positive CT scans in the sense that if there is a tissue density difference demonstrated by the scan, there will be tissue differences in that location. There is, of course, no guarantee that tissue of disc density is in fact disc, but a space-occupying lesion will be present. False-negative scans do occur, but that is not a problem since the examination is not performed to decide whether or not the patient requires surgery, but rather to indicate where the surgery should be conducted. Since a negative CT scan does not

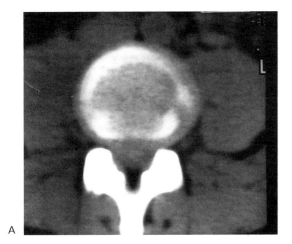
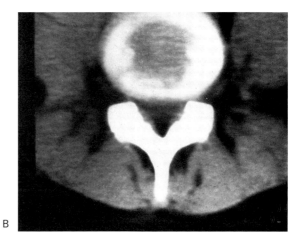

Fig. 10.5   A huge hernia (**A**) is still a cause of false-negative CT scanning and it is important to recognize the difference in density between the massive hernia in (**A**) and the normal dura as shown at another level (**B**).

answer the question, further investigation is clearly necessary.

There are some problems using CT scanning for prediscectomy assessment.

Large hernias. CT scanning is excellent for the diagnosis of small but significant disc hernias (Fig. 10.7b) but the huge herniation can still be missed. Note in Figure 10.5 how the massive disc hernia mimics a normal dural sac and does not seem to extend behind the limits of the normal dural sac. The interpreter has to be alert to the fact that there is a subtle difference in the density of the dural sac at the level of the massive hernia in comparison with the level above, and that there is no epidural fat anterior to the dural sac. It is not difficult in cases of doubt to set the machine to highlight tissue of dural density which will leave the disc density as a negative, or to highlight the psoas and ligamentum flavum density which is the same as that of the disc in order to highlight the disc hernia (Fig. 10.6).

Too many hernias. Finding several disc hernias is not as good as finding one, because the purpose of the procedure is not to diagnose the presence of a disc hernia but rather to indicate the level of the lesion. The finding of three disc hernias in a patient does nothing more than place him in the 98% of patients whose lesions are at any one of the lower three disc levels. Although Wilberger and Pang (1983) have shown that large hernias

almost always become symptomatic, it is not accepted practice to perform prophylactic discectomy at an asymptomatic level in order to prevent future disability.

Asymptomatic/wrong side. Sometimes an unequivocal disc hernia will be demonstrated on the asymptomatic side or at the wrong level, or both. One might focus on the asymptomatic but impressive lesion (Fig. 10.7a) and ignore the unimpressive but clinically significant smaller lesion at a different level (Fig 10.7b). We should remember that disc hernias are usually present before they become symptomatic, and we can then understand why the occasional patient will have a large disc hernia which is not compatible with the clinical findings. Once again it may be tempting to carry out a prophylactic discectomy at an asymptomatic level at the same time as treating the symptomatic lesion, but there is no scientific support for such an action.

If CT scanning does not answer the question of where to operate, what should we do next?

Both myelography and MRI have the ability to demonstrate the rare intradural tumour which mimics discogenic nerve pain. However, MRI has the added advantage of demonstrating nerve roots well beyond the edge of the vertebral canal. With the sophisticated new software described in

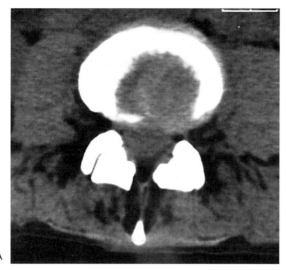
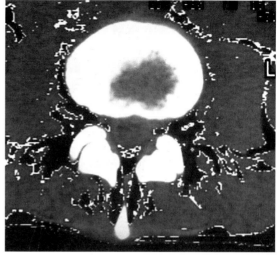
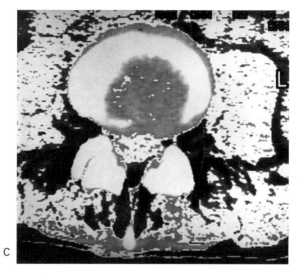

Fig. 10.6   If there is doubt about the presence of a massive disc hernia (**A**) the CT scanner can be set to highlight tissue of dural density (**B**) or disc density (**C**) which is the same as psoas muscle and ligamentum flavum to clarify the situation.

Chapter 11, individual nerves can be followed for a significant distance into the retroperitoneal space. This can demonstrate physical interference with, and possibly chemical change in, the nerve which hitherto was impossible to assess by other methods.

Discography can be a useful investigation, but it has been largely superseded by other methods of imaging. It is still useful as a pain-provocation procedure in the patient with multiple hernias to help decide which is symptomatic. Unfortunately,

discography does not always reproduce sciatica reliably, and one is then dependent on assessing which is the most sensitive hernia.

Fusion

Back pain which is due to segmental instability, and which is causing sufficient disability, is treated by fusion. The radiological investigation would therefore seem to be easy — demonstrate abnormal mobility. Unfortunately, it is extra-

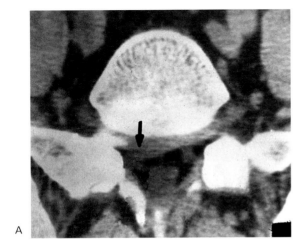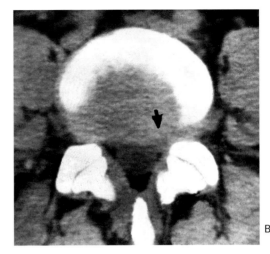

A   B

Fig. 10.7   An obvious hernia at the wrong level and the wrong side (**A**) may distract one from the clinically significant but less obvious lesion at another level on the correct side (**B**). (Reproduced with the permission of St James's University Hospital, Leeds.)

ordinarily difficult to do so. In very specific circumstances where a single level is to be assessed, flexion and extension films (Fig. 10.8) can be used. However, coupled movement causes rotation as well as flexion which simulates instability. Carefully controlled films such as horizontal beam laterals with the patient being placed over an obstacle are useful for the thoracic spine, but it is not usually helpful to use mobility films to assess lumbar instability. It is possible to demonstrate abnormal mobility with some accuracy, but it is difficult to relate such abnormal mobility to a patient's clinical picture, and the concept of segmental instability is still one with little practical application.

There are many clues which suggest abnormal mobility on standard films. If a disc degenerates then there must be abnormal mobility. Subluxation may occur at the degenerate level, reaching its epitome with degenerative spondylolisthesis. Osteoarthritis of the facet joint is an equally good indicator of abnormal mobility. On the other hand, traction spurs have been seen with normal discs (Quinnell & Stockdale 1982) and with only minimal degeneration (Milgram 1990). It is difficult to match the radiological evidence of abnormal mobility with the clinical picture. Can there be instability without degeneration? It is quite clear that some patients have one level that

is excessively mobile, yet no evidence that it is degenerate on standard film. Disc degeneration might sometimes follow rather than be a cause of instability. In these patients, flexion and extension films might be useful.

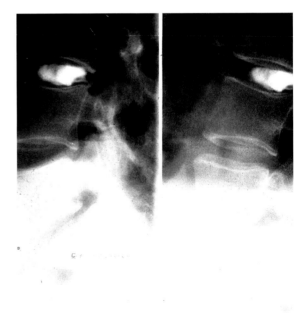

Fig. 10.8   Flexion (right) and extension (left) in lateral radiograph suggest excessive movement at L4/5.

Discography has much to offer in both multiple and single level disc pathology. If a patient is to be treated surgically for back pain, if that pain can be reproduced by injecting a single level in the spine and the pain can be relieved by anaesthetizing that level, then it is that level which requires surgery. This is the purpose of discography — not to show that discs need surgery or that discs are degenerate, but to show which is the symptomatic disc (Fig. 10.9). It has been used to show that a disc above the level to be fused should be included in the fusion because it is badly degenerate and could become a source of symptoms. However, McCall (1986) has shown that the symptomatic results of fusion do not seem to depend on the integrity of the disc above the level fused. The single severely degenerate disc in a young patient, particularly above L4/5, is usually symptomatic, but it is much more difficult to assess whether a single level is significant in a patient with several pathological degenerate levels.

Decompression

Spinal stenosis compressing nerve tissue and causing claudication is the usual indication for decompressive laminectomy, facet undercutting or foraminal enlargement. Stenosis can be demonstrated by CT scanning, whether it is concentric, lateral recess, foraminal, or extravertebral (Fig. 10.10). It is much more difficult to decide if the stenosis is significant. Stenosis can be profound in patients who are entirely asymptomatic provided the stenosis has been gradual and is at a single level (see Ch. 17). It is not surprising, therefore, that the results of surgical treatment of stenosis are so variable (Dickson 1987).

Combined CT scanning and myelography is useful for lateral recess stenosis and its variants. The use of MRI in spinal stenosis is discussed in the following chapter.

Special mention should be made of degenerative spondylolisthesis. It is the commonest overlooked and under-treated cause of debilitating back pain and spinal claudication in older patients. Their complaints are often ignored and one of our patients become faecally incontinent before stenosis was recognized. Degenerative spondy-lolisthesis displaces the posterior elements forwards as far as the displacement of the vertebral body, and if the canal is already small, a complete cauda equina block can readily occur with a minor degree of displacement (Fig. 10.11).

Ganglia from osteoarthritic facet joints constitute a specific type of stenosis which can be seen readily with CT scanning. Frequently they contain gas (Fig.10.12), and then the diagnosis is certain.

OTHER DIAGNOSTIC PROBLEMS

Facet pain

Facet arthrography has as many antagonists as proponents. However, if a patient's pain has been provoked by an injection of contrast medium into a facet joint, and it is relieved by the injection of local anaesthetic into that joint, it is reasonable to treat the patient with local anaesthetic and long-term anti-inflammatory drugs. Joint fusion is, however, another question. Soft tissue injections diffuse a great distance and can affect remote structures. It is essential, therefore, that facet injections are contained within the joint capsule, and quantities greater than 1 ml should not be used diagnostically or therapeutically, because they will extend beyond the confines of the joint capsule. If the injected material enters the epidural space, precise localization of the origin of the symptoms becomes impossible.

The post-laminectomy spine

The radiological investigation of the post-laminectomy back has changed completely with the introduction of MRI and gadolinium, and it is now difficult to justify using any other technique. In the symptomatic patient following laminectomy, one is attempting to differentiate scar tissue from a recurrent disc hernia. Contrast-enhanced CT scanning was previously used for this problem, but was often unrewarding; the technique may distinguish vascularized scar tissue from disc, but tissue that does not enhance could be scar, nerve root or disc hernia. Disc hernias can be covered with a thin layer of enhancing scar (Fig. 10.13), and if this does not enhance to the point that it is visible, measurement of the density of the mass

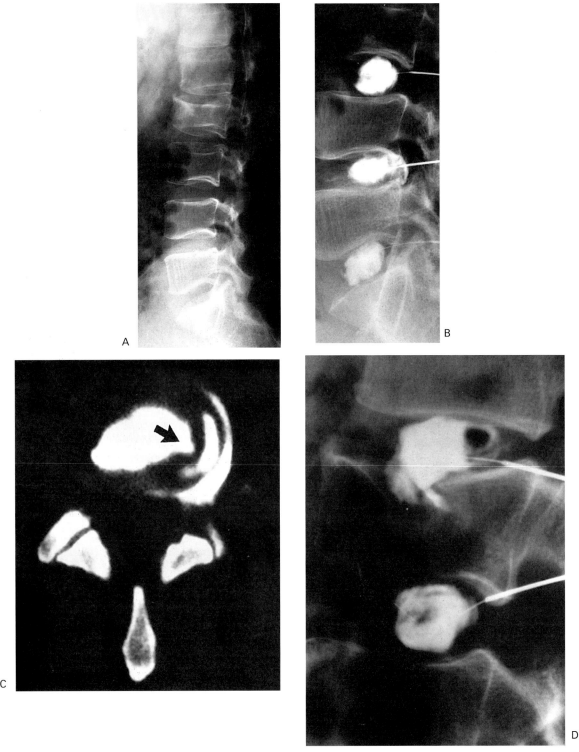

Fig. 10.9   A young man who fell at work and fractured L1 (**A**) presented with the gradual onset of incapacitating low back and left sacroiliac pain. Although the discogram (**B** and **C**) showed that the L4/5 disc had an annulus rupture with left-sided extravasation of contrast medium, the injection at this level was asymptomatic and the abnormality was an incidental finding. On the other hand, discography at L1/2 (**D**) reproduced the patient's pain faithfully and local anaesthetic relieved his pain. This was the symptomatic level.

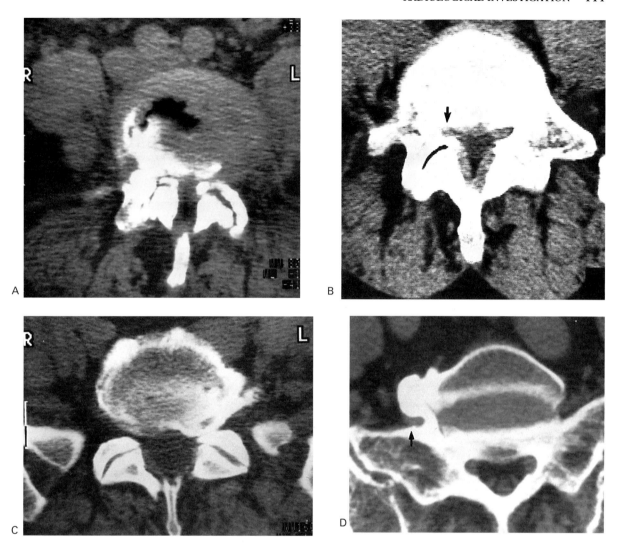

Fig. 10.10 Spinal stenosis is readily demonstrated by CT scanning whether it is concentric (**A**), lateral recess (**B**), foraminal (**C**), or virtually extravertebral (**D**). The critical observation is demonstration of physical interference with nerve tissue such as the flattened nerve root in (**D**), and even then correlation with clinical findings may be difficult. One should not be surprised if a patient with a stenosis as shown in (**A**) is entirely asymptomatic. (Fig. 10.10 (B) reproduced with the permission of St James's University Hospital, Leeds.)

with cursors will give a false reading, suggesting that the entire mass and not just the rim is enhanced. This is a significant cause of error in the interpretation of the post-laminectomy CT scan.

Assessment post-fusion

That a fusion is solid can sometimes be demonstrated by either steep oblique tomography (similar to the projection used for spondylolysis) or by an inclined frontal tomogram of the lower lumbar region. However, it takes CT scanning to show that the solid graft is anchored to the spine. If frontal or oblique tomograms demonstrate continuous solid bone, and CT scanning shows that it is firmly attached to the posterior elements, the fusion is sound. Reformatting of CT images in a curved plane following the fusion mass can present a single picture of the entire

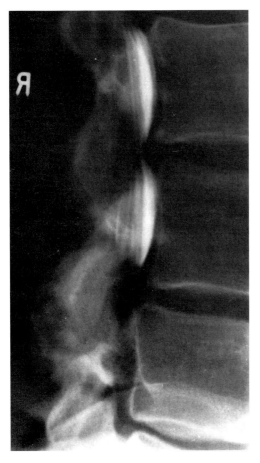

Fig. 10.11 A minor degree of degenerative spondylolisthesis can cause complete cauda equinal block in a patient whose spinal canal is small to start with. Because the deterioration is slow the patients may develop profound neurological disturbance before the cause is appreciated. The patient, for example, developed faecal incontinence before the significance of the spondylolisthesis was recognized. (Reproduced with the permission of St James's University Hospital, Leeds.)

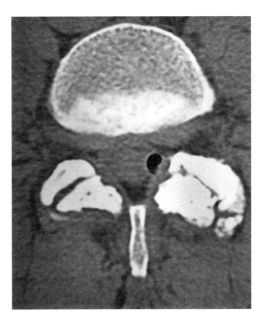

Fig. 10.12 Ganglia associated with osteoarthritic facet joints can cause compression of the dural sac. When they are air-filled as in this example or have a calcified wall the diagnosis is straightforward. (Reproduced with the permission of St James's University Hospital, Leeds.)

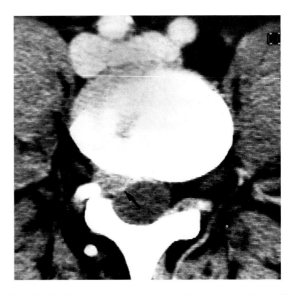

Fig. 10.13 Contrast medium injected in large quantities will enhance the scar tissue that forms around a disc hernia. This will not present diagnostic difficulties if the enhancement is sufficient to be seen, but if it is not, then a measurement of enhancement in the area will suggest that the entire mass is enhancing granulation tissue rather than enhancement of a coating on a recurrent disc hernia. This is a major cause of incorrect diagnosis in the post-laminectomy spine.

mass, which is better than either oblique or frontal tomography.

Bone scintigraphy is also useful in assessing fusion. Fused bone should lose its scintigraphic activity 2 years after fusion, and persistence of high levels of activity indicates persistent pseudoarthrosis. Flexion/extension films are unhelpful.

Broken metal indicates that at some stage the fusion mass had broken, but the fusion can have repaired subsequently.

Without a careful and rational clinical assessment of the patient, radiographs are likely to present the clinician with dangerous pitfalls of misdiagnosis. However, as a supplement to sound clinical judgement, radiography will help identify the site of significant pathology and simplify surgical procedures. Dialogue between clinician and radiologist is essential.

REFERENCES

Bell G R, Rothman R H, Booth R E, Cukler J M, Garfin S, Hekowitz H et al 1984 A study of computerised axial tomography. 2. Comparison of metrizamide myelography and CT in the diagnosis of herniated lumbar disc and spinal stenosis. Spine 9: 552–556

Booth R E, Cuckler J M, Gayin S, Bell G R, Rothman R H 1984 A study of computerized axial tomography and metrizamide myelography. Spine 9: 552–556

Dickson R A 1987 The surgical treatment of low back pain. Current Orthopaedics 1: 387–390

McCall I W 1986 Radiological assessment of back pain. Seminars in Orthopaedics 1: 71–85

Milgram J W 1990 Radiologic and histologic pathology of non-tumorous disease of bones and joints. In Milgram J W (ed) Northbrook Publishing, Hong Kong, p 537

Nachemson A C 1983 Work for all. Clinical Orthopaedics and Related Research 179: 77–85

Pennel R G, Maurer A H, Noakdapour A 1985 Stress injuries of the pars interarticularis. Radiological classification and indications for scintigraphy. American Journal of Roentgenology 145: 763–766

Quinnell R C, Stockdale H R 1982 The significance of osteophytes on lumbar vertebral bodies in relation to discographic findings. Clinical Radiology 33: 197–203

Rothman R H, Wiesel S W, Bell G R 1986 Editorial: On CT scanning and metrizamide myelography. Spine 11: 1

Stewart H D, Quinnell R C, Dann N 1987 Epidurography in the management of sciatica. British Journal of Rheumatology 26: 424–429

Wiesel S N, Tsour N, Feffer H L, Citrin C M, Patronas N 1984 A study of computerised axial tomography. 1. The incidence of positive CAT scans in an asymptomatic group of patients. Spine 9: 549–552

Wilberger J E, Pang D 1983 Syndrome of the incidental herniated lumbar disc. Journal of Neurosurgery 59: 137–141

11. Magnetic resonance imaging (MRI) in the investigation of patients with back pain

J. A. McCulloch

INTRODUCTION

Magnetic resonance imaging (MRI) will soon be the imaging modality of first choice for the investigation of patients with low back pain. In centres where it is readily available it is quickly displacing myelography (radiculography) and CT scanning as the first investigation when an imaging study is indicated (Fig. 11.1). Its superior delineation of soft tissue morphology and chemistry, its ability to cut slices in any plane (routinely, sagittal slices as well as axial are provided) and its ability to show the entire lumbar spine (including the conus) cause us to ask how CT scanning can ever remain a priority test in the investigation of patients with back pain. However, in the growing enthusiasm for MRI we must not forget its weaknesses: it does not show bony detail as well as CT and it is so sensitive a modality that many patients with so-called abnormal MRIs are in actual fact suffering from some other cause of symptoms than the lesion seen on MRI (Boden et al 1990).

Roentgen introduced X-ray 100 years ago; 20 years ago the MRI was first proposed for human use (Bloch et al 1946, Purcell et al 1946, Damadian 1971); and only 10 years ago the first high quality, clinically useful image of the brain was generated at Hammersmith Hospital in London (Doyle et al 1981). Today, clinicians are obtaining high quality images of spinal structures, yet much is still to be achieved in radiological science. The rate of advancement in software and hardware is bewildering, but for the spinal clinician it is important to grasp some basics (Sprawls & Peterson 1988).

From the most basic physical perspective, the MR image is a display of radio-frequency signal intensities emitted by tissues. A bright area is appropriately described as having a high signal intensity. Contrast is present in an image because the various tissues emit signals with different intensities.

PHYSICS

A grasp of the basic physics is helpful to the clinician in appreciating the potential for growth in MRI.

Definitions

Magnetic

There are two magnets essential to MRI:

1. The external magnet, i.e. the magnet that is part of the imaging machine. Its strength is described in tesla (T) and the most common sizes are 0.5, 1.0 and 1.5 T, the strongest magnets in the world. (In contrast, the earth's magnetic field is 0.5×10^{-4} T.)
2. The internal magnets, i.e. the miniature magnet of the hydrogen atom contained in the body.

Resonance

A resonating system is one that oscillates between high and low energy states. Radio-frequency waves of an appropriate wavelength, when transmitted through the body, can cause the hydrogen atoms to resonate (change their vector).

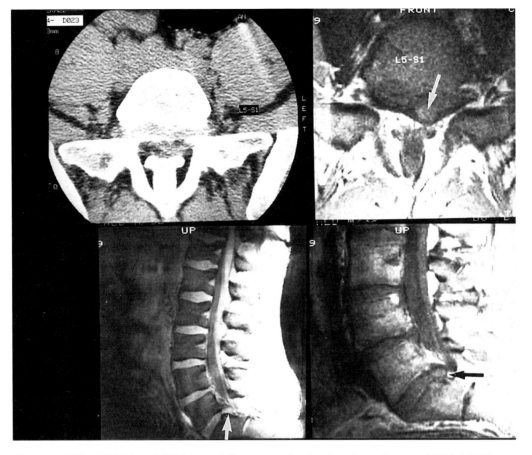

Fig. 11.1   CT vs MRI. The axial CT (upper left) suggests a herniated nucleus pulposus at L5/S1, left. There is no doubt on axial MRI (upper right) and sagittals (lower left and right).

The atom

An atom is the smallest unit of a chemical element that retains its chemical identity. It is composed of a nucleus around which electrons orbit. The nucleus comprises almost all of the mass of an atom, but because of the orbiting electrons comprises less of the actual size of an atom. A nucleus is made up of protons with a single positive electrical charge, and neutrons with no charge. The number of protons in the nucleus is the atomic number of the atom or element. Atoms with uneven atomic numbers have spin and charge, giving them angular momentum, so that they act like small magnets. Examples of nuclei with uneven atomic numbers are H (1), Na (23), and P (31).

The original designation of this modality,

'nuclear magnetic resonance', was quite appropriate — i.e. nuclei being realigned by a magnet and resonated with radio-frequency waves.

Hydrogen

The atom used for MRI is the hydrogen (^{1}H) atom because it is abundant in the body and capable of giving off a strong signal when resonated. It is a simple element with one proton in the nucleus, no neutrons and no orbiting electrons. It is the hydrogen ion in body water that is available for resonating. To a lesser extent, the hydrogen ion of lipids will resonate and contribute to the MRI signal, with protein and nucleic acid H^+ ions offering nothing to the signal.

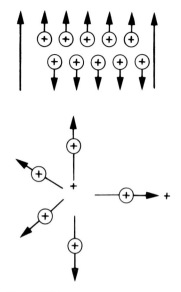

Fig. 11.2 (Top) Within the external magnet, the hydrogen protons will line up as shown. (Bottom) Outside the influence of the MRI magnet, the hydrogen protons are randomly oriented with 'no net magnetic vector'.

The hydrogen atom is positively charged and possessed of spinning or angular movement. This movement produces an internal mini magnetic field around each of the multitude of hydrogen atoms in the body. Normally, at any one moment, the hydrogen ions are randomly oriented in the body with a net magnetic effect of 0 (or neutral magnetic effect).

Alignment

The hydrogen atom magnet is randomly oriented in the body, but when placed in an external magnetic field it will align itself parallel to the magnetic field, producing a net magnetic vector (Fig. 11.2).

TECHNIQUE OF PERFORMING MAGNETIC RESONANCE IMAGING

The steps involved

Step 1

The patient is placed in the magnetic coil gantry of the scanner and the magnet turned on. (The magnet is, in fact, constantly turned on.) The magnetic field across the body will cause each hydrogen atom (and other magnetic atoms) to line up with the external magnetic field producing the net magnet vector (Fig. 11.2).

Step 2

A radio-frequency wave is broadcast into the body tissue (Fig. 11.3). The pulsating radio-frequency wave will be of a predetermined frequency, such that its most significant effect will be on the hydrogen atom. The predetermined frequency is called the 'pulse sequence'. Some of the hydrogen magnets will absorb some of the energy from the series of radio wave energy and tilt over (Fig. 11.4). The 'excited' hydrogen atoms have absorbed the energy from the radio-frequency (RF) and in their tilted position are said to be at a higher energy level, resulting in an overall change in direction of the net magnetic vector.

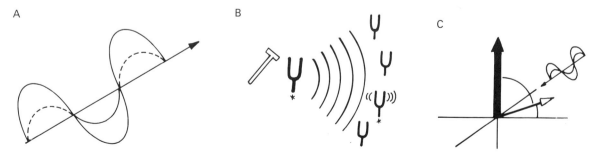

Fig. 11.3(A) A radio-frequency wave is a pulsating electromagnetic force travelling as a wave in the direction of the arrow. **(B)** If the radio-frequency wave is of the correct frequency it will resonate the hydrogen ions most, and other ions least (just as a tuning fork with * frequency will only resonate a tuning fork of a similar frequency (*). **(C)** The hydrogen proton (and its magnetic vector) are deflected away from its aligned position of Fig. 11.2 (from closed arrow to open arrow).

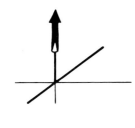

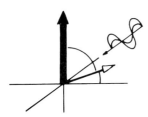

Fig. 11.4 (Top) All of the hydrogen protons are under the influence of the external magnet and the result is a magnetic vector (heavy closed arrow). (Bottom) With the correct radio-frequency wave some of those hydrogen ions are deflected and end up in a higher energy state resulting in a different magnetic vector (open-ended arrow).

The series of the RF pulse are repeated in cycles of finite time known as 'repetition time' (TR).

Step 3

During a gap in the pulsatile RF wave, the hydrogen magnets (atoms) will attempt to re-orient themselves in the magnetic field, returning the net magnetic vector to its original magnetized non-resonated position. In doing so, the hydrogen atoms will release energy by rebroadcasting the RF signal they absorbed on deflection. This re-broadcast radio-frequency wave can be picked up with an antenna just as a car radio picks up a broadcast signal. By 'tuning in' to a particular frequency, the echo of the RF signal can be detected. The time in the gap in the RF wave when 'tuning in' is done is known as the echo time (TE). The TE can be altered by altering the time when the detection antenna is turned on (Fig. 11.5).

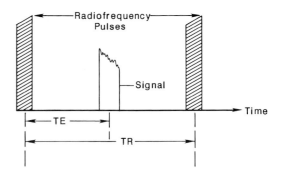

Fig. 11.5 TR and TE. The time to listen for the signal being given off is known as TE.

Step 4

As the net magnetic vector returns to its original position, the rebroadcast signal is detected by an antenna in the form of a surface coil applied to the patient's spine (the patient is actually lying on the coil). As explained later, the use of surface coils in spinal imaging has resulted in much improved images. The signal is detected as a magnetic resonance signal. Different RF signals from different regions of the sample are recorded by the computer as digital data of varying signal intensity. The computer, in turn, converts this digital data into varying shades of grey to produce an image. The image is easily transferred to a film just like a CT scan image where a strong signal appears white, a weak signal black and in-between signals are various shades of grey (Fig. 11.6).

Hardware

It is at this level of imaging physics that the clinician will get lost trying to understand what the MRI machine can do. It is important to recognize that MR technology is changing rapidly and the use of MRI is very dependent on a radiologist being constantly on top of these changes; it is impractical for a clinician to own or operate an MRI without a radiologist. Further, the production of quality MR images is very operator-dependent. It is possible, but unexpected, for an average X-ray technician to produce a poor X-ray or CT image; it is easy for an average technician

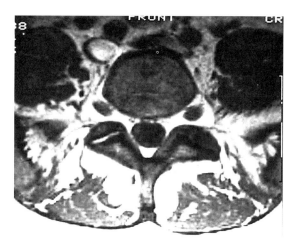

Fig. 11.6   Axial spin echo T_1 image (designated as SE 900/22 i.e. TR of 900 ms and TE of 22 ms using spin echo technique). The thecal sac and nerve roots are of low intensity signal, surrounded by high intensity (white) fat. The facet joint bone is of low intensity signal and the cartilage cleft on the right has high intensity signal.

to produce a poor MR image. It is important that supervision provide direction on the appropriate coil, imaging plane and matrix, slice thickness, number of excitations, pulse sequence parameters (TR), and echo time (TE), all terms with which clinicians are not familiar.

Field strength

MRI machines are built with varying magnet sizes measured in tesla (T). The strength of the magnet is many times the earth's gravitational pull and is capable of twisting aneurysm clips, pulling hairpins out of the head, moving wheelchairs and decoding credit cards.

Magnet sizes commonly used in medicine today are 0.5 T (mid-field), 1 T (high field) and 1.5 T (highest field strength). It is not necessarily true that the bigger magnet is better, but imaging of difficult areas, such as the posterior fossa and base of the brain, is better with the higher field strengths. Although the manufacturers state that it is possible to get good spinal images from the lower field strength machines, the author's early experiences would suggest that the most consistently good spinal images come from the machines with the highest field strength (Egerter 1991).

Pulse sequence

In reading about MRI, clinicians will see the term 'pulse sequence' mentioned often. There are two types of pulse sequences commonly used today: one (spin echo) was used exclusively for clinical imaging of the spine in the original proto-

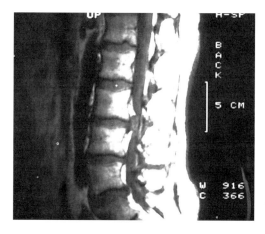

Fig. 11.7(A)   Sagittal T_1 (SE 600/22). Note the lack of contrast differentiation between the back of the disc space and the dural sac. A large disc rupture is present at L3–4 and a small herniated nucleus pulposus is present at L5/S1.

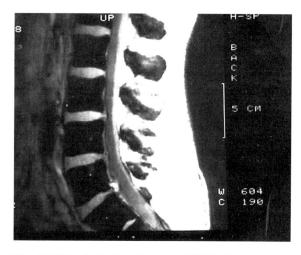

Fig. 11.7(B)   Sagittal gradient echo (GE 200/11 flip angle 60°). Note the clear difference in signal intensity at the disc/dural junction.

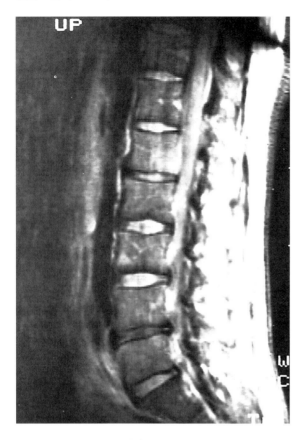

Fig. 11.10   Proton density image (SE TR 2500/TE 15, a rarely used protocol). Note lower signal intensity from bone and ligament vs higher signal intensity from CSF. The dural sac is dark but not as dark as in sagittal T_1 (see Fig. 11.7(A)).

response to MR is no different than electron density determining the grey scale in CT. The superior soft tissue depiction comes not from proton density but from T_1 and T_2 relaxation effects. This is because many substances with similar proton and electron densities will emanate different signal intensities on MR due to the marked differences in T_1 and T_2 values (Table 11.1). Note that water (CSF) has the longest T_1 and T_2 relaxation times, whereas fat protons have a short T_1 and intermediate T_2 relaxation time. These relaxation times can easily be altered by binding the H^+ proton with protein macromolecules; i.e. fluids (water) can have a variety of signals (appearances) based on their protein content.

It should be noted that:

- Substances with the *shortest* T_1 relaxation time give off the brightest signal (fat, lipid-containing molecules or proteinaceous fluid)
- Substances with the *longest* T_1 relaxation time (oedema, CSF, pure fluid, tumours (benign and malignant)) give off a low signal and appear greyer (Fig. 11.11).

By selecting a scanning protocol with a short TR and TE the image is weighted to emphasize these T_1 characteristics, but weighting too heavily will ruin the image by invoking other physics equations that affect signal to noise ratios, scan time and so on, a subject far beyond this chapter. Just the correct amount of TR and TE is needed to produce a useful T_2 image.

A protocol that lengthens TR and lengthens TE (Fig. 11.9) is called a T_2-weighted image, in which the reverse signal characteristics occur — i.e. the longer the T_2 relaxation time the brighter the signal (remember the longer the T_1 relaxation time the greyer the picture) (Fig. 11.12).

Substances with a short T_2 relaxation time include muscle and tendons. Substances with a long T_2 (brighter image) include water and CSF, oedema and inflammation. Thus many common disease processes become conspicuous on T_2-weighted images because the increased free water of oedema and inflammation gives a brighter (whiter) signal.

The T_1- and T_2-weighted images are summarized in Figure 11.13 and Table 11.2.

Gradient echo imaging

Spin echo imaging techniques as discussed above take time and are thus expensive. The longer the patient has to remain in the gantry for a study, the poorer the efficiency of the million(s) dollar

Table 11.1 T_1 and T_2 values of various tissues (mid-field strength magnet).

Tissue	T_1 (ms)	T_2 (ms)	
CSF (water)	2000	250	Long
Fat	150	150	↓
Muscle	450	64	Short

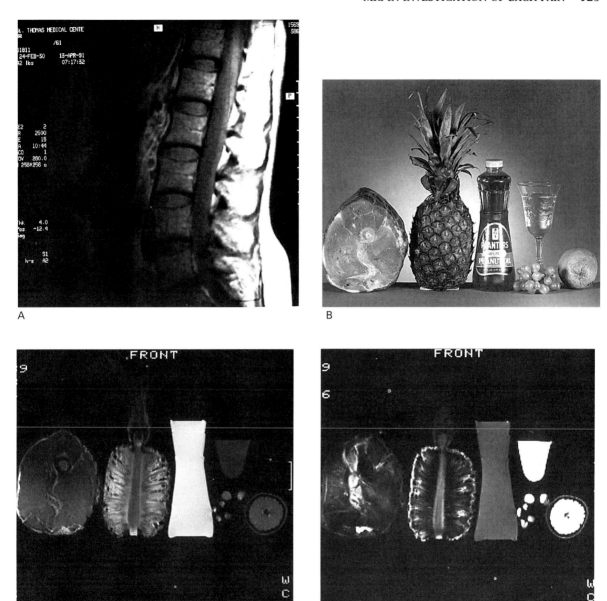

Fig. 11.11(A)   The Grey scale. (B) A ham (muscle), pineapple (fibre), peanut oil (fat), grapes (water), water, orange (water). (C) T_1 (SE 800/22). Compare fat and water to the T_2 image (D). On T_1 weighting, fat has a high (white) signal intensity, while water is intermediate. Next look at muscle (ham) which is also intermediate signal. Bone has no signal on T_1 and is black. The only other high signal intensity (like fat) comes from the external surface of the ham. Although parts of the pineapple have whiter or higher signal intensity than water it is still not equivalent to fat. (D) T_2 (SE 2500/90). Now fat (oil) has an intermediate signal intensity and water is brighter. Compare the orange and the grapes — they have followed water in signal intensity or whiteness, i.e. they are predominantly water. The part of the pineapple that has the most water (whiteness) is its skin! Bone is still black, with no signal intensity at all. These three figures show how to use the grey scale to determine tissue composition. (Exercise courtesy of Dr Edward Bury, Neuroradiologist, Akron City Hospital, Akron, Ohio.)

Brightest image = Short T_1 and long T_2 relaxation time in tissues

↓   ↓

Darkest image = Long T_1 and short T_2 relaxation time in tissues

Fig. 11.12 The Grey scale.

Table 11.2 The Grey scale in various tissues.

	T_1 weighted	T_2 weighted
CSF	black	white
Grey matter	grey	white
White matter	white	grey
Marrow	grey	whiter
Disc nucleus	grey	white
Disc annulus	less grey	black
Fat	bright	grey
Subacute haemorrhage	bright	grey
Gadolinium-enhanced tissues	very white	grey
Muscle	grey	grey

investment in hardware. This had led to the development of gradient echo imaging which speeds up image acquisition time by using less than 90° angle deflection of the proton magnetic field (Fig. 11.7). The following points are of note:

1. It takes less time to acquire images using gradient echo techniques (and thus the expensive hardware becomes more efficient).
2. The more the angle of flip approaches 90° the more the image will resemble (but not be identical to) a T_1-weighted spin echo image.

A

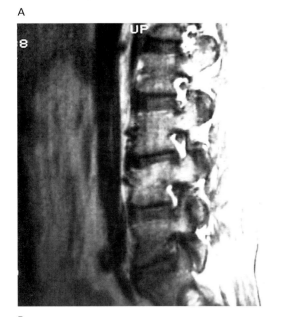

B

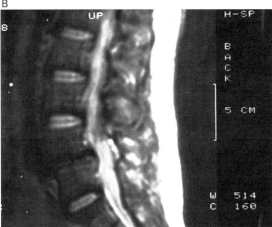

Fig. 11.13 (A) T_1 (SE 60/22) parasagittal cut through the foramen. The nerve root (intermediate signal intensity) appears surrounded by fat (high signal intensity). The foramen L5 is occupied by the superior facet of S1. (B) T_2 (SE 2000/60) median sagittal showing the high signal intensity CSF and discs except for the L4–5 disc which has lost its signal intensity through degeneration at the slip level.

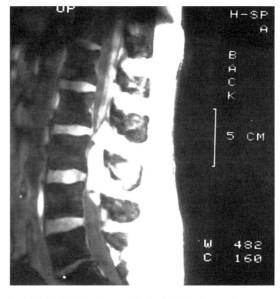

Fig. 11.14 GE 20/11 — sagittal which is close to but not quite like a spin echo T_2 weighted — the discs have high signal intensity, but the CSF is intermediate. The lymphoma visible in the canal behind L3 was missed on CT until the patient presented with paralysis.

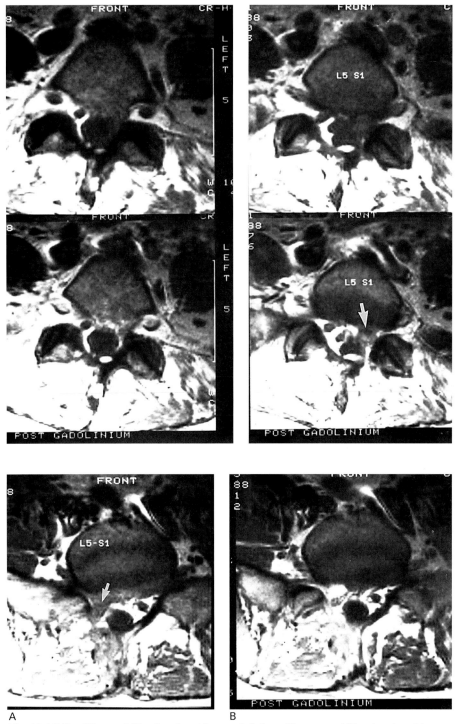

Fig. 11.15(A)   (Top row) T_1 spin echo without gadolinium; (Bottom row) T_1 spin echo with gadolinium. The image to the left shows that all the tissue anterior and lateral to the thecal sac enhances — no disc material is present. The bottom right (arrow) shows a non-enhancing recurrent fragment of disc. (B) The reverse of (A). Without gadolinium is the mass (arrow) scar or recurrent disc? After injection of gadolinium, it is obviously scar.

3. The more the flip angle approaches 10° the more the image will resemble a T_2-weighted image (Fig. 11.14).

4. The physics is far beyond this chapter but terms such as FLASH and GRASS signify the various programmes used to obtain the gradient echo image. The shortening of time to gather a clinically useful image is a significant advantage in MRI and clinicians will be seeing more and more gradient echo images.

Gadolinium-enhanced MRI

As for CT, there is a contrast agent to enhance the image (Haughton 1988). Gadolinium, when injected intravenously, will deposit in aqueous solutions (provided they have a blood supply) and brighten the water protons on T_1-weighted images (Fig. 11.15). Gadolinium itself does not throw off a signal but rather affects the water-bound hydrogen protons such that they throw off a much higher signal; this results in highlighting of scar tissue, separating it from a recurrent fragment of disc. The advantages of gadolinium are:

— It is non-allergic (no anaphylactic reactions reported to date)

— It is safe (hundreds of thousands of IV gadolinium injections have been given with no side-effects)

— It brightens water H^+ protons on T_1-weighted images

— The higher the field strength of the unit, the more pronounced is this paramagnetic effect.

MAGNETIC RESONANCE IMAGING OF THE SPINE

Imaging hardware

Figure 11.16 shows the set-up for lumbar MRI including the surface coil in the table which is directly over the area of study. As a scanning technique, body coil sagittal imaging (without the surface coil) can be done (Fig. 11.17) to screen for metastases and then axial

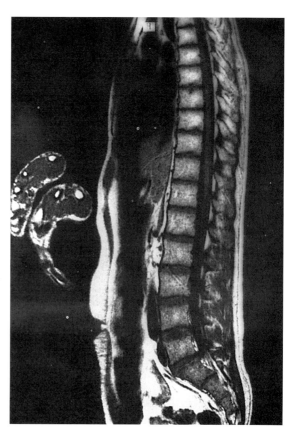

Fig. 11.17 Body coil image showing upper thoracic to lower lumbar. This technique is a good scan seeking secondary deposits in the vertebrae and/or when cord compression is present with some question as to level.

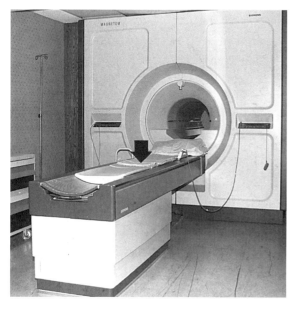

Fig. 11.16 A Seimens 1.5 tesla unit (Somatom ®) with surface coil (arrow).

images, using the surface coil, can be concentrated in the area picked up as abnormal on the body coil sagittals.

Protocols

Imaging protocols for lumbar MRI on the machine in our centre (Siemens Somotom 1.5 T) include (approximations):

- T_1 sagittals with TR of 600 ms and TE of 20 ms
- T_2 sagittals with TR of 2000 ms and TE of 60 ms
- Gradient echo sagittals with flip angle of 60°
- T_1 axials with a TR of 1000 ms and TE of 20 ms

Slices are 4 mm thick with a 2-mm gap between slices. No angling of the gantry is used so that no part of the spinal canal is left unexamined (Fig. 11.18).

Patient precautions in preparation for MRI

The primary patient problem in MRI is the claustrophobia experienced by about 3% of the patients in the MRI tunnel or gantry that covers the patient head to toe (Haughton 1988). The best approach to this phenomenon is to give the patient limited information about MRI and then ask if they have had any claustrophobic experiences in the past. Giving too much information about the machine will frighten some patients. Most adult patients who will experience serious claustrophobia precluding an MRI examination have had other claustrophobic experiences in the past and will say so. Those patients can be sedated, some needing considerable doses of intravenous relaxant and pain medication. The MRI scan is such an important investigative tool that it is worth the extra effort on the part of the technologists, the clinician, the radiologists and the patient to accept that claustrophobia will be a problem, and use whatever sedative routine is necessary to accomplish the investigation.

The second most common patient complaint about the scanner is the noise created during the examination. Simply warning the patient about this beforehand will control this problem.

There are certain patients who cannot have an MR scan because of the power of the magnet. These include patients with pacemakers, middle

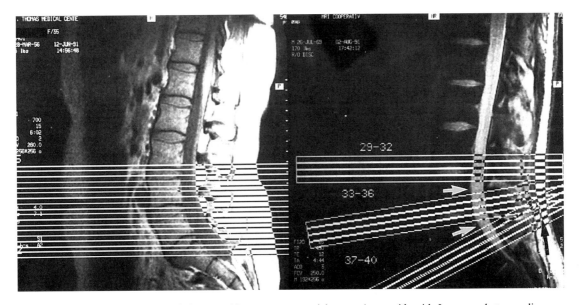

Fig. 11.18 (Left) The recommended protocol in our centre: straight cuts, 4 mm wide with 2 mm gap between slices. (Right) Angled cuts cause two problems: areas of the spinal canal behind the vertebral bodies are not demonstrated (arrows); and the overlap (dark arrow) causes cross-resonance and decreases image resolution.

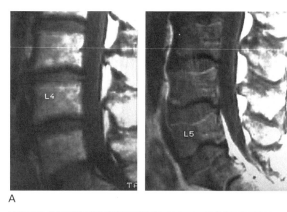

A

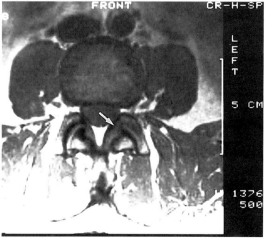

C

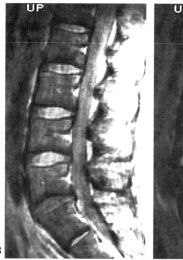
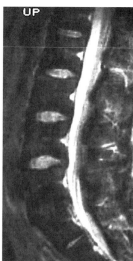

B

Fig. 11.19(A)   A normal sagittal T_1 weighted (T_1 SE). Note the short dural sac on the left that, on myelography, would not show an L5/S1 disc. (B) A normal sagittal T_2 weighted (T_2 SE) (right); a normal sagittal gradient echo (left). (C) A normal axial T_1 weighted (T_1 SE). The arrow points to the ligamentum flavum.

ear prostheses, some heart valves and any patient who may have inadvertently received a metal sliver in the eye. Some old aneurysm clips cannot be placed in the scanner (newer clips are not ferromagnetic).

As a precaution, patients are asked not to bring into the scanner room such items as analogue watches, hairpins, credit cards, keys or any object that might be snatched up by the magnet. Fortunately most orthopaedic implants are non-ferromagnetic or are so well fixed that it is not dangerous for the patient to be scanned. Obviously if the metal is centred in the area of the study it will produce a poor quality image.

Weight restrictions

There is a patient weight restriction of approximately 135 kg. This has as much to do with the size of the gantry (tunnel) as with the ability of the table to carry a heavy patient. Taller patients a little heavier than 135 kg may fit into the tunnel and shorter patients weighing less than that amount may not fit into the tunnel.

Normal MR anatomy

Figure 11.19 shows normal sagittal T_1-weighted, sagittal T_2-weighted, gradient echo and axial T_1-weighted images of a normal lumbar spine.

Lumbar pathology

Degenerative disc disease

Degenerative discs. Evident on T_1- and T_2-weighted images (Fig. 11.20) will be disc degeneration, disc space narrowing, osteophytes and Knuttson's phenomenon (Jenkins et al 1985, Murphy et al 1991, Panagiotacopulos et al 1987). Note that on T_1 images (Fig. 11.20) the disc/CSF interface is less distinct because both have low signal intensity. Gradient echo images

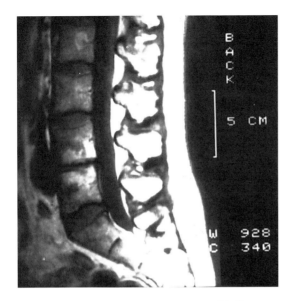

Fig. 11.20   Degenerative disc disease L4–5 with disc space narrowing and adjacent fatty infiltration of vertebral bodies.

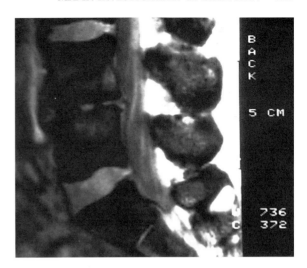

Fig. 11.21   Gradient echo in the same patient; note the difference in the disc/CSF interface between T_1 and GE images.

(Fig. 11.21) give a more distinctive image of this interface (Modic et al 1984, 1986).

Sagittal slicing laterally depicts the foramina clearly so that pathology lateral to the pedicle can be detected (Fig. 11.22).

Modic and colleagues (1984) have classified end-plate changes into three distinct types (Fig. 11.23):

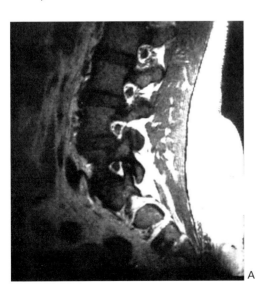

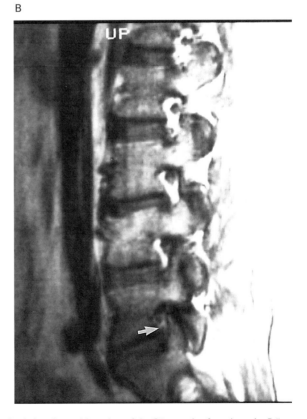

Fig. 11.22(A) T_1 sagittals showing normal foramina. (B) T_1 sagittal showing subluxation of the S1 superior facet into the L5 foramen (arrow).

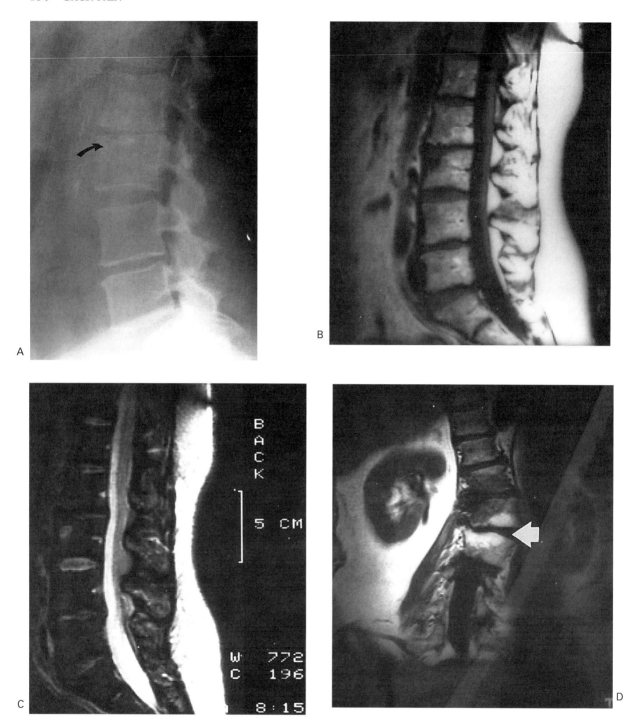

Fig. 11.23(A)   Modic type 1 degenerative disc disease — plain X-ray. (B) On T_1 image the area is dark. (C) On T_2-weighted image it is white. (D) Modic type 2 degenerative disc disease (arrow); note the type 1 changes at the disc space above. (See text for description.)

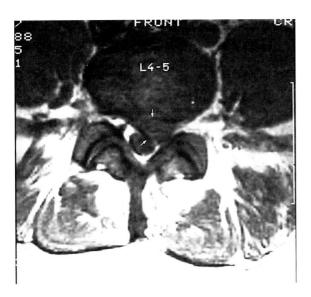

Fig. 11.24 T_1-weighted axial image of herniated nucleus pulposus with the annulus torn. Arrows are at each edge of torn annulus.

1. Type I — fibrovascular changes in the end-plate decrease the signal on T_1-weighted images and increase signal intensity on T_2-weighted images. Similar changes may occur in osteomyelitis but the lack of involvement in the intervertebral discs on T_2-weighted images rules out infection.
2. Type II — when yellow marrow replaces type I changes the signal intensity increases on T_1-weighted images and an iso-intense signal occurs on T_2-weighted images.
3. Type III — end-plate sclerosis results in a decreased signal on both T_1- and T_2-weighted images.

Disc herniations. The soft tissue definition of MRI is so good that it is often possible to see the rent in the annulus (Fig. 11.24) signifying an extruded or sequestered disc. Axillary and foraminal discs, impossible to detect on radiculography, are readily seen on MRI (Fig. 11.25). Disc pathology must not be confused with arachnoid cysts (Fig. 11.26), synovial cysts (Fig. 11.27) and conjoined nerve roots (Fig. 11.28).

Canal stenosis. Spinal canal and subarticular stenosis and the number of segments involved are readily seen on MRI (Fig. 11.29). The distinction between congenital or global stenosis (Fig. 11.30) and acquired or intra-segmental stenosis

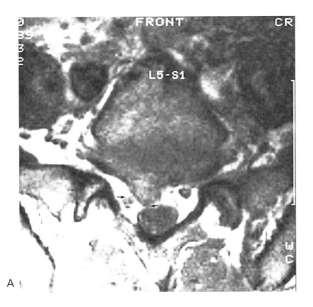

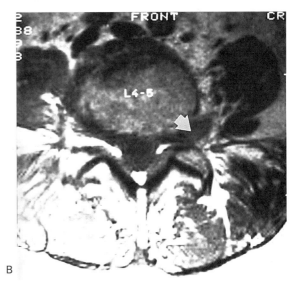

Fig. 11.25(A) T_1-weighted axial image of axillary disc herniation L5/S1 right. The disc fragment is medial to the nerve root and its posterior extension is beyond the posterior border of the nerve root (arrows). **(B)** T_1-weighted axial of foraminal herniated nucleus pulposus L4–5 left (arrow).

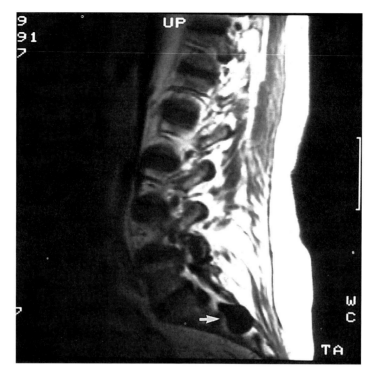

Fig. 11.26 T_1-weighted sagittal of arachnoid or Tarlov cyst (arrow). Note that it is of the same signal intensity as CSF.

(Fig. 11.29) is also readily apparent. The next development in MRI assessment of spinal stenosis will be flow studies using fast imaging techniques to show alteration in CSF flow.

Miscellaneous defects. Figure 11.31 shows spondylolysis and spondylolisthesis. There is no better way to assess the postoperative lumbar spine in a patient with recurrent or persistent symptoms than with gadolinium-enhanced MRI (Fig. 11.15). Ross and colleagues (1987) have shown various stages of arachnoiditis on MRI (Fig. 11.32).

Trauma

Although plain film radiography and CT continue to be the corner-stones in radiological assessment of spinal trauma, valuable information can be obtained from MRI in these patients (Fig. 11.33). All too often in the older age group the distinction between tumour and osteoporotic compression fractures can only be made with MRI (Fig. 11.34).

Neoplasia

The soft tissue sensitivity of MRI makes it the superior modality for assessing all forms of spinal neoplasia. The extent of bone marrow replacement and both the number of vertebral bodies involved and the tumour replacement of each body are readily apparent (Fig. 11.35). The interface between the skeletal and neurological tissue is readily assessed on MRI (Fig. 11.36).

Primary tumours of the lumbar spinal canal are best assessed with MRI. The once-in-a-lifetime case of a puzzling sciatica that turns out to be a conus tumour (Fig. 11.37) is convincing evidence of the value of the routine sagittal images that always demonstrate the conus.

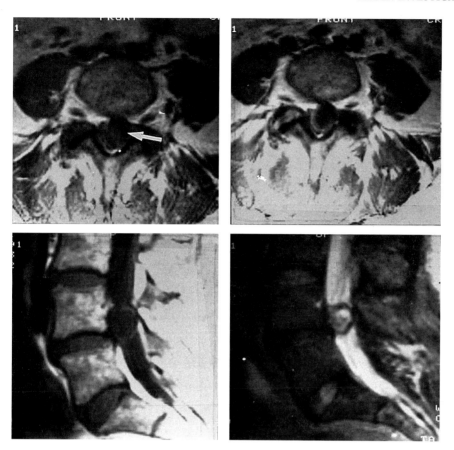

Fig. 11.27 Synovial cyst. (Top left) Axial T_1 cyst (arrow) is isointense to CSF. (Top right) Post-gadolinium, cyst has halo around it and almost obliterates the thecal sac. (Bottom left) A hyperintense rim is noted on T_1 sagittal after gadolinium injection. (Bottom right) The sagittal with hypointense rim thought to be calcification or haemorrhage and hyperintense cyst (T_2 spin echo).

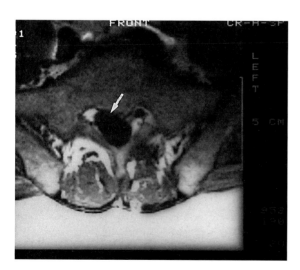

Fig. 11.28 Conjoined nerve roots. T_1 axial showing conjoined nerve roots that are isointense with dural sac, attached to dural sac, and surrounded by enlarged spinal canal (arrow).

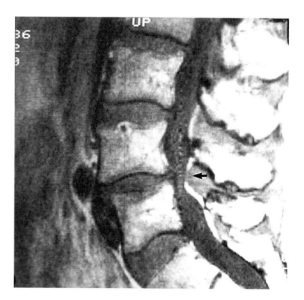

Fig. 11.29 Sagittal T_1 of acquired spinal stenosis with degenerative spondylolisthesis. Note that ligamentum flavum infolding is significant part of lesion (arrow).

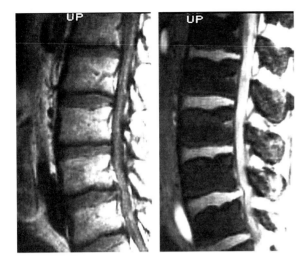

Fig. 11.30 Congenital (global) stenosis on T_1 and gradient echo sagittals — the entire canal (not a segment as in Fig. 11.29) is narrowed.

Fig. 11.31 Lytic spondylolisthesis. (Top left) The lytic defect on CT. (Top right) Equivalent MRI T_1 axial showing lytic defect (arrow). This is not as clear as on CT — a weakness of MRI in revealing bony detail. (Bottom left) Sagittal T_1 MRI showing lytic defect (arrow). (Bottom right) A normal facet joint for comparison to lytic defect characteristics above.

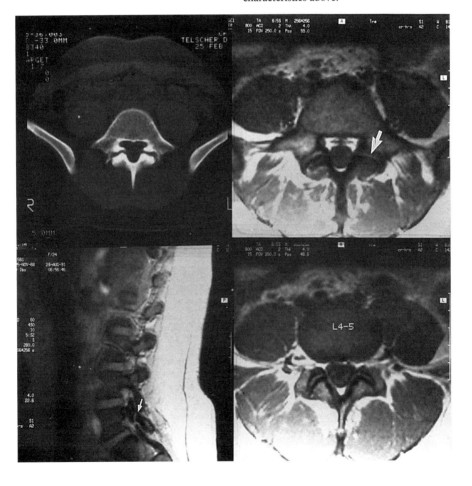

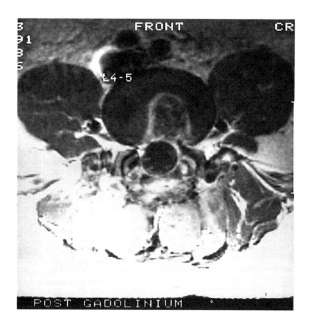

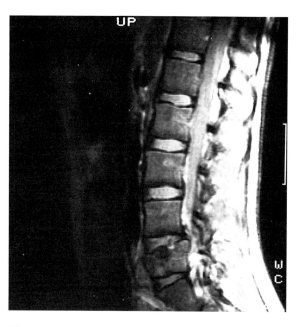

Fig. 11.32   Arachnoiditis: T_1 axial with gadolinium enhancement shows nerve roots clumping around edge of dura. Intradiscally is a poor attempt at an interbody fusion.

Fig. 11.33   A gradient echo sagittal slice of a burst fracture L5 showing fragment in canal.

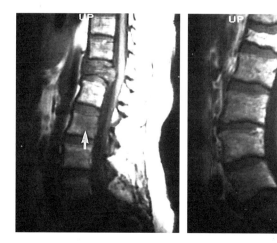

Fig. 11.34   Malignant vs benign compression fracture. (Left) T_1 sagittal of compression fracture secondary to metastatic deposit. Marrow of compressed vertebra has low signal intensity from tumour replacement. A second metastatic deposit is present in uncompressed vertebra (arrow). (Right) Compression fracture in osteoporotic bone. The bone has higher signal intensity from fatty (non-tumour) replacement of marrow.

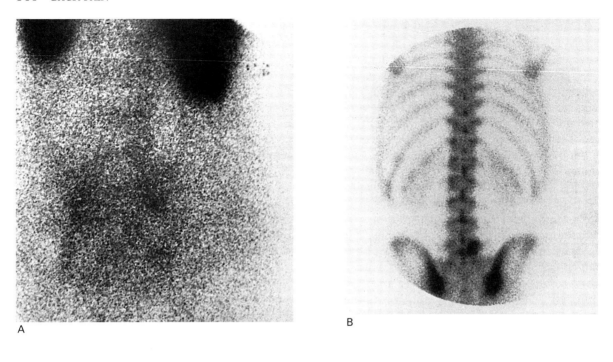

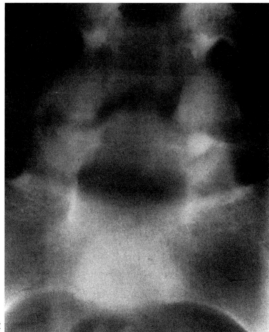

Fig. 12.4 Osteoid osteoma of the right pedicle of L5: (**A**) blood pool (**B**) bone scan (**C**) X-ray tomogram.

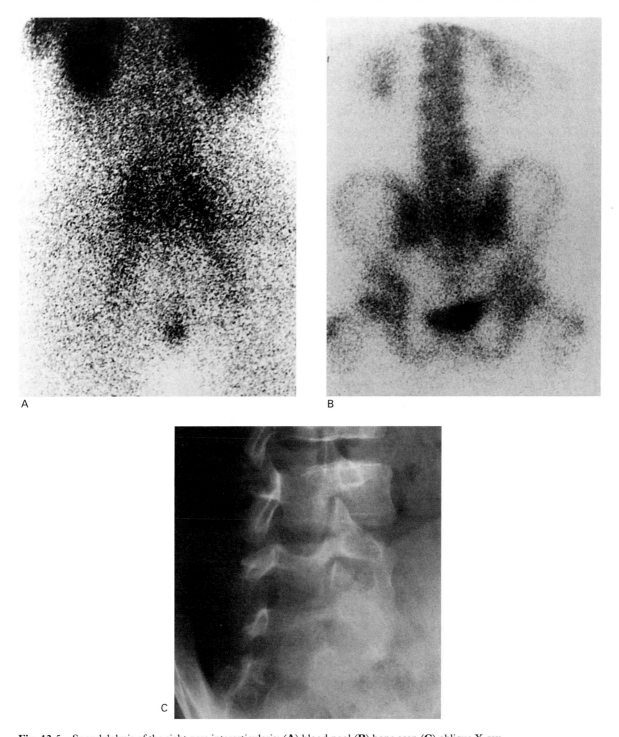

Fig. 12.5 Spondylolysis of the right pars interarticularis: (**A**) blood pool (**B**) bone scan (**C**) oblique X-ray.

Metastatic malignant disease

Perhaps the most common indication for bone scanning is the investigation of bone metastases in patients with a known or suspected primary carcinoma. It is often possible to demonstrate the presence and extent of such lesions. It has been well recognized for over 20 years that radionuclide bone scans can demonstrate bone metastases long before they are visible on X-ray. Osteoblastic metastases show as areas of high uptake in bone (Fig. 12.6) and, whilst their appearances are usually non-specific for the nature of the primary tumour, it is often possible to be specific about secondaries from prostatic carcinoma. The uptake in bone metastases from prostatic carcinoma is very dense, often with a uniform uptake in each vertebral body (Fig. 12.7). The appearance may vary from three or four discrete deposits of high uptake to uniform involvement of the entire skeleton, the so-called superscan. It may be difficult to differentiate prostatic metastases from Paget's disease when only the vertebral bodies are involved, since both conditions show exceptionally high uptake of ^{99m}Tc-MDP. When other bones such as the pelvic bones, skull or long bones are

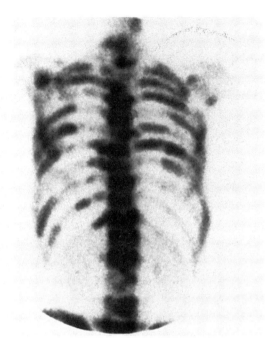

Fig. 12.7 Widespread metastatic disease from prostatic carcinoma.

also affected by Paget's disease the differentiation from metastases is easier (Fig.12.8), though the two conditions may coexist. The bone scan will demonstrate osteoblastic metastases earlier than X-rays, and also give a more accurate description of their number, size and activity.

One or two areas of increased uptake, even in patients with known primary malignancy, may be caused by pathology other than metastatic disease. X-rays of these areas should be carefully examined to exclude fracture, active degenerative change or Paget's disease.

The false-negative rate of bone scans in detecting bone metastases is small, mainly in patients with highly anaplastic carcinoma, or in those with slow-growing tumours with relatively little osteoblastic reaction. Osteolytic metastases are not usually discernable until they are more than 2–3 cm in diameter, when they show areas of absent uptake of ^{99m}Tc-MDP (Fig. 12.9). Bone scanning is therefore not recommended in the search for osteolytic carcinoma metastases or multiple myeloma because small deposits may not be demonstrated. Even with widespread multiple myeloma the bone scan may appear entirely normal.

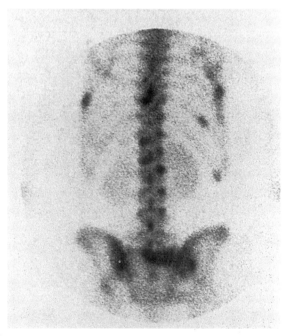

Fig. 12.6 Multiple small metastases from a primary breast carcinoma.

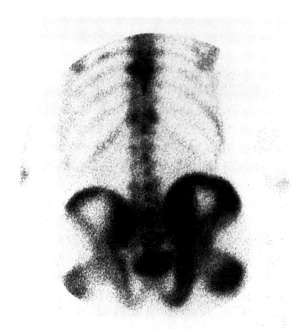

Fig. 12.8 Paget's disease of D9, D12, the right hemipelvis and right femur.

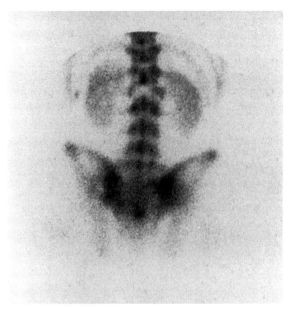

Fig. 12.9 Large osteolytic metastasis in the body of L1 showing absent uptake.

Trauma

Compression fractures

Fractures of the vertebral bodies give positive images on bone scans which usually appear as linear areas of increased uptake (Fig. 12.10). The concentration of the tracer increases for 6 months at the sites of recent fractures, but then slowly decreases as healing progresses. Thus, recent fractures less than 6 months old show a more intense uptake than older ones. The bone scan is a valuable method for determining the age of vertebral compression fractures in osteoporotic patients, but it cannot distinguish between benign and malignant causes of vertebral body compression.

Spondylolysis

A bone scan can clearly demonstrate stress fractures as areas of increased bone activity. Recent and healing fractures are well demonstrated at 4 h but do not show on the blood pool image, whereas osteoid osteomas, haemangiomas and infection show on both. A negative scan does not

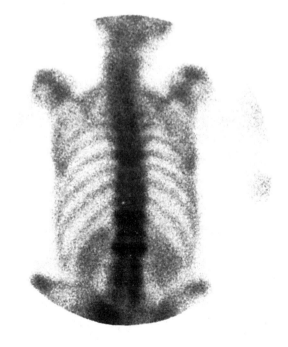

Fig. 12.10 Recent compression fractures of D8, D12 and L2 showing as linear areas of high uptake.

exclude an established spondylolisthesis, but it excludes stress fracture. A positive scan suggests potential for healing. It is particularly valuable in the early lesion of spondylolysis. The patient should be treated as having a stress fracture in order to prevent an established spondylolisthesis and possible long-term disability.

Infection

Osteomyelitis of the spine can be demonstrated by bone scanning. It shows both increased uptake in the blood pool images as a result of increased blood flow to the infected bone, and also intense uptake in the later images (Fig. 12.11). When both blood pool and late views are made the diagnosis is usually not in doubt. If, however, only late images are made then it is necessary to correlate the clinical history and X-rays with the bone scan to differentiate infection from other pathology. Osteomyelitis can be distinguished from cellulitis by using both blood pool and late images. Osteomyelitis generally shows increased

vascularity and increased bone activity appearing in both phases of examination, whilst cellulitis shows increased vascularity adjacent to bone in the blood pool phase, and little or no increase in bone uptake in the late images.

Occasionally acute osteomyelitis does not show as an area of high uptake but as a 'cold' area. This paradoxical appearance is not understood, but may be due to thrombosis of medullary vessels and relative ischaemia. This finding is seen only in the first few days of the disease. It is commoner in young children and is unusual in the spine, probably because the diagnosis of vertebral osteomyelitis is sometimes delayed.

Arthritic and degenerative conditions

Osteoarthritis

Because bone scanning can demonstrate increased vascularity and increased bone activity, it has a place in the investigation of degenerative joint disease. It can define the extent of active disease,

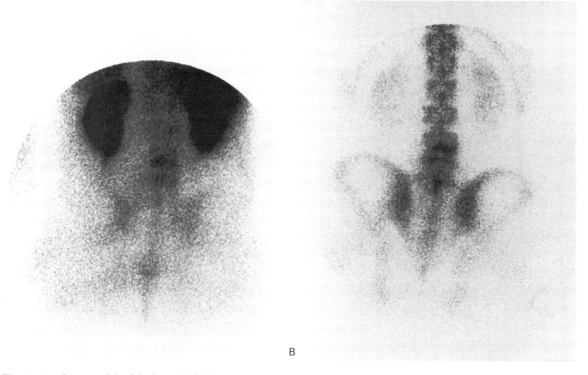

A   B

Fig. 12.11   Osteomyelitis of the lower half of L4 and upper part of L5 following laminectomy. (**A**) blood pool (**B**) bone scan.

and distinguish between acute active and chronic degenerative changes. Chronic osteoarthritis appears as an ill-defined loss of definition of the joint space. Active disease shows an ill-defined boundary but also a diffuse increase in activity (Fig. 12.12). This is less intense than is seen in healing fractures, malignancy or infection. Bone scanning can document the early presence of arthritis and assess serial changes in the disease, but it has not been tested in facet joint arthritis.

Ankylosing spondylitis

In the active phases of the disease certain characteristic features may be seen on a bone scan. There is often an increase in uptake in the costovertebral joints of the dorsal spine giving the so-called 'pine tree' appearance (Fig. 12.13). This is not usually seen during remission. There may also be a significant increase in uptake in the sacroiliac joints. Attempts to assess the severity of disease by quantifying this increased uptake have not shown practical value.

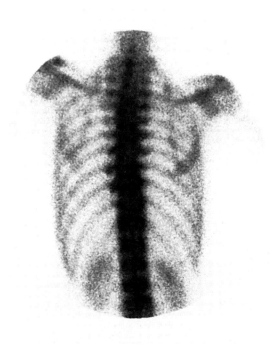

Fig. 12.13   Ankylosing spondylitis. Posterior view of the dorsal and lumbar spine showing increased uptake in all the vertebrae with loss of joint spaces at the costovertebral joints of the upper dorsal spine.

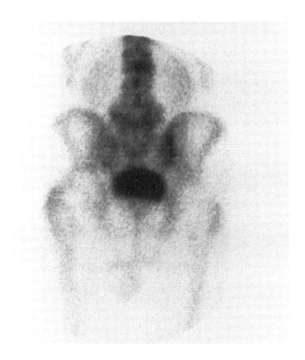

Fig. 12.12   Osteoarthritis of the lower lumbar spine.

Sacroiliitis

Sacroiliitis is better diagnosed by bone scan than X-ray, since radiographs are seldom positive at an early stage in this disease. Both blood pool and later images are positive (Fig. 12.14), but it may be difficult to differentiate an infective from an inflammatory condition. In osteitis condensans ilii the bone scan will not be positive, which will help to differentiate it from sacroiliitis.

Scheuermann's disease

Patients with Scheuermann's disease do not show bone scan abnormality at any stage of the disease. An abnormal bone scan would suggest some other disease process.

Metabolic bone disease

The precise role for bone scanning in metabolic bone disease has not been defined. However,

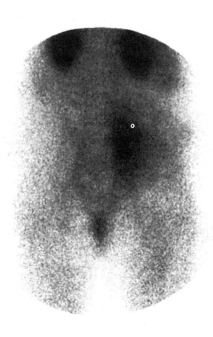

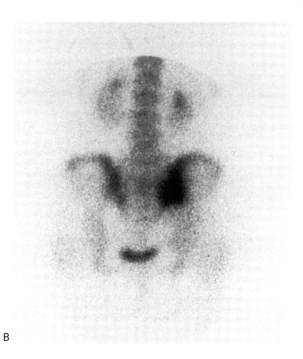

A

B

Fig. 12.14 Unilateral infected sacroiliitis, posterior view: (**A**) blood pool (**B**) bone scan.

there are certain characteristic features which, if seen during the scanning of patients with un-explained back pain, might suggest metabolic bone disorder. Primary and secondary hyper-parathyroidism may both produce increased osteoblastic activity. It may be demonstrated as a generally high uptake throughout the entire skeleton, with increased bone to soft tissue con-trast. Alternatively there may be increased uptake in the end-plates of the vertebrae mimicking the radiographic 'rugger jersey' appearance. These changes should lead to an examination of the chest and skull. The later is likely to show increased calvarial uptake and the sternum to show a higher uptake than the ribs, the so-called 'tie' sign. There will also be an absence of the normal renal activity. Brown tumours do not accumulate ^{99m}Tc-MDP.

No significant abnormality in bone uptake is seen in patients with primary osteoporosis because the bone scan is not sensitive enough to show any general decrease in uptake. However, focal ab-normalities may be seen in these patients as a result of everyday minor trauma and microfractures.

In osteomalacia there is a rapid uptake of tracer after injection and a high bone to soft

tissue ratio. Fractures and pseudofractures show as small areas of intense activity and must be differentiated from metastatic disease. This is not difficult because in osteomalacia the rib lesions tend to involve a number of adjacent ribs in line.

Other bone disorders

The bone scan is sensitive but non-specific in detecting osteoblast activity. Positive bone scans will be found in fibrous dysplasia (Fig. 12.15), non-ossifying fibroma, osteochondroma, benign osteoblastoma, lymphoma, haemangioma, sar-coma, eosinophilic granuloma, the healing phase of avascular necrosis and fractures in patients with os-teogenesis imperfecta or the child abuse syndrome.

No increase in uptake will be seen in bone islands. Focal areas of decreased or absent uptake can be seen if they are relatively large. They may be present in metastatic malignancy, early post-traumatic aseptic necrosis, bone infarct, sickle cell crisis (Fig. 12.16), myeloma and eosinophilic granuloma, leukaemia and following radiotherapy.

Bone scanning with ^{99m}Tc-labelled phosphates thus provides a sensitive, non-invasive method for

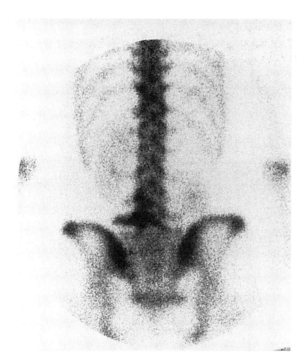

Fig. 12.15 Fibrous dysplasia involving and enlarging the left transverse process of L5 and to a lesser extent L4.

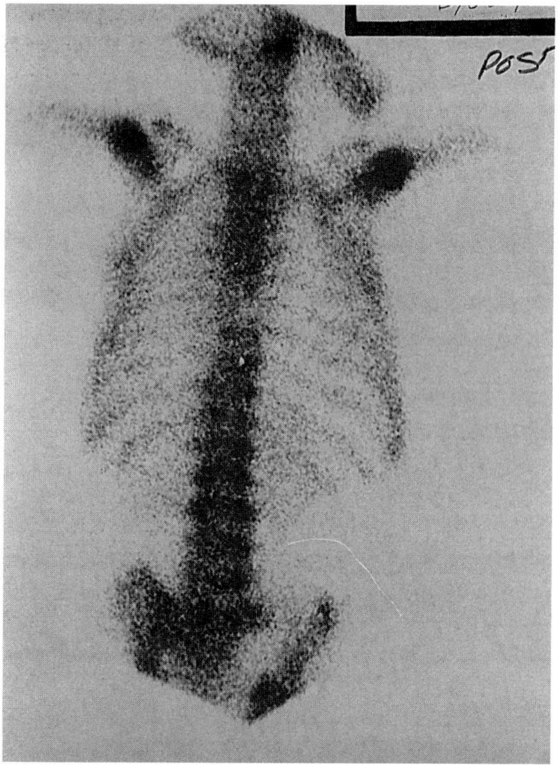

Fig. 12.16 Infarction of D7–9 and the right sacroiliac region due to sickle cell anaemia in a 4-year-old child.

the detection of a wide variety of diseases affecting the spine. These include traumatic, inflammatory, neoplastic, metabolic and degenerative causes. The bone scan will show osteoblastic changes long before X-rays will show any increase in calcium content, and will detect many diseases weeks or months before any changes are evident radiologically. The relatively poor resolution of the bone scan adds to its poor specificity and X-rays are essential for accurate diagnosis. Bone scan complements X-rays, and is a diagnostic procedure which should be considered in patients with back pain.

REFERENCES

Borak J 1942 Relationship between the clinical and roentgenological findings in bone metastases. Surgery, Gynaecology and Obstetrics 75: 599–606

Gilday D L, Ash J M 1976 Benign bone tumours. Seminars in Nuclear Medicine 6: 33–46

Simon G 1973 In: Principles of bone X-ray diagnosis. Butterworths, London

Smith F W 1989 In: Sharp P F, Gemmell H G, Smith F W (eds) Practical nuclear medicine. IRL Press, Oxford. p 245–264

Smith F W, Gilday D L 1980 Scintigraphic appearances of osteoid osteoma. Radiology 137: 191–195

Subramanian G, McAfee J G, Blair R J, Kallfetz F A, Thomas F D 1975 Technetium -99m-methylene diphosphonate — a superior agent of skeletal imaging: comparison with other complexes. Journal of Nuclear Medicine 16: 744–755

Vieras F, Boyd C M 1975 Diagnostic value of renal imaging incidental to bone scintigraphy with ^{99m}Tc-phosphate compounds. Journal of Nuclear Medicine 16: 1109–1114

Winter P F, Johnson P M, Hilal S K, Feldman F 1977 Scintigraphic detection of osteoid osteoma. Radiology 122: 177–178

13. Ultrasound in spinal investigation

Meire (1978) and Suarez and colleagues (1975) used ultrasound to display echoes from the lumbar vertebral canal, scanning through the abdomen. In the same year, Campbell and associates (1975) were able to demonstrate fetal spina bifida with ultrasound. A method of measuring the oblique sagittal diameter of the vertebral canal from the posterior aspect was introduced in 1978 (Porter et al 1978) and we have now examined many thousands of patients and volunteer subjects. The technique does produce an impressive two-dimensional display of echoes — the B-scan (Fig. 13.1) demonstrating vertebral body and lamina echoes.

The distance between the reflecting surfaces of these echoes can be measured from the B-scan with electronic callipers (Asztely 1983) or more precisely from an A-scan display at any one particular level (Fig. 13.2). There has been much debate about the accuracy, repeatability and relevance of the measurements.

ACCURACY

It has been suggested that it is not technically possible to use ultrasound to measure to an accuracy of less than half a wavelength. Using a

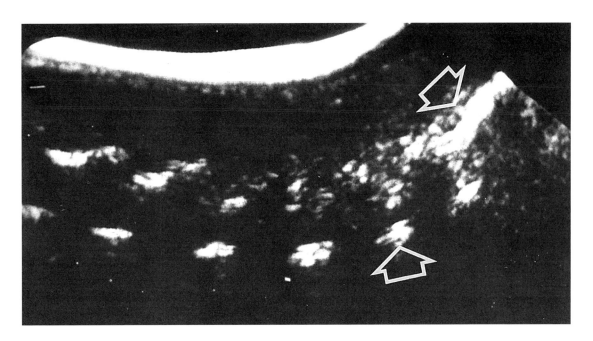

Fig. 13.1 B-scan display of a lumbar spine showing the vertebral body and lamina echoes, and the 'silent' vertebral canal. Arrows indicate echoes from the fifth lumbar vertebral body and echoes from the sacral laminae.

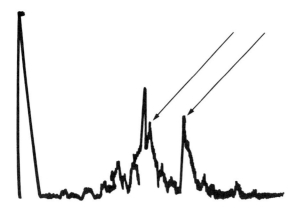

Fig. 13.2 A-scan display indicates the echoes believed to be reflected from the boundaries of the vertebral canal, the first arrow from the cranial lip of the lamina, and the second from the posterior surface of the vertebral body.

1.5 Mhz transducer, half a wavelength is 0.5 mm, and this is the range resolution. It is not possible to differentiate two surfaces closer together than this. The accuracy of the technique is therefore said to be questionable when measuring to a decimal place of a millimetre. The limitations of range resolution, however, do not mean that the measurement between two widely separated surfaces is also limited by the range resolution. In practice, the accuracy of the diasonograph using a 1.5 Mhz transducer allows for detection of 0.05 mm movement of a reflecting surface fixed to a micrometer screw gauge. This was confirmed by Hammond (1984) who was able to measure movement of an interface with an accuracy of 0.05 mm. Such precision is highly acceptable for spinal measurement.

Table 13.1 Inter-observer error of ultrasound measurement between a trainee and an experienced ultrasonographer during the 2nd and 3rd weeks, and during the 4th and 5th weeks of training.

| Level | Mean (cm) SD | |
	2nd and 3rd week (n = 34)	4th and 5th week (n = 36)
L1	0.042 (0.037)	0.038 (0.037)
L2	0.041 (0.032)	0.043 (0.044)
L3	0.052 (0.042)	0.045 (0.041)
L4	0.048 (0.040)	0.050 (0.040)
L5	0.066 (0.054)	0.047 (0.043)

REPEATABILITY

Some have criticized the method on the grounds of poor repeatability (Stockdale & Finlay 1980, Finlay et al 1981), though with care and time we have been able to obtain a mean repeatability of 0.5 mm (Hibbert et al 1981, Table 13.1). Others have found less acceptable mean repeatability of up to 1.29 mm (Legg & Gibbs 1984, Hammond 1984). A discrepancy of 0.5 mm is not inconsiderable when we are interested in a vertebral canal range from 11 to 18 mm. The repeatability is probably adequate for epidemiological studies (Battié et al 1986).

ANATOMICAL RELEVANCE

We confess we are unsure about the exact origin of the echoes. Our first and present impression is that they are from the cranial aspect of the posterior surface of the vertebral bodies and from the posterior margin of the canal at the cranial lip of the lamina (Fig. 13.3). Much of the sound must enter the canal through the ligamentum flavum. We are not convinced that we can identify echoes

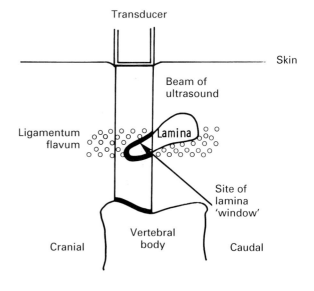

Fig. 13.3 Diagram to show the site of the ultrasound beam in the 15° oblique sagittal plane and the probable origin of the echoes.

from soft tissues. On the other hand Asztely (1983) and Kadziolka and colleagues (1981) conclude from cadaveric work that the echoes they measure originate from the boundaries between the dural sac and surrounding tissues at the level of the intervertebral disc. This may indeed be the echo from the posterior boundary, where the dura and the cranial lip of the lamina are closely opposed, but if the dura were the echo from the anterior boundary, we would have expected to recognize gross reduction of measurements with a large disc herniation. It would indeed be helpful to identify the site of the disc indenting the dura, but this is not our experience. Hammond (1984) concluded that the echoes arise from both bony and soft tissues of the spine, and that the operator can accentuate or diminish the echoes by altering the scanning plane or signal processing. Kamei and co-workers (1990), using a 3.5 Mhz transducer, found ultrasound of value in diagnosing disc protrusion and identifying its level. The ultrasound beam is an area of sound varying with the focus of the transducer and must inevitably average to a point measurement. This adds a further question as to which point is actually being measured.

CLINICAL RELEVANCE

There is no debate about the clinical relevance of the shallow vertebral canal. Following the early papers of Sarpyener (1945), Verbiest (1954) and Van Gelderen (1958), others have confirmed that a variety of back pain syndromes are related to spinal pathology in the presence of an already small canal. What is at issue is whether ultrasound is sufficiently accurate and repeatable to be useful clinically. Howie and colleagues (1983) discard the technique because the preoperative measurements bear no relationship to the observed level of pathological problem found at surgery. If indeed bony parameters are being measured, it is unlikely that ultrasound will show the clinical level of significant pathology, which is more often a combination of bone and soft tissue encroachment. They noted, but failed to comment upon, the fact that half their operated patients had vertebral canals in the bottom 10% of their 'normal values' from healthy volunteers.

Forsberg and Wallöe (1982) reported that B-scan measurements for their patients who had made a poor recovery from disc surgery were narrower than for those who had recovered uneventfully. We have found ultrasound measurements to be meaningful in certain clinical situations, and the results of population studies to be valuable epidemiologically. The uncertainties of ultrasound, however, have meant that the criticisms have been largely accepted and it is not a diagnostic aid that has yet received general acceptance.

APPLICATION

For patient management

The attraction of ultrasound as a diagnostic tool lies in its simplicity and safety for the patient (Figs 13.4 and 13.5). We have routinely scanned every patient with back pain and, recognizing the margin of error in the results, we are usually able to comment on the significance of space in the vertebral canal when talking to the patient at the end of the consultation. It is possible to explain to the patient with recurrent episodes of back pain, who frequently finds himself listing to one side and yet has never had sciatic pain, that though he may have a disc producing back pain,

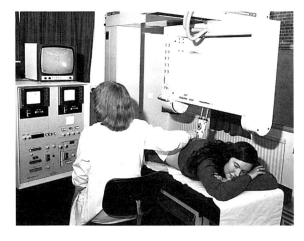

Fig. 13.4 Photograph of the diasonograph providing both B-scan and A-scan echoes. The gantry is fixed at 15° to the sagittal plane.

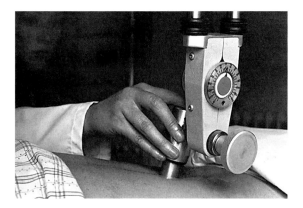

Fig. 13.5 The transducer is moved along the lumbar spine, a few cm lateral to the spinous processes.

he is fortunate to have an adequate vertebral canal protecting the nerve root. For the next young patient with leg pain and poor straight leg raising, the narrow canal is discussed as a persisting vulnerability, with need for a great deal of respect.

A narrow canal with an unstable segment makes discussion about dural pain sensible. So many patients with rising expectations about health want to know as much as possible about the source of pain, and ultrasound does give that opportunity to answer some of their questions in a logical manner.

Neurogenic claudication

There are many factors responsible for the symptoms of neurogenic claudication in addition to the shallow vertebral canal, including soft tissue encroachment, segmental movement and vascular insufficiency. The small canal, however, is an essential factor (Fig. 13.6). If the possibility of surgery is contemplated, myelography or a CT scan is essential, but there are some patients not sufficiently disabled for surgery, or with inappropriate signs, where one would withhold invasive investigations. An ultrasound scan in the upper percentiles would suggest a diagnosis other than neurogenic claudication (Figs 13.7 and 13.8). Tervonen and Koivukangas (1989) have used transabdominal ultrasound and found it well suited for diagnosing central spinal stenosis.

Pulsations from the cerebrospinal fluid or dura can be identified by Doppler ultrasound at each interlamina level in healthy patients (Hammond 1984). Changes in these pulsations in relation to posture and exercise may prove to have diagnostic value in neurogenic claudication, where one of the vexing problems is to determine at which of several levels is the pathological process responsible for the symptoms. Unnecessarily extensive surgical decompression may then be avoided.

A

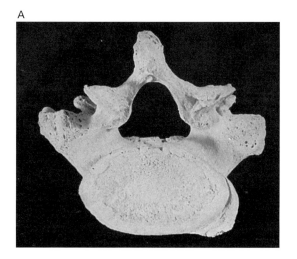

B

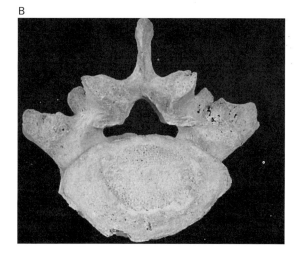

Fig. 13.6 Examples of fifth lumbar vertebrae: (**A**) with a large dome-shaped vertebral canal, and (**B**) with a shallow trefoil-shaped canal. The latter is compatible with neurogenic claudication if there is multiple-level pathology.

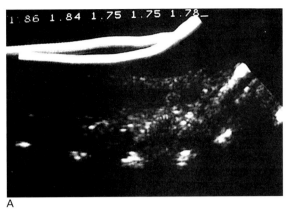

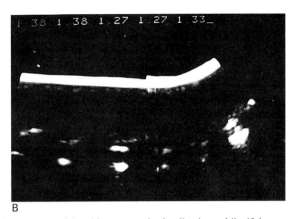

A   B

Fig. 13.7   Examples of ultrasound B-scans. The wide canal (**A**) is not compatible with neurogenic claudication, whilst if the patient (**B**) has claudication symptoms, MRI or CT and myelography are indicated.

Isthmic spondylolisthesis

Forward displacement of the proximal vertebral body is usually obvious from the B-scan echoes (Fig. 13.9). The displacement may be more apparent on ultrasound than radiologically, perhaps because it is accentuated by the forward rotation of the body. The canal measurements are generally wider than in patients without a lysis, partly because the displaced lamina increases the sagittal diameter, and also because the canal in spondylolisthesis is usually dome-shaped and rarely trefoil.

Hammond (1984) attempted to identify the unstable spondylolysis by measuring the sagittal diameter of the canal by ultrasound before and

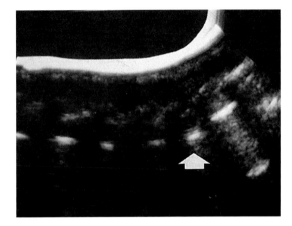

Fig. 13.9   B-scan display of a patient with isthmic spondylolisthesis, showing the forward displacement of the echo from the body of L5.

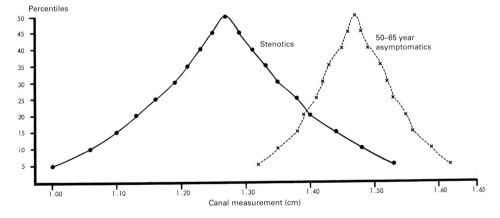

Fig. 13.8   Graph showing the quintile ultrasound measurements at L5 for a series of patients with neurogenic claudication, compared with quintiles for 124 subjects without back pain (50–65 years of age).

after torsion or flexion of the lumbar spine, but his results were equivocal.

Ultrasound has its limitations, even if one accepts a fair degree of accuracy, repeatability and anatomical relevance. It has not been shown to help in the prediction of outcome of an episode of back pain, in the likelihood of a recurrence within 12 months (Drinkall et al 1984), nor will it make the diagnosis of the level of significant pathology. It does make us think about space in the vertebral canal, however, and if we understand its limitations it can be a useful tool.

Intraoperative ultrasonography

Ultrasound has been used intraoperatively to investigate extradural cord or root impingement and intradural and intramedullary spinal cord pathology (Dohrmann & Rubin 1982, Knake et al 1983, Morse et al 1984, Quencer et al 1984, Eismont et al 1984). After laminar excision the wound is filled with Ringer's lactate solution and the spine examined with a real-time machine, the sterile probe being covered with sterile lubricant within a plastic cover.

Following spinal trauma the degree of anterior bony encroachment and stenosis can be identified. The technique helps to locate the hidden fragment of a sequestrated disc, and for the neurosurgeon, to demonstrate extramedullary masses and intra-medullary cavities; ultrasound permits the optimal access.

Endoscopic ultrasonography is a further extension of this principle, and with an ultra-sound transducer incorporated into the tip of a myeloscope it may soon be possible to examine the contents of the vertebral canal from within with improved accuracy.

Epidemiology

Epidemiologically our ultrasound results suggest that the depth of the vertebral canal is an important factor in most patients with back pain. In a general practice study (Drinkall et al 1984), we found that patients attending with back pain had significantly smaller measurements than a randomized group of matched controls without any previous attendance with back pain. Patients attending hospital with back pain, when compared with volunteers of similar age, tended to have narrower canals, 39% of clinic patients, 43% of those admitted and 46% of those having spinal surgery being below the 10th percentile of the volunteers.

An industrial study showed that 37% of the days lost from work by a group of coal miners over 50 years of age was by the 10% of men whose canals were the narrowest (MacDonald et al 1984) (Fig. 13.10). In the 3 years after measurement, the men who took early retirement had significantly narrower canals than those who stayed at work. It seems that the canal size as measured by ultrasound has some value in predicting those most vulnerable to back pain.

Population studies using ultrasound in three distinct back pain syndromes throw some light on their pathogenesis. Of our patients with symptomatic disc lesions, 41% had canal measurements below the 10th percentile for asymptomatic volunteers, suggesting that for many the canal size is an important factor in the pain mechanism. This is more significant in our older patients with neurogenic claudication, 57% of whom were below the 10th percentile. In root entrapment syndrome, where the lesion is more lateral in the root canal, only 30% had central canal measurements below the 10th percentile.

In back pain syndromes associated with vertebral displacement, the canal size as measured by ultrasound seems to have variable significance. It assumes greater importance when pain is associated with retrolisthesis or rotationary displacement (43% below the 10th percentile), some importance in degenerative spondylolisthesis, and less in isthmic spondylolisthesis.

Ultrasound measurements of the cervical vertebral canal are useful in population studies, where a non-invasive method is preferable to radiographs. We have measured many young volunteers and shown a good correlation between cervical and lumbar canals, especially at the lower cervical and lumbar levels. This may be one factor in the common association between symptomatic cervical and lumbar spondylosis (Edwards & La Rocca 1985).

Ultrasound gives us the opportunity to investigate the growing vertebral canal. Children

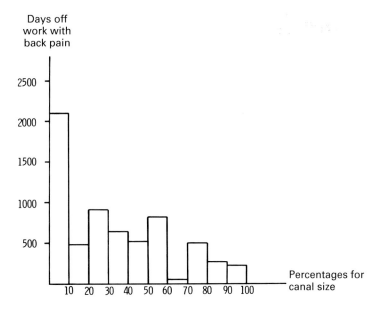

Fig. 13.10   Histogram of the days lost from work due to back pain by 191 miners over 50 years of age, according to canal size; 32% of days lost were by men with canals below the 10th percentile.

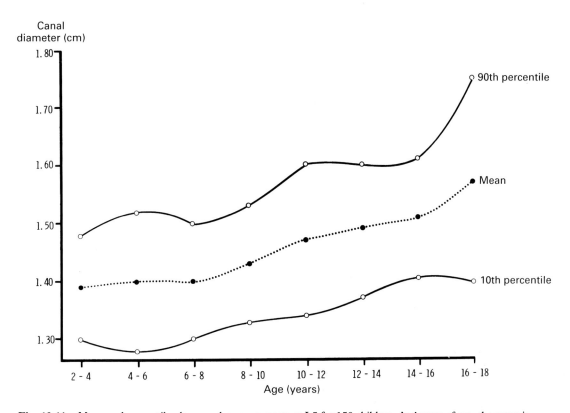

Fig. 13.11   Mean and percentile ultrasound measurements at L5 for 150 children. At 4 years of age, the mean is wider than the 10th percentile of the adult population.

are easier to measure than adults and Figure. 13.11 shows the mean and percentiles for 150 children. The relatively large sagittal diameter of the infant's canal indicates that its growth is accomplished early in development and this measurement may be a marker in later life of infantile malnutrition. The canal could prove to be an indicator of health status, and its measurement by non-invasive technique valuable (Clark et al 1985).

There is no question at all that space within the vertebral canal is of great clinical significance. An individual with a shallow canal, and especially a trefoil-shaped canal at L5, has a highly vulnerable back and is a subject at risk. The question still to be answered is whether this individual can reliably be identified by ultrasound.

REFERENCES

Asztely M 1983 Lumbar sonography: a comparative radiological study. Theses: Departments of Diagnostic Radiology and Orthopaedic Surgery, University of Goteborg, Sweden

Battié M C, Hanson T H, Engel J M, Zeh J, Bigos S, Spengler D M 1986 The reliability of measurements of the lumbar spine using ultrasound B-scan. Spine 11: 144–148

Campbell S, Pryse-Davies J, Coltart T M, Sellor M, Smith J D 1975 Ultrasound in the diagnosis of spina bifida. Lancet 2: 1336

Clark F A, Panjabi M M, Wetzel F T 1985 Can infant malnutrition cause adult vertebral stenosis? Spine 10: 165–170

Dohrmann G J, Rubin J M 1982 Intra-operative ultrasound imaging of the spinal cord; syringomyelia, cysts, and tumours — a preliminary report. Surgical Neurology 18: 395–399

Drinkall J N, Porter R W, Hibbert C S, Evans C 1984 The value of ultrasonic measurement of the spinal canal diameter in general practice. British Medical Journal 288: 121–122

Edwards W C, La Rocca S H 1985 The developmental segmental sagittal diameter in combined cervical and lumbar spondylosis. Spine 10: 42–49

Eismont F J, Green B A, Berkowitz B M, Montalvo B M, Quencer M, Brown M J 1984 The role of intra-operative ultrasonography in the treatment of thoracic and lumbar spine fractures. Spine 9: 782–787

Finlay D, Stockdale H R, Lewin E 1981 An appraisal of the use of diagnostic ultrasound to quantify the lumbar spinal canal. British Journal of Radiology 54: 870–874

Forsberg L, Walløe 1982 Ultrasound in sciatica. Acta Orthopedica Scandinavica 53: 393–395

Hammond B R 1984 The detection of spondylolysis using lumbar sonography. Thesis, University of Surrey

Hibbert C S, Delaygue C, McGlen B, Porter R W 1981 Measurement of the lumbar spinal canal by diagnostic ultrasound. British Journal of Radiology 54: 905–907

Howie D W, Chatterron B E, Hone M R 1983 Failure of ultrasound in the investigation of sciatica. Journal of Bone and Joint Surgery 65-B: 144–147

Kadziolka R, Asztely M, Hanai K, Hansson T, Nachemson A 1981 Ultrasonic measurement of the lumbar spinal canal. Journal of Bone and Joint Surgery 63-B: 504–507

Kamei K, Hanai K, Matsui N 1990 Ultrasonic level diagnosis on lumbar disc herniation. Spine 15: 1170–1174

Knake J E, Chandler W F, McGillicuddy J E 1983 Intra-operative ultrasonography of intra-spinal tumours: initial experience. American Journal of Neuroradiology 4: 1019–1021

Legg S J, Gibbs V 1984 Measurement of the lumbar spinal canal by echo ultrasound. Spine 9: 79–82

MacDonald E B, Porter R, Hibbert C, Hart J 1984 The relationship between spinal canal diameter and back pain in coal miners: ultrasonic measurement a screening test? Journal of Occupation Medicine 26: 23–28

Meire H B 1978 Diagnose des diskusprolaps — altraschallmetrode enkwickelt. Med Tribune 30 Oct 5

Morse B M M, Quencer R M, Green B A 1984 Intra-operative ultrasonography in spinal trauma. Radiology 153: 125–134

Porter R W, Wicks M, Ottewell D 1978 Measurement of the spinal canal by diagnostic ultrasound. Journal of Bone and Joint Surgery 60-B (4): 481–485

Quencer R M, Morse B M M, Green B A, Eismont F J 1984 Intra-operative spinal sonography of soft tissue masses of the spinal cord and spinal canal. American Journal of Neuroradiology 5: 507–515

Sarpyener M A 1945 Congenital stricture of the spinal canal. Journal of Bone and Joint Surgery 27: 70–79

Stockdale H R, Finlay D 1980 Use of diagnostic ultrasound to measure the lumbar spinal canal. British Journal of Radiology 53: 1101–1102

Suarez T R, Marich K W, Holzemer T F, Talnzer J, Green P S 1975 Biomedical imaging with SRI ultrasonic camera. Acoust. Holog 6: 1–13

Tervonen O, Koivukangas J 1989 Transabdominal ultrasound measurement of the lumbar spinal canal. Spine 14: 232–235

Van Gelderen V 1958 Ein orthotisches (lordotisches) kauda syndrom. Acta Pyschiatrica Neurologica Scandinavica 23: 57

Verbiest H 1954 A radicular syndrome from developmental narrowing of the lumbar vertebral canal. Journal of Bone and Joint Surgery 36-B: 230

14. Diagnostic pain provocation

With a contribution by J. Shepperd

Improved spinal imaging has revolutionized the investigation of back pain, but identifying pathology is not the same as identifying the source of pain. Asymptomatic disc herniation is common in the young adult, occult spinal stenosis frequent in the elderly, and spondylolisthesis is present in many an unsuspecting athlete. The clinician's dilemma when faced with these lesions is whether they are significant or whether such common pathology is coincidental. Diagnostic pain provocation techniques can help resolve the problem.

ROOT INFILTRATION

Local anaesthetic root block can be used to distinguish referred from root pain (Haueisen et al 1985), and nerve root infiltration can help to identify which root is affected (Macnab 1971, Akkerveeken 1989, Stanley et al 1990). Contrast is injected into the epiradicular space to ensure correct placement, and the patient is asked whether the sharp pain they experience is identical to the symptomatic pain, and then if it is abolished by local anaesthetic.

FACET JOINT INJECTIONS

Pain provocation with arthrography of the apophyseal joint might suggest this is a pain source. Injection of 0.5 ml of contrast is sufficient; 2 ml risks capsular rupture as a spurious cause of pain (Dory 1981). The obliquity of the joints can cause placement difficulty (Carrera et al 1980), and it probably helps to introduce the needle vertically (Destouet et al 1982). Because of placement difficulty and the spill-over effect of

anaesthetic, the diagnostic value of facet joint injections is still unresolved.

DISCOGRAPHY

Discography has been strongly supported as a useful diagnostic test (North American Spine Society 1988). There is no doubt that it can help to distinguish various stages of disc degeneration (Adams et al 1986, Vanharanta et al 1987), though magnetic resonance imaging (MRI) is probably now a superior investigation for disc pathology. Discograms can show ruptures that mimic the experienced pain (Gibson et al 1986). However, the interpretations can be false (Yasuma et al 1988), probably because of the intricate multiple-level nervous supply to the outer annulus and posterior longitudinal ligament which can be reached by injected irritants. Discography can also produce back pain in previously pain-free subjects, and we cannot at present state that pain from a degenerate disc caused by injection means that the particular disc is the cause of the patient's problem (Nachemson 1989).

DIAGNOSTIC SPINAL PROBING

As an extension of the injection techniques, J. Shepperd has introduced diagnostic spinal probing. It can assist other techniques to identify whether a facet joint is painful, if a root is sensitive to pressure, and when considering fusion, whether one particular segment is painful.

The patient is investigated as a day patient in theatre by the nurse, anaesthetist and surgeon. Midazolam achieves amnesia, and the sedation requirements are carefully assessed by the anaes-

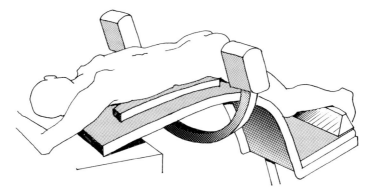

Fig. 14.1   A Knight spinal table adaptor for universal radiographic screening, allowing optimal position also for posterior surgery, with minimal venous congestion.

thetist. A table adaptor permits universal screening with a C-arm image intensifier (Fig. 14.1), and the patient is placed with the spine centred and discs parallel in all planes.

The superior border of the posterior superior iliac spine is palpated and infiltrated with lignocaine, the needle serving as a radiological marker that the point of entry is appropriate. The skin is then penetrated with a sharp 1.5-mm cannula (Fig. 14.2), and after penetrating the lumbar fascia, the trochar is changed to a blunt version.

The disc is approached first from the periosteum over the posterior ileum, to the inferior surface of the superior facet. The pain response is noted as the probe passes through the posterior muscles, and then the facet joint is probed and manipulated. The posterior longitudinal ligament and the disc annulus are examined (Fig. 14.3). The edge of the disc is recognized by its characteristic rubbery resilience. Pressure at this site generally produces a pain response, particularly at the lateral expansion of the posterior longitudinal ligament. Shepperd, who has conducted over 1700 diagnostic probings, believes that this area of the outer annulus is the most potent generator of pain in the back. The patient is asked about the character of the pain, its severity and its distribution.

Using a straight or curved needle, the disc is entered and discography performed with Niopam

400, using a digitized duplicator image. If the discogram is abnormal, 20 mg depomedrone and 40 mg gentamycin are injected, followed by distension with 2–5 ml of 0.7 marcaine. Alteration in disc height is noted and the patient's pain response is recorded. The needle is removed and the disc edge again probed.

If the facet joint is thought to be a pain source, it is examined also by facet arthrography, with instillation of anaesthetic and depomedrone.

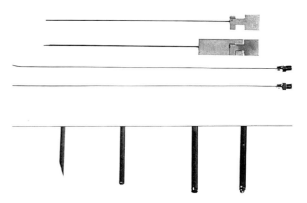

Fig. 14.2   Instruments for spinal probing: (**A**) blunt trochar fitting into a 1.5-mm cannula (**B**); straight or curved long spinal needles (**C**) for disc or facet injection; Close-up view of sharp trochar (**D**), blunt trochar (**E**), 1.5-mm cannula (**F**) and the coupled trochar and cannula (**G**).

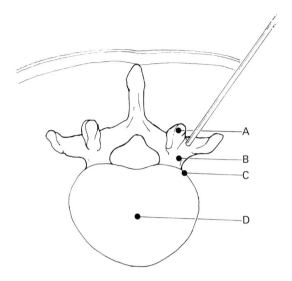

Fig. 14.3 Structures examined by probing: (**A**) the facet joint, (**B**) the subfacet perineural root region, (**C**) the edge of the disc at the lateral part of the posterior longitudinal ligament, and (**D**) discography with distension by Marcain.

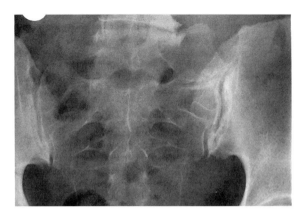

Fig. 14.4 Radiograph of hemisacralized L5. The articulation can be a nociceptive source.

Other segments are investigated if there is multiple level pathology, including hemiarticulations which can be a nociceptive source (Fig. 14.4).

After returning to the ward, the patient is encouraged to mobilize and undertake the activities that would normally produce pain. Under the supervision of a nurse, they record their own response. Then, returning home, they record on an analogue scale their level of pain over a 2-week period. Such probing has limitations but as an adjunct to other procedures it can be a useful aid to diagnosis. Not least, a number of patients have lasting benefit from what is primarily intended as a diagnostic procedure.

REFERENCES

Adams M A, Dolan P, Hutton W C 1986 The stages of disc degeneration as revealed by discograms. Journal of Bone and Joint Surgery 68-B: 36–41

Akkerveeken P F 1989 Lateral stenosis of the lumbar spine. Thesis, University of Utrecht

Carrera G F, Haughton V M, Syvertsen A, Williams A L 1980 Computed tomography of the lumbar facet joints. Radiology 134: 145–148

Destouet J M, Giyula L A, Murphy W A, Monsees B 1982 Lumbar facet joint injections: indication, technique, clinical correlation, and preliminary results. Radiology 145: 321–325

Dory M A 1981 Arthrography of the lumbar facet joints. Radiology 140: 23–27

Gibson M J, Buckley J, Mawhinney R 1986 Magnetic resonance imaging and discography in the diagnosis of disc degeneration: a comparative study of 50 discs. Journal of Bone and Joint Surgery 68-B: 369–373

Haueisen D C, Smith B S, Myers S R, Pryce M L 1985 The diagnostic accuracy of spinal nerve injection studies.

Clinical Orthopaedics and Related Research 198: 179–183

Macnab I 1971 Negative disc exploration. Journal of Bone and Joint Surgery 53-A: 891–903

Nachemson A 1989 Editorial comment. Lumbar discography — where are we today? Spine 14: 555–557

North American Spine Society 1988 Position statement on discography. Spine 13: 1343

Stanley D, McLaren M I, Euinton H A, Getty C J M 1990 A prospective study of nerve root infiltration in the diagnosis of sciatica: a comparison with radiculography, computed tomography, and operative findings. Spine 15: 540–543

Vanharanta H, Sachs B L, Spivey M A, Guyer R D, Hachschuller S H, Rashbaum R F, Johnson R G, Ohnmeiss D, Mooney V 1987 The relationship of pain provocation to lumbar disc degeneration as seen by CT/discography. Spine 12: 295–298

Yasuma T, Ohno R, Yamauchi Y 1988 False-negative lumbar discograms; correlation of discographic and histological findings in postmortem and surgical specimens. Journal of Bone and Joint Surgery 70-A: 1279–1290

Diagnosis and management

15. Herniated nucleus pulposus — pathology, diagnosis and management

PATHOLOGY

Mixter and Barr (1934) first described the clinical significance of disc herniation and the results of surgical excision. The diagnosis became so fashionable that almost all backache was attributed to the intervertebral disc. It has now taken its rightful place as a common source of acute and chronic disability, but even when responsible for symptoms it is only one factor amongst many.

The torn annulus and loose fragment

Disruption of the inner fibres of the posterior annulus alone will not cause the nucleus to bulge, even when loaded. In vitro studies suggest that there must also be a loose fragment of annulus, which in association with the torn annulus results in a space-occupying protrusion into the anterior aspect of the vertebral canal (Brinkmann et al

1992). If the outer fibres of the annulus are intact it is a protrusion, but if more peripheral fibres of the annulus are also torn or separated, the protrusion will increase in size and finally rupture through the outer fibres as a nuclear hernia. A disc is extruded when the displaced nuclear material within the vertebral canal is still connected to material within the disc (Fig. 15.1). It is sequestrated when nuclear material escapes into the vertebral canal as one or more free fragments. The posterior longitudinal ligament and the fascial extension laterally generally prevent the disc material from rupturing freely into the canal (Fig. 15.2), but this can occur, and free fragments migrate to other locations. A central protrusion is more effectively resisted by the strong posterior longitudinal ligament than a more lateral lesion. A far lateral lesion is also uncommon, but there can be considerable variation in both the site and the size of the lesion.

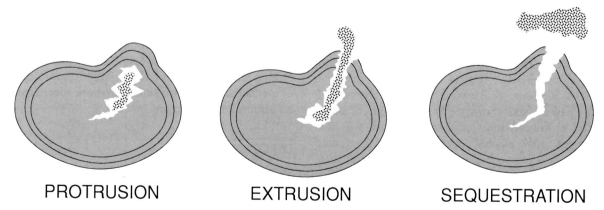

PROTRUSION   EXTRUSION   SEQUESTRATION

Fig. 15.1 Diagram showing a disc protrusion where there is a loose fragment and a fissure. There is a bulge of the annulus but some of the outer annular fibres remain intact. A complete annular fissure results in an extrusion when a loose fragment is partly within and partly outside the annulus. The loose fragment is sequestrated when it is outside the annulus.

Number of patients

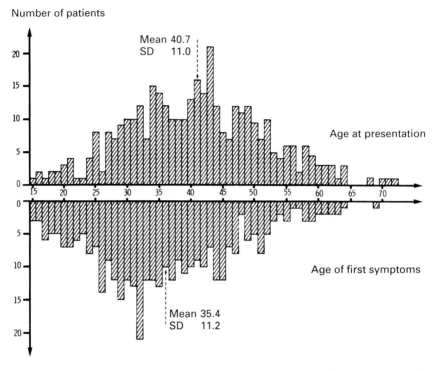

Fig. 15.5 Histogram showing the age of patients attending hospital with a symptomatic disc protrusion, and the age of the same patients when they first experienced back pain.

Root pain

Pain in the lower back is usually the first symptom, but it is root symptoms and signs that make the diagnosis. Pain spreads or is replaced by pain first in the buttock, thigh, posterior calf and ankle. In an L5 lesion, there may be pain or numbness in the big toe, and with an S1 lesion, in the outer foot. Its intensity is variable.

Root pain, of course, can result from many different pathologies, but root pain from disc protrusion is classically worse with coughing, sneezing, laughing or straining. This is quite distinct from the root pain of lateral canal stenosis (Ch. 16) where the root pain is not affected by coughing or laughing. Coughing may not aggravate the pain when a far lateral disc affects the nerve beyond the dural sleeve. Perhaps it is the sudden rise in CSF pressure which is responsible for this symptom rather than a rise in disc pressure.

The characteristics of root pain from disc herniation are also different from root entrapment.

The leg pain is severe in the upright posture because the tension of a protrusion is greater in a loaded disc. Perhaps this difference is not so apparent when the disc is sequestrated. And the root pain of a disc is often relieved by lying down, in contrast to root entrapment pain which is severe at night. In the younger patients the symptoms are less marked than the signs. Many a young man will remain at work with a large lumbar disc lesion, with few symptoms other than stiffness of the back and legs.

Many patients with disc protrusion complain that they have difficulty getting dressed in the morning. Shoes and socks are a particularly awkward problem; either they need help with dressing, or they lie on the bed in order to reach to their toes (Fig. 15.6). This is a root tension symptom correlating well with straight leg raising. For a patient with good straight leg raising, the 'sock test' is inappropriate.

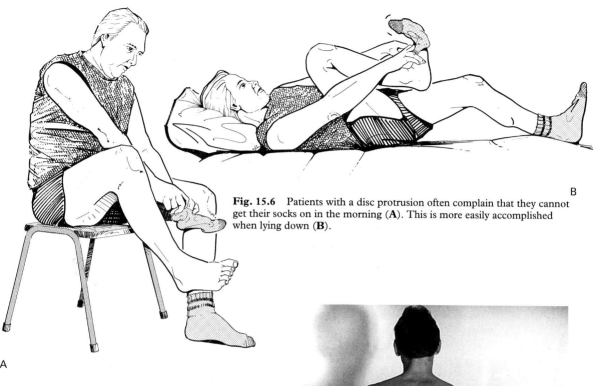

Fig. 15.6 Patients with a disc protrusion often complain that they cannot get their socks on in the morning (**A**). This is more easily accomplished when lying down (**B**).

A

Trunk list

An interesting phenomenon that accompanies a disc protrusion in about one-third of the patients is gravity-induced list. Nearly 50% of patients having disc surgery will have a trunk list (Khuffash & Porter 1989). The pelvis remains horizontal with the floor, but the lumbar spine deviates to one side with a 'wind-swept' appearance (Fig. 15.7). The list is abolished by lying down and by hanging on a bar (Fig. 15.8). It is not known if it serves a useful function, but it does shift the centre of gravity from the central plane, altering the weight distribution when standing (Figs 15.9 and 15.10). The reflex spasm can be abolished only by lying down.

The psoas is the muscle probably mainly responsible for the list (Grieve 1983), but the spinal mechanism is not understood. The list is almost always associated with a disc protrusion (Scott 1983). We observed such a list in 5.6% of patients attending a back pain clinic. Of 100 listing patients, 71 had pain in a sciatic distribution

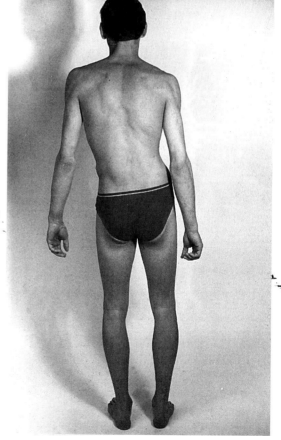

Fig. 15.7 The 'wind-swept' appearance of a patient with a lower lumbar disc protrusion, listing to the left.

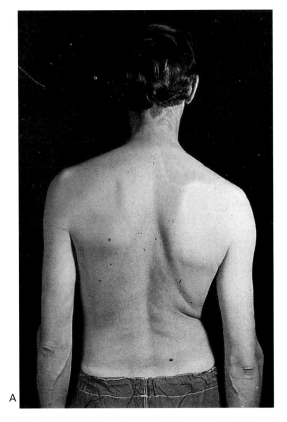
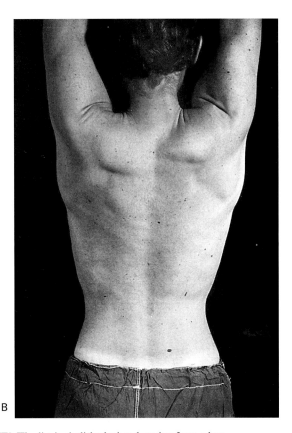

A   B

Fig. 15.8(A)   The author, unable to correct a list when standing. **(B)** The list is abolished when hanging from a bar.

below the knee, and 49 fulfilled McCulloch's criteria (1977) for a symptomatic lumbar disc lesion; 20 subsequently had surgical excision of the disc. It is interesting that no patient with a list had isthmic spondylolisthesis, when either disc protrusion is less common or the wide canal of spondylolisthesis is significant.

It has previously been suggested that a list has functional value, easing the root away from a protruding disc (Bianco 1968, Patzold et al 1975, Scott 1983), but in our series of 20 listing patients who required disc surgery, there was no consistent topographical relationship between the disc, the root and the side of the list. It has also been suggested that a list is likely to occur with a disc lesion at L5/S1 because of the powerful restraint of the iliolumbar ligaments, but this was not our experience. In fact, 12 had excision of

the L5/S1 disc, six excision of L4/5 and two of the L3/4 disc.

The fact that almost twice as many patients list to the left (66 compared with 31 to the right) suggests that a dominant reflex may be responsible for the laterality and there is evidence to support this (Porter & Miller 1986) (Fig. 15.11). A few patients can demonstrate an alternating list (Remak 1881, Carpenter 1933), listing first to one side and then to the other. Some patients have coupled movements, rotating and listing to one side when bending forwards, an unusual sign apart from a disc herniation.

Lumbar flexion and extension are limited probably because of dural irritation and correspond to the limitation of straight leg raising. Lateral flexion is unaffected.

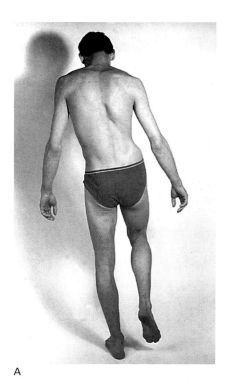

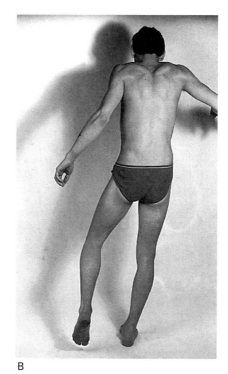

A

B

Fig. 15.9(A)
Photograph of the patient
in Fig. 15.7, now standing
on the left leg. The list
remains. **(B)** Now
standing on the right leg,
the list seems to be
corrected (but see Figs
15.10 (A) and (B)).

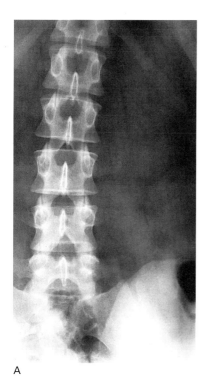

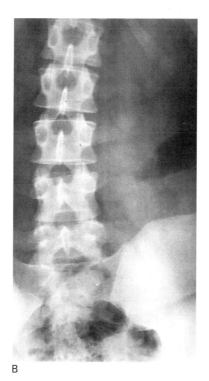

A

B

Fig. 15.10(A)   AP radiograph
of a patient with symptomatic
disc lesion, listing to the left
when standing. The centre of
gravity is shifted to the left.
(B) Radiograph of the same
patient now standing on the right
leg alone. The left psoas is
bulging and contracted as the leg
is raised. The centre of gravity is
now over the mid-line, but the
scoliosis is uncorrected.

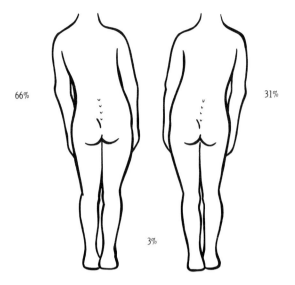

Fig. 15.11   In a series of 100 consecutive patients with a list, 66 were to the left, 31 to the right, and three alternating.

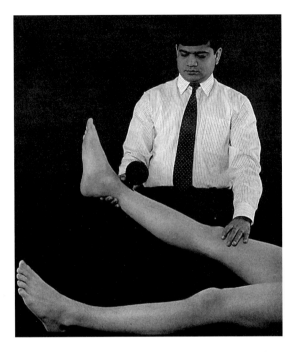

Fig. 15.12   Straight leg raising should be measured with a precision goniometer with the patient lying on a firm surface with one small pillow. The knee is supported and care taken to ensure that the pelvis does not rotate.

Degrees of change of S.L.R. from base level
after at least 8 hours in bed

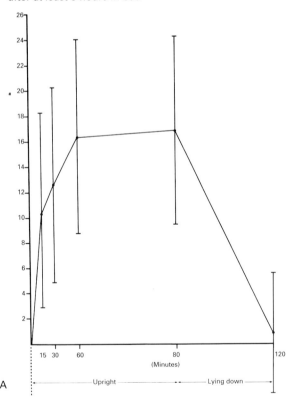

Degrees of change of S.L.R. from base level
after at least 8 hours in bed

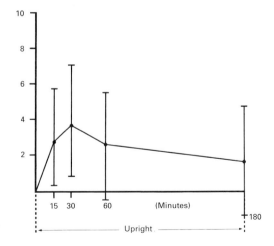

Fig. 15.13   The mean changes in straight leg raising and standard deviation during 180 min in the upright posture following recumbency, and then during 120 min recumbency, for 20 patients who had more than 10° of change (**A**) and for eight patients (**B**) who had less than 10° of change. (Reproduced with the permission of Doncaster Royal Infirmary.)

Straight leg raising

The straight leg raising test is perhaps the most important sign for diagnosis of disc herniation. Its limitation is a sign of root tension and it is rarely encountered in any other condition. Limitation of straight leg raising may in fact be a reflex to prevent root tension (Ismaiel & Porter 1992). Straight leg raising of 50° or less is almost pathognomonic of a disc lesion. Some care and some clinical experience are necessary to elicit and evaluate the sign (Fig. 15.12), and modifications of straight leg raising can reinforce its value. Cross-leg pain particularly has prognostic significance. A positive femoral stretch test is common in lateral protrusions at the L4/5 level (Christodonlides 1989). Cross-leg femoral stretch pain has not been described — why not?

When straight leg raising is limited, it can change diurnally (Fig. 15.13). The diurnal straight leg raising test (Porter & Trailescu 1990) is used as a test of the competence of the disc, to distinguish whether there is a tense protrusion or a complete rupture of the annulus. If there is a complete through and through tear of the annulus, with a loose fragment extruded or sequestrated, there will be no change in the root tension after recumbency or after being upright. However, if the outer fibres of the annulus are intact, the disc is still competent and its changing fluid content will affect the root tension signs. After 2 h of recumbency or a night in bed, the bulging disc will be tense, and the straight leg raising limited to, say, 60–30°. After being upright for 1 or 2 h the hydrostatic pressure of increased spinal load will cause fluid to be extruded from the disc, and when lying down for a further test of straight leg raising, the reduced disc tension will permit an improved straight leg raising to say 70–50° (Figs 15.14, 15.15 and 15.16).

Supplementary signs

Other signs may be helpful but are not pathognomonic. Tenderness will usually be localized to the level of the disc lesion. The root responsible may be suggested from diminution of a knee or ankle reflex, motor weakness, wasting and sensory impairment but this does not necessarily help to distinguish either the root involved or the pathology affecting that root. A disc lesion at the L4/5 level can cause L4, L5 or S1 root symptoms, and a disc at L5/S1 can affect either the L5 or S1 root; and the same signs of neurological impairment can occur in disc herniation and in root entrapment syndrome. It is not the signs of neurological impairment, but root tension symptoms and signs that suggest a disc protrusion.

One can confidently make the diagnosis of a lumbar intervertebral disc lesion with such a

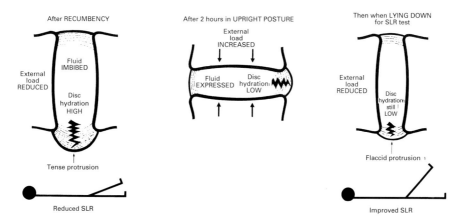

Fig. 15.14 Diagram showing how diurnal changes in the disc hydration might affect nerve root tension signs. After recumbency the disc has imbibed fluid, a protrusion will be tense, and straight leg raising very limited. After being upright for 2 h, fluid has been extruded. Then when lying down for the straight leg raising test, the external load is reduced and the protrusion is flaccid, with improved straight leg raising.

Disc protrusion

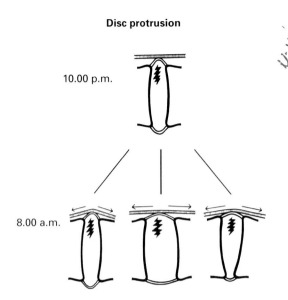

10.00 p.m.

8.00 a.m.

Fig. 15.15 Diagram to show how hydration of a disc might increase root tension signs by an increased bulge kinking the root (bottom, left) or a widened disc space stretching the root (bottom, centre) or an angled disc space stretching the root (bottom, right).

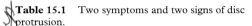

Table 15.1   Two symptoms and two signs of disc protrusion.

Root pain aggravated by coughing
Difficulty putting on shoes and socks
A trunk list
Limited straight leg raising

history and collection of abnormal signs (Table 15.1) even if it is not possible to identify the level. If they persist over a few weeks, it is unusual to find a myelogram, CT or MRI examination normal.

Presumptive lower lumbar disc herniation

There are occasions when the diagnosis cannot be made with such confidence. The diagnosis is only presumptive, and yet symptoms and signs suggest a disc protrusion. Such a patient may have back pain associated with a gravity-induced list but no nerve root involvement and no root

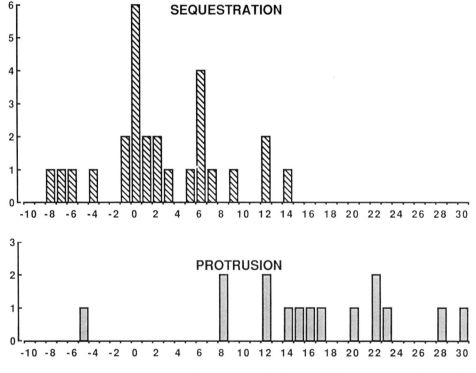

Fig. 15.16   The preoperative improvement (degrees on the horizontal axis) in straight leg raising after 2 h in the upright posture in 41 patients having discectomy; 12 of the 15 protrusions had more than 10° improvement, compared with only three of the 26 sequestrated discs.

signs; or there may be a minimal root lesion with pain to the ankle, straight leg raising slightly reduced and no abnormal neurological signs. One would not over-investigate for the sake of a diagnosis unless this was likely to affect management, and the diagnosis will remain only speculative.

MANAGEMENT

Conservative management

The best place to recover from an acute disc lesion is in bed. It has not been shown that anything is better. Some may work it off, others may be fortunate enough to have it manipulated away, but in the acute attack, a short period of bed rest is the treatment of choice. For many patients the severity of the pain leaves no alternative. A pillow under the knees can help, but the patient usually finds the most comfortable position for themselves. Food is taken in sandwich form, and a straw or a feeding cup prevents the spilling of fluids. Initially analgesics may be needed around the clock but they should be reduced as the pain settles, at least during the day.

There is, however, a price to pay for too much rest in bed. There is a rapid weakening of the locomotor system, in addition to cardiovascular and psychological change. Even initially, bed rest need not be strictly imposed and as improvement permits, graduated activity is encouraged. Improved straight leg raising is the best sign, remembering, however, that it can alter diurnally by as much as 30°, and the posture in the previous hour must be known. If straight leg raising is still very limited after 2 weeks, specialist help is needed.

There is a place for inpatient bed rest. It is difficult to account for the therapeutic effects of a hospital bed, but it is better than rest at home. Many an obdurate disc will settle with 2 weeks of inpatient care. Bed rest, letting the patient find their own position of comfort, or lying supine with the hips and knees flexed, is probably as good as traction. The common denominator for conservative inpatient treatment is an adequate period spent in the horizontal position.

There has been no satisfactory study comparing the effects of inpatient traction with bed rest alone for patients with acute disc herniation. If traction is applied, pelvic traction is preferable to Pugh's leg traction when there is the possible complication of deep venous thrombosis. Pelvic traction also has its complications, with pain or numbness in the outer thigh from compression of the lateral femoral cutaneous nerve. It calls for repositioning or removal of the corset. Lower abdominal pain, possibly from tension on the rectus muscles, is relieved by flexing the hips on a couple of pillows. No more than 2 pounds per stone body weight is necessary. Traction could alter the fluid dynamics of the disc, or at best it may only keep the patient in bed.

The best prognostic sign is improvement in straight leg raising, and it should return to almost 90° before the patient is allowed home. One regrets allowing a patient home in less than 2 weeks, even if there appears to be a rapid recovery.

Patients at this stage can be arbitrarily divided into three groups. The first are obviously better, with little discomfort, good straight leg raising and no abnormal neurological signs. They can go home, stay off work a few weeks and expect a good result in the short term. They want to know how much exercise and how much rest are necessary, their future limitations, and how recurrences can be prevented. A 'Back School' programme is helpful at some time during the recovery phase (Ch. 26), ideally beginning in the recumbent period.

A second group are not better, but have made some progress. Straight leg raising may have increased from 20/70 to 60/80. Some abnormal neurological signs may have resolved, but perhaps sensory impairment remains. The experience of Weber (1983) is that these patients ultimately do as well treated conservatively as by operation. Even if imaging has shown a disc herniation with root involvement, good long-term results with conservative management can be expected (Alaranta et al 1990). These patients can go home to have periods of rest, gradually increasing their activity over the weeks; 3 months in a lightweight corset can help. Recovery may be slow, with further recurrences. They do not appear to develop perithecal or perineural fibrosis (Saal et al 1990). Surgery does not offer a better prognosis. Experience with percutaneous techniques for this group is as yet insufficient to identify their role.

A third group fail to improve and require active

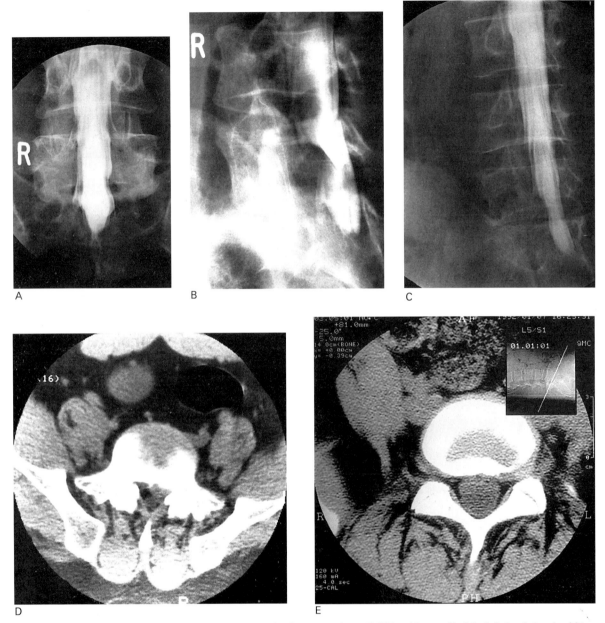

Fig. 15.17(A)   The classical myelographic appearance of a disc protrusion at L5/S1, with cut-off of the left dural sheath of S1.
(B) A massive disc herniation at L5/S1 distorting the dural sac. Both discs (**A**) and (**B**) were easily removed through a small fenestration.
(C) Dural cut-off sign of the S1 root on the left at L5/S1.
(D) CT scan of the same patient showing large left-sided disc protrusion.
(E) CT scan showing a far lateral disc protrusion in the left root canal. (Fig. 15.17 (A), (C) and (D) reproduced with the permission of Doncaster Royal Infirmary.).

treatment, either by surgically excising the disc or by percutaneous techniques. If after 3 weeks in a hospital bed, straight leg raising is 50° or less, it is worth identifying the disc by MRI, CT or a radiculogram (Fig. 15.17) and treating it actively. Continuing cross leg pain and persistent motor weakness at this stage also predict a probable failure of further conservative treatment.

One may be tempted to abandon conservative management if there is gross weakness of dorsiflexion of the foot or of the peronei. If, however, there is some motor improvement, patience may be rewarded by full recovery.

Surgery

Indications

1. It is negligent to delay surgical treatment when bladder dysfunction follows a massive disc prolapse. A neurogenic bladder is the price of delay. A patient who is incontinent or unable to pass urine needs urgent and careful neurological assessment, emergency imaging and rapid surgical excision of the massive disc.

2. Early surgery may be appropriate on other occasions. Some clinical factors suggest inevitable failure of conservative management, and although not constituting an emergency, delay is unjustified. A history of steadily increasing symptoms over several months with progressive restriction in straight leg raising suggests a disc herniation that will not improve with bed rest.

Mr JA, a 37-year-old executive, attended with a 10-week history of pain in the left thigh and calf, and some paraesthesia in the outer foot. He had not been able to rest but kept at work taking six analgesic tablets most days. Straight leg raising was 80/70. A month later, although he put into practice the advice of the 'Back School', symptoms remained and straight leg raising was further reduced to 70/40. MRI showed a disc herniation at L4/5 and the following day an extruded fragment was removed. With slow progression of symptoms and signs the disc was unlikely to resolve by conservative means, and bed rest would have been inappropriate.

3. There are also a number of signs that suggest a patient is likely to require surgery:
   a. *Trunk list*: the presence of a list increases the chances of a patient with disc symptoms requiring surgery (Khuffash & Porter 1989).

Of our patients with disc symptoms and a trunk list, 40% eventually required surgery, compared with 20% of patients without list.
   b. *Cross-leg pain*: this sign is a predictor of the failure of conservative management (Eismant & Currier 1989). Of our patients with disc symptoms and cross-leg pain, 51% required discectomy, compared with 15% of patients who did not have cross-leg pain (Khuffash & Porter 1989). These two signs in combination are strong predictors.
   c. *Diurnal change in straight leg raising*: this is also a predictor of outcome. A competent disc, where intact peripheral annular fibres contain a protrusion, may be associated with diurnal changes in straight leg raising by as much as 30°. However, diurnal change is unlikely when a free fragment has extruded or sequestrated through an annular tear, and there is then a poor prognosis for conservative treatment (Porter & Trailescu 1990).

The degree of limitation of straight leg raising is no predictor of outcome. Many patients with straight leg raising of 30/20 will improve with 2 weeks' bed rest and avoid surgery. Neither is the presence of abnormal neurological signs (areflexia, motor weakness, wasting or sensory loss) a predictor of outcome, these can recover. Similarly, the identification of a disc lesion by imaging with MRI, CT or myelography is no reason to operate.

Symptoms and signs associated with a failure of conservative management are summarized in Table 15.2.

Only when the decision to operate has been made is imaging requested. With MRI or CT the site of the lesion is identified, the choice of imaging modality depending on resources. Using imaging as a 'fishing trip' to make a diagnosis is bad

Table 15.2 Symptoms and signs associated with failure of conservative management; SLR = straight leg raising.

Objective evidence of a steady reduction in SLR over a few weeks
Failure of SLR to improve with 2 weeks' bed rest
A trunk list
Cross-leg pain
No diurnal change in SLR

practice. It is likely to reveal disc protrusions that can be clinically irrelevant.

Surgical procedures

The principles of disc surgery are to reduce the disc pressure on the nerve root, with its resultant pain, disability and neurological deficit, and to avoid immediate and late complications. To achieve these aims, there has been an unprecedented expansion of surgical choice, from percutaneous techniques, microdiscectomy and minimal intervention to traditional fenestration, wide exposure and combined fusion.

Fenestration discectomy The patient lies prone on an operating frame with the abdomen dependent avoiding an increase in venous pressure. Semiflexion makes the operation easier by increasing the interlaminar space. An incision is made over the spinous processes of L4 and L5 or L5 and S1, and subcutaneous bleeding is minimized by keeping strictly to the mid-line. Paraspinal muscles are separated from the spinous processes and laminae, and the tendinous insertions of multifidus divided. Self-retaining retractors provide both a good exposure and haemostasis. The fifth lumbar vertebra is identified by grasping the spinous processes with bone holders and noting the relative mobility of L5 compared with S1. Lumbarization or sacralization should not cause confusion if this has previously been identified radiographically. If the site of the disc lesion has been confidently identified by MRI, CT or radiculography, and this corresponds with the clinical assessment, only one disc space need be exposed. A small window of the caudal aspect of the lamina above is removed with rongeurs and a square of ligamentum flavum is excised.

As the dura is gently displaced medially, a bulging disc is first felt with a dissector and then seen as a white protrusion. The displaced nerve root, responsible for the sciatica and tension signs, is identified and carefully retracted medially away from the protrusion. It can be flattened like a ribbon over the disc material, and unless recognized, an apparent incision into the disc can cut the root or, in a far lateral disc, the ganglion. It is important to consider the possibility of a conjoint root. It is an anomaly that occurs in at least 8%

of the population (Hasue et al 1983, Kadish & Simmons 1984) and makes the nerve root vulnerable to surgical injury. If the nucleus is extruded or sequestrated, it may be forced into the wound by the process of teasing away of the nerve root. The disc material can then be extracted in one piece (Fig. 15.18). A blunt dissector is inserted through the rent in the annulus into the nuclear space. Other fragments of nucleus are removed with a disc extractor. When a disc is protruding, with some outer fibres of the annulus intact, it is necessary to make a cruciate incision in these fibres, and then extract the nuclear material. The limit of the nucleus is recognized by the feel of the tissue, but the remaining annulus should not be penetrated by the extractor. Generally, one or two large fragments are removed, and several smaller pieces. If all the loose fragments are not removed from within the annulus, there is a possibility of late recurrence. It is not necessary to remove disc material which is not loose. Extravagant excision of disc material will result in disc space narrowing and late sequelae.

At the end of the operation the dura should be free and the nerve root mobile. If the root is still tight then some sequestrated material remains and further exposure is necessary, perhaps into the root canal (Kunogi & Hasue 1991). Provided the disc protrusion is unequivocal and the root is free, there is no need to explore the other side or

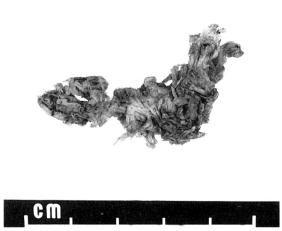

Fig. 15.18 Sequestrated nucleus pulposus.

other levels. When the vertebral canal is particularly narrow and trefoil in configuration, it is worth decompressing the central canal and sometimes decompressing the root canal in addition to removing the prolapsed disc. There is no place for surgical exploration of the vertebral canal as a diagnostic procedure. If at the time of operation no disc pathology is recognized, there has been an error of clinical judgement, and if the vertebral canal is of adequate dimensions it is preferable to do no more. It is unjustifiable to incise or to excise a normal disc or decompress an adequate canal.

Careful closure and haemostasis, with or without suction drainage, avoids haematoma with its risk of subsequent infection and scar tissue formation.

Microsurgical discectomy   Williams in 1986 first reported the use of the operating microscope for discectomy. With minimal trauma to the tissues, disc material is removed and the root decompressed (Hudgins 1983). It reduces operating time, morbidity, blood loss and hospital stay, with an early return to work (Andrews & Lavyne 1990). The medial portion of the facet may be removed for exposure. Extradural fat is not disturbed, and only as much disc material as necessary is removed to relieve the nerve root from visible compression.

Because of limited exposure, it should not be used in the presence of spinal stenosis nor in the previously operated patient (Williams 1986). Dural tears and postoperative discitis are probably as common as with the traditional approach. One might argue that what is gained by the advantages of precise surgery is lost by what is sometimes inadequate exposure. Of patients with disabling disc symptoms, 55% have vertebral canal diameters below the 10th percentile for asymptomatic subjects (Porter et al 1978); this narrowing is not easily recognized before surgery, nor with monocular vision at the time of operation. Spinal stenosis has been blamed for 19% of failures after microsurgical discectomy, and this cannot be predicted with confidence by preoperative imaging (Williams 1986).

The reported success rates of microdiscectomy are probably comparable with traditional surgery. Early morbidity is less, but complications are higher, especially when the surgeon is learning the technique.

Minimal intervention   This technique was developed by J. Shepperd. Under general anaesthetic, using X-ray control to be sure of the level of operation, the disc is approached through a vertical 2-cm incision, just lateral to the mid-line. Two purpose-designed hooked retractors and a fibre optic suction root retractor provide adequate exposure with a dry and illuminated field (Fig. 15.19).

Using an image intensifier, a needle is placed in the mid-line to identify the precise placement of the skin incision. It is directed posterior and in line with the disc to be explored. An incision is then made 1 cm proximal and 1 cm distal to the needle, through the superficial fat to the lumbar fascia. The fascia is incised vertically and, keeping close to the spinous process, a plane is developed between the bone and the erector spinae down to the lamina. The position is again checked on the image intensifier. Specialized lever retractors are placed over the facet joint, again confirming the position radiologically. The ligamentum flavum is cleared with pituitary rongeurs under direct vision, using the sucking root retractor as a light source. The ligamentum flavum is divided using a No. 15 blade on a long handle, and a flap excised using one of a range of four 45° Love Kerrison upcut punches, which vary from 1 to 6 mm. Through a small fenestration particularly at L4/5 the disc and nerve root are inspected. The

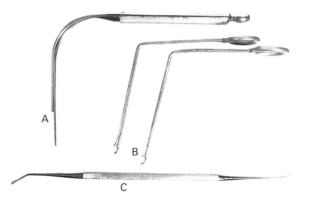

Fig. 15.19 Shepperd's instruments for minimal intervention surgery: (**A**) Root retractor incorporating a fibreoptic light and sucker (**B**) Facet joint hook retractors (**C**) Elongated Watson Cheyne probe for examining the root and disc.

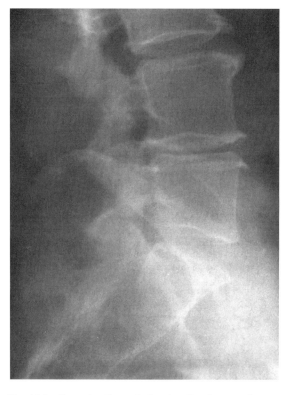

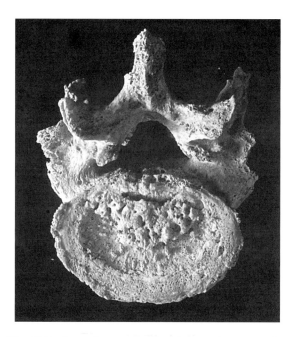

Fig. 16.3   Osteophyte encroaching the posterior aspect of the left root canal at L5.

Fig. 16.2   Lateral radiograph showing disc degeneration at L4/5 with some retrolisthesis, and posterior vertebral bar formation. The L4 root is vulnerable in the root canal, and the L5 root in the central canal between the vertebral bar in front, and the cranial aspect of the lamina behind.

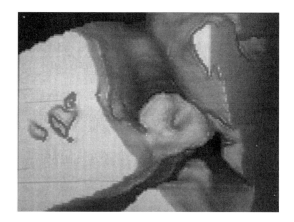

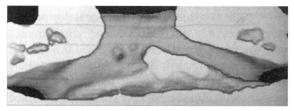

Fig. 16.4   Three-dimensional reconstruction of a cadaveric specimen of a spinal osteochondroma (top) encroaching into the entrance of the root canal. The patient had been asymptomatic, apart from having a back strain 6 years before. A coronal section through the pedicles at L5/S1 shows patency of the root canal (bottom) (by courtesy of Graeme Smith).

always preserved (Fig. 16.4). It may be reduced, but never occluded. If a CT scan should give the impression that the canal is non-existent, this is but an artefact of the mathematical display. CT measurements underestimate the size of the root canal (Smith 1991, Smith et al 1992).

Soft tissue involvement adds to the bony encroachment. Organization of an annulus after a disc protrusion, or fibrosis of extruded or sequestrated nucleus, reduces the available space for the root. The posterior longitudinal ligament can thicken, the ligamentum flavum infold (Towme & Reichert 1931), the apophyseal joint capsule hypertrophy or bulge with synovial hyperplasia (Rauschning 1987), and soft tissue of a lytic pars proliferate until space for the nerve root is at a premium. A foraminal cause of entrapment has been attributed to the corporotransverse ligament. This ligament is rarely mentioned in books of anatomy or pathology but it is generally present in the lumbar foramen, and may at times be implicated in root entrapment (Church & Buchker 1991, Olsewski et al 1991) (Fig. 16.5). Venous engorgement in the root canal with oedema and fibrosis may further restrict space. Epidural fibrosis follows the trauma of surgery, whether from haematoma, infection, foreign body reaction, or rough handling of tissues. Some individuals with defective fibrinolysis may be prone to develop fibrosis (Poutain et al 1987). The dorsal root ganglion which is situated in the root canal inferior to the pedicle of the vertebra is prone to compressive ischaemia in degenerative spines (Rauschning 1987).

Segmental movement adds a dynamic component to root canal stenosis (Panjabi et al 1983, Penning & Wilmink 1987, Penning 1992). Extension and rotation reduce available space encroaching onto the nerve root complex and radicular vessels. Extension and rotation are both limited in patients with root entrapment syndrome. This becomes particularly significant when there is posterior or rotational displacement of the vertebrae (Fig. 16.6) (Krayenbuhl & Benini 1979); degenerative spondylolisthesis can produce the same symptoms. Postural movement, especially extension, can compromise the root and precipitate symptoms.

Walking can produce root pain both by segmental rotationary movement and by epidural venous engorgement associated with exercise. When there is coexistent central canal stenosis at

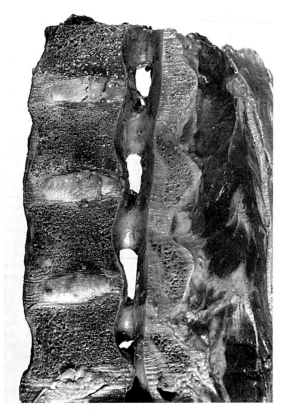

Fig. 16.5 A photograph of a sagittal section of a cadaveric spine showing the central and root canals from L1 to L4. There is posterior vertebral bar formation at the lower border of L4 with soft tissue thickening from a degenerate disc, and a thickened ligamentum flavum. The corporotransverse ligament is seen at the lower aspect of each foramen (by courtesy of Graeme Smith).

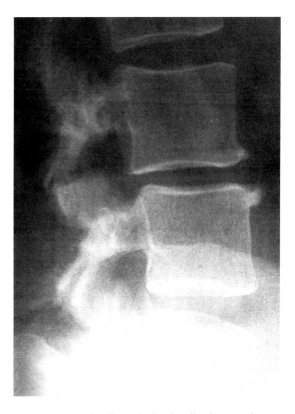

Fig. 16.6 Lateral radiograph showing disc degeneration at L3/4. A double shadow of the posterior aspect of L3 suggests a rotational displacement. Excessive segmental movement can affect one of the roots at the foramina if already in a restricted space.

the segment above, a two-level venous block is probably responsible for unilateral claudication, with no leg pain at rest but pain when walking causing the patient to stop. However, the patient with root entrapment pain from acute exacerbation of a single level root stenosis has pain at rest (as distinct from root claudication). This pain can be made worse by walking but it does not necessarily make them stop. The root itself is pathological as a result of trauma in the root canal, and the dynamic factors of normal root extension in walking and bending assume clinical significance.

Just as the tunnel is never occluded, the root is never trapped. There is some excursion, even if at operation the root gives the impression of being tight. The lumbar roots normally have an excursion of a few millimetres limited by proximal and distal attachments (Spencer et al 1983). These attachments probably make the root vulnerable to traction symptoms in the presence of pathological change. A mobile root in a restricted space will produce root irritation and oedema. Local friction on a tethered root or anomalous root with limited excursion will have similar results (Kadish & Simmons 1984). The root then becomes considerably thicker, harder and inelastic with perineural fibrosis.

Wiltse and colleagues (1984) described an unusual cause of root entrapment syndrome when gross displacement of an isthmic spondylolisthesis compresses the L5 root between the fifth lumbar transverse process and the alar of the sacrum — 'the far out syndrome'. Spinal tumours (Royster et al 1991) and extraspinal tumours and aneurysms can also present as lumbar root neuropathy.

There are thus many pathological changes that can cause lumbar root pain in the middle-aged and older patient. The most common site of these changes is in the root canal, related to disc pathology of a previous decade (Figs 16.7 and 16.8).

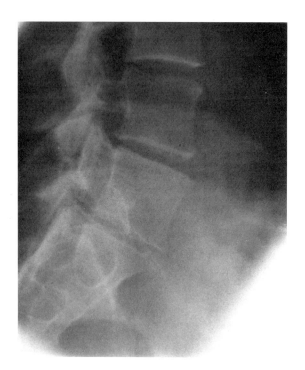

Fig. 16.7 Lateral radiograph of a degenerate L4/5 disc with posterior osteophytes, producing root pain many years after the start of the original pathology.

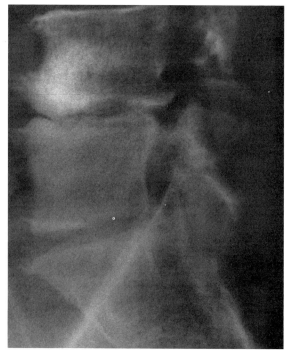

Fig. 16.8 Gross disc degeneration at L4/5 with retrolisthesis and posterior vertebral bar formation. The affected root may be L4 ot L5. (Reproduced with the permission of Doncaster Royal Infirmary.)

CLINICAL PRESENTATION

Though the pain from root entrapment is in the same distribution as the sciatica from a disc lesion — from the buttock, thigh, calf to the foot — its character is different. It is described as a severe pain often unremitting day and night. Whilst the pain from a disc is frequently relieved by lying down, this pain is so troublesome at night that the patient will walk about. Sitting is uncomfortable, and they sit in a chair asymmetrically avoiding weight on the affected buttock. Driving far is impossible, as though the whole length of the sciatic nerve is over-sensitive. Unlike root pain of disc origin it is unaffected by coughing and sneezing. These patients never have a trunk list, and they do not complain about being locked in the stooped position after washing their face or cleaning their teeth (common symptoms with disc protrusion). Getting dressed in the morning presents no difficulty, as flexing forward increases space in the root and central canal.

The periodicity of the pain is variable. One patient may experience constant severe pain, and present at the consulting room after many sleepless nights. Another may have mild pain with episodes of severe pain in relation to posture, especially to sitting or standing for long. Another may say that walking aggravates the pain. If only walking produces pain one should suspect root claudication from a two-level stenosis (see page 205), but in root entrapment syndrome, rest pain is the main complaint.

The past history is also variable. There has usually been previous disc pathology. A previous disc protrusion may have been either classical, with root pain, or have produced only back pain; the symptoms may even have been entirely occult. The degree of original disc symptoms years before depends much on the size of the central vertebral canal. There may have been no symptoms at all from a disc protrusion into a wide dome-shaped central canal, but with disc space narrowing over the years, bony and soft tissue degeneration and perhaps slight vertebral displacement, the root becomes compromised. The very first symptom of the silent lesion years before, it now causes severe root pain from root canal entrapment. The root affected by root canal

stenosis, however, is usually the root proximal to the root previously affected by disc protrusion. For example, a protrusion at L5/S1 will commonly involve the S1 root, whilst the degenerative change which follows the protrusion will affect the L5 root in the root canal (Fig. 16.9). There may, of course, be disc degeneration which has followed disc pathology in the absence of any protrusion, and any previous disc symptoms.

The progress of the root pain once it has developed is unpredictable. It can develop and subside in weeks, months or years, and patients may therefore present with long or short histories. It has no typical pattern, sometimes being severe and gradually resolving, and at other times getting steadily worse, requiring surgery.

The abnormal signs are few. In a series of 249 patients, we found that 32% could reach down to touch the floor with straight knees. Lumbar extension, however, was considered to be full in only 12%. Straight leg raising was 80° or more in 74%. Reflexes were normal in 84%, sensation normal in 82%, and muscle wasting and weakness recorded in less than 5%. Only one-third of Getty's patients with root entrapment (1981) had significant restriction of straight leg raising, and this was similarly recorded by Macnab (1977). There is a greater incidence of abnormal neurological signs in those patients who have had previous surgery, and in those referred for surgery

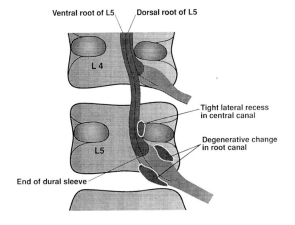

Fig. 16.9 Diagram to show that a disc protrusion at L5/S1 will generally affect S1 root, whilst two decades later a degenerate disc space at L5/S1 will tend to involve L5 root.

from other units because of the intensity and duration of root symptoms. For many patients with little to find clinically, the diagnosis therefore begs a good history. Most patients have some radiological evidence of degenerative change, reduction of L5/S1 disc space being the most consistent finding.

MANAGEMENT

Most patients presenting to an orthopaedic surgeon with root entrapment syndrome can be managed by a careful explanation of the cause of pain, and advice; 81% of our patients were managed in this way (Porter et al 1984). They certainly need to be given time to discuss the probable cause of the pain, and to understand that if aggravating factors can be avoided, it will probably settle. If sitting for long and standing increase the symptoms, the position should be quickly changed. The mechanical stress on the spine should be kept to a minimum, and if this is not understood, it is reinforced with a back school programme. The patient is told that symptoms will probably remain for a long time, but will reduce in intensity and eventually settle.

Of our patients with root entrapment treated in this way, 187 described their symptoms after 2 years. Three-quarters of them still had some root pain but it was less troublesome, and only 12% had either returned in those 2 years or sought help elsewhere.

For some patients the pain is so intense that it is not reasonable to offer advice only. It is difficult to obtain statistical evidence that an epidural injection is better than placebo (Klenerman et al 1984), but there is strong circumstantial evidence that this is the best indication for an epidural. Although it may not always be effective, many patients admit that the epidural is the start of improvement, whilst others obtain immediate and complete relief of pain. A solution of 40 cc of normal saline with 2 cc of steroid and local anaesthetic injected epidurally at the level of the lesion can produce good results.

For a few patients, surgical decompression of the root canal is essential. Careful patient selection is vital to obtain a good result. The diagnosis

must be correct and the symptoms sufficiently severe and not resolving by conservative means. The diagnosis can be difficult, and supplementary evidence from investigations is essential. Myelography is generally unhelpful, the lesion being too far lateral to be detected (Euinton et al 1984), but it will exclude other pathology in the severely disabled patient.

There has been a rapid development in new electrophysiological tests which help to identify radiculopathy (Watanabe & Tanaka 1990, Williamson 1991, Dvorak et al 1991). Dermatomal somatosensory evoked potentials are the most sensitive (Tokuhashi et al 1991). However, these methods are not universally available.

In expert hands, electromyography can provide objective evidence of impaired root function and it will sometimes identify the root affected. (Leyshon et al 1980, Wilbourn 1992). However, this investigation will not predict which nerve roots are responsible for symptoms (Merriam et al 1982), probably because of the variable anatomy of root innervation. Electrodiagnostic methods can complement other investigations and help in the overall evaluation but probably have limited value, especially after previous laminectomy (Eisen & Hoirch 1983). Thermography has been disappointing, identifying neither the site nor the side of the lesion (So et al 1989, Hoffman et al 1991).

A CT scan or MRI is imperative before intervention therapy. Transverse imaging has revolutionized the planning of surgery for root entrapment syndrome (Fig. 16.10) and three-dimensional CT is a most valuable adjunct (Fig. 16.11). Furthermore, CT or MRI which includes the abdomen and pelvis will occasionally show extraspinal causes of radiculopathy, occult malignant tumours, haematoma or aneurysms (Kleiner et al 1991). These techniques are most helpful in demonstrating the bony contours of the central and root canal, and the degree of encroachment by bone and ligamentum flavum. When facet degenerative change is a significant factor, the extent of undercutting of the superior facet can be predicted. Gadolinium enhancement is useful if there has been previous surgery, differentiating epidural scarring from degenerative disc material.

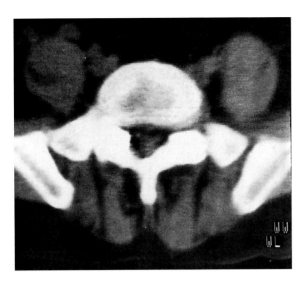

Fig. 16.10 CT scan of a patient with severe root pain, showing asymmetrical canal and overhanging facet.

Sophisticated imaging can never provide us with a diagnosis of root entrapment syndrome. Symptomless degenerative pathology is so common in the middle-aged and elderly population that one cannot make the diagnosis on imaging alone. The decision to operate depends on the history and examination, with imaging only directing the surgeon to the significant level.

How can we assess the severity of the pain? We can only observe the patient's behaviour in response to pain, and unfortunately the degree of the root pathology is not always related to the patient's behaviour to that pathology. Exaggerated signs are associated with exaggerated symptoms.

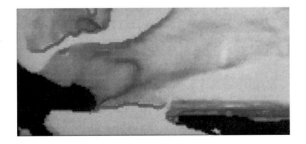

Fig. 16.11 Three-dimensional reconstruction of CT images of the root canal produces clear and representative pictures of the anatomy, though the actual dimensions of the canal are underestimated (by courtesy of Graeme Smith).

The root pathology may not be as gross as the symptoms suggest, and the subsequent results of surgery a disappointment. In a condition where symptoms outweigh the abnormal signs, a preoperative psychological assessment is a useful supplement to the clinical examination. It may indicate an abnormal profile with a poor prognosis.

Diagnostic nerve root infiltration can help identify the pathological root (Macnab 1971, Akkerveeken 1989, Stanley et al 1990). An 18-gauge 6-inch spinal needle is introduced to the nerve root, and the patient is asked to describe whether the sharp pain they experience is identical to the symptomatic pain, and whether it is abolished by local anaesthetic. It is probably most useful for the patient who has had previous surgery.

Before considering surgery, there should also be an adequate period of observation over several weeks lest the condition resolve either naturally or with the help of one or more epidural injections. When the diagnosis is clear, the pain severe and of long duration, when it is not settling and there is no evidence of exaggeration, surgical decompression of the root can be rewarding. Getty and colleagues (1981) recorded early relief of leg pain in 68% of their operated patients.

Decompression of the root requires adequate exposure of the root over the length at risk (Scoville & Corkhill 1973). The site of compression may be suspected preoperatively by conventional radiography, by CT scan, MRI or occasionally by myelography. Electrical studies may help to identify the root. The area is exposed surgically and the root followed proximally and distally until there is no question at all that it is free and mobile. There is sometimes, however, uncertainty about the area of pathology and about the root which is involved, and it may be necessary to explore the lower lumbar central canal and two root canals fairly extensively. The confidence with which one views the investigations will determine the extent of surgical exploration. Many feel that a wide decompression is generally necessary, removing half the lamina at L5, occasionally at L4 if the 4th lumbar root is suspect, and following the L5 root well into the root canal undercutting the lamina to ensure complete freedom for the root. The L5 root may be obviously thickened and tough with perineural fibrosis, and there is then no doubt about the root involved. Bony hypertrophy in the 5th lumbar root canal should not cause us to automatically suspect that root. The S1 root may be the cause of the symptoms, and removal of the upper sacral lamina may in fact reveal compression under the cranial lip.

Others more confident of the site of the lesion may be happy to perform a limited decompression, removing the window of lamina and part of the apophyseal joint, undercutting the lamina and removing ligamentum flavum (Getty et al 1981). There are obvious advantages in a more limited exposure provided the decompression is adequate. Most patients experience early postoperative relief of the severe leg pain but many have symptoms which persist, varying in degree, perhaps the result of irreversible root pathology.

Root entrapment which develops proximal to a previous fusion is treated by root decompression, with or without extending the fusion. The presence of root symptoms with a degenerative spondylolisthesis at L4/5 requires root decompression and fusion. When a pars lysis is responsible for root pain, opinions differ about decompression and fusion, or fusion alone (see Ch. 19). A trial of conservative management for all these patients can be rewarding.

REFERENCES

Akkerveeken P F 1989 Lateral stenosis of the lumbar spine. Thesis, University of Utrecht

Church C P, Buchker M T 1991 Radiographic evaluation of the corporotransverse ligament at the L5 intervertebral foramen: a cadaveric study. Journal of Manipulative and Physiological Therapeutics, 14: 240–248

Crock H V 1981 Normal and pathological anatomy of the lumbar spinal nerve root canals. Journal of Bone and Joint Surgery 63-B: 487–490

Dvorak H, Herdmann J, Theiler R 1991 Magnetic transchemical brain stimulation: painless evaluation of central motor pathways. Spine 15: 155–160

Eisen N A, Hoirch M 1983 The electrodiagnostic evaluation of spinal root lesions. Spine 8: 98–106

Euinton H A, Lock T J, Barrington N A, Getty C J M, Davies G K 1984 Radiological diagnosis of bony entrapment of lumbar nerve roots using water soluble radiculography. Presented to the International Society for the Study of the Lumbar Spine, Montreal

Getty C J M, Johnson J R, Kirwan E O'G, Sullivan M F 1981 Partial undercutting facetectomy for bony entrapment of the lumbar nerve root. Journal of Bone and Joint Surgery 63-B: 330–335

Hoffman R M, Kent D L, Deyo R A 1991 Diagnostic accuracy and clinical utility of thermography for lumbar radiculopathy. Spine 16: 623–627

Kadish L J, Simmons E H 1984 Anomalies of the lumbosacral nerve roots; an anatomical investigation and myelographic study. Journal of Bone and Joint Surgery 66-B: 411–416

Kleiner J B, Donaldson W F, Curd J G, Thorne R P 1991 Extraspinal causes of lumbo sacral radiculopathy. Journal of Bone and Joint Surgery 73-A: 817–821

Klenerman L, Greenwood R, Davenport H T, White D C, Peskett S 1984 Lumbar epidural injections in the treatment of sciatica. British Journal of Rheumatology 23: 35–38

Krayenbuhl H, Benini A 1979 Die enge des recessus lateralis in lumalen bereich der wirbelsaule als ursa che der nervenwurzelkompression bei bandscheibenvers chamlerung. Zeitschrift für Orthopadie 117: 167–171

Leyshon A, Kirwan E O'G, Wynn Parry C B 1980 Is it nerve root pain? Journal of Bone and Joint Surgery 62-B: 119

Macnab I 1971 Negative disc exploration. Journal of Bone and Joint Surgery 53-A: 891–903

Macnab I 1977 Backache. Williams and Wilkins, Baltimore

Merriam W F, Smith N J, Mulholland R C 1982 Lumbar spinal stenosis. British Medical Journal 285: 515

Olsewski J M, Simmons E H, Kallen F C, Mendel F C 1991 Evidence from cadavers suggestive of entrapment of fifth lumbar nerves by lumbosacral ligaments. Spine 16: 336–347

Panjabi M M, Takata K, Geol U K 1983 Kinematics of lumbar intervertebral foramen. Spine 8: 348–357

Penning L 1992 Functional pathology of lumbar spinal stenosis. Clinical Biomechanics 7: 3–17

Penning L, Wilmink J T 1987 Posture-dependent bilateral compression of L4 or L5 nerve roots in facet hypertrophy. Spine 12: 488–500

Porter R W, Hibbert C, Evans C 1984 The natural history of root entrapment syndrome. Spine 9: 418–422

Poutain G D, Keegan A L, Jayson M I V 1987 Impaired fibrinolytic activity in defined chronic back pain syndromes. Spine 12: 83–86

Rauschning W 1987 Normal and pathologic anatomy of the lumbar root canals. Spine 12: 1008–1019

Royster R M, Kujawa P, Dryer R F 1991 Multi-level osteochondroma of the lumbar spine presenting as spinal stenosis. Spine 16: 992–993

Scoville W B, Corkhill G 1973 Lumbar disc surgery: technique of radical removal and early mobilisation. Journal of Neurosurgery 39: 265–269

Shepperd J A N 1984 Anatomy of the L4/L5 and S1 nerve roots and their associated thecal sheaths: cadaver studies. Personal communication

Smith G 1991 CT measurements of the root canal. Thesis, University of Aberdeen

Smith G, Aspden R, Porter R W 1993 Comparison between measurements from CT reconstruction and direct measurements of the root canal. Spine (in press)

So Y T, Arminoff M J, Olney R K 1989 The role of thermography in the evaluation of lumbosacral radiculopathy. Neurology 39: 1154–1158

Spencer D L, Irwin G S, Miller J A A 1983 Anatomy and significance of fixation of the lumbosacral nerve roots in sciatica. Spine 8: 672–679

Stanley D, McLaren M I, Euinton H A, Getty C J M 1990 A prospective study of nerve root infiltration in the diagnosis of sciatica: a comparison with radiculography, computed tomography and operative findings. Spine 5: 540–543

Tokuhashi Y, Satoh K, Funami S 1991 A quantitative evaluation of sensory dysfunction in lumbosacral radiculopathy. Spine 16: 1321–1328

Towme E B, Reichert F L 1931 Compression of the lumbosacral roots of the spinal cord by thickened ligamenta flava. Annals of Surgery 94: 327–336

Watanabe J, Tanaka H 1990 Identification of alpha-motor nerve fibre potentials in lumbar epidural space and its clinical significance. Spine 15: 1131–1137

Weinstein P R 1983 Diagnosis and management of lumbar stenosis. Clinical Neurosurgery 30: 677–697

Wilbourn A J 1992 The electromyographic examination. In: Rothman, Simeone (eds) The Spine. W.B. Saunders, Philadelphia

Williamson J B 1991 Percutaneous stimulation of the cauda equina. A new diagnostic method in spinal stenosis. Spine 16: 460–462

Wiltse L, Guyer R, Spencer C, Glenn W, Porter I 1984 Alar transverse process impingement of the L5 spinal nerve. (The far out syndrome). Spine 9: 31–41

17. Neurogenic claudication — its clinical presentation, differential diagnosis, pathology and management

The term 'claudication of the spinal cord' was first used by DeJerine (1911) when describing three patients with claudication symptoms but normal peripheral pulses. Van Gelderen (1948) reported a patient with symptoms of lumbar root compression which appeared on walking and were relieved by rest, which he thought was due to thickening of the ligamentum flavum. Bergmark (1950) described 'intermittent spinal claudication', attributing a neurospinal origin to the walking pains of two patients. It was Verbiest in 1954 who recognized that structural narrowing of the vertebral canal could compress the cauda equina and produce claudication symptoms, and since that time there have been numerous publications on the subject (Gathier 1959, Brish et al 1964, Dyck & Doyle 1977, Bowen et al 1978, Blau & Logue 1978, Porter 1986).

CLINICAL PRESENTATION

History

This intriguing syndrome usually affects men over 50 years of age who have been heavy manual workers. They complain of discomfort in the legs when walking affecting both legs equally or one alone, usually in the thighs, calves and feet. Bilateral symptoms occur with a male to female ratio of 8 to 1, whilst the ratio in unilateral claudication is 3 to 1. Describing the discomfort is difficult, but they describe the legs as feeling 'heavy' or 'tired', as though it is difficult to drag one leg after another. One man says his legs felt like those of a deep sea diver, another as though he had cricket pads on his legs (Table 17.1).

There is usually a threshold distance when the discomfort develops, and a tolerance distance when the patient has to stop walking, and the tolerance is about twice the threshold. The distance can vary during the day, from one day to the next, and even during one stretch of walking. The second period of walking can be longer than the first after a short rest. Often the patient gradually reduces the walking speed and stoops forwards until they finally stop — the stoop test (Dyck 1979). They will lean forwards on a wall, or stoop forwards and tie up a shoelace to save embarrassment, and after a few minutes the feeling in the legs recovers sufficiently for them to start walking again. The flexed position seems to relieve the discomfort and for that reason they may be able to walk better up a hill leaning forwards, than down a hill leaning back. Extending the spine in the standing position can precipitate symptoms in the severely disabled patient. They may be able to cycle for miles and climb a ladder and stairs, but not come down stairs easily. As the condition progresses, the walking distance reduces sometimes to only 20 yards, but inability to walk at all is uncommon. It is probably not neurogenic claudication if a man can walk more than a mile at a reasonable pace without having to stop. Some patients complain of mild leg symptoms even at rest, but for the majority rest will relieve the discomfort.

Nights are usually troublesome, with sleep being disturbed by restless legs and night cramps, and

Table 17.1 Symptoms of neurogenic claudication.

No significant leg pain at rest
Pain in one and/or both legs walking
Symptoms above and below the knee
Walking limited to less than 500 m
History of back pain

they will often get up and walk about at night. Back pain is a common but not an invariable accompaniment. There is usually a long history of back pain, sometimes with previous surgery, and claudication symptoms for a number of years before they seek help.

EXAMINATION

Apart from the spinal posture, the examination is remarkable for its lack of gross abnormality. The patient may be able to flex well forward with extended knees though lumbar extension is usually absent. In fact, it may be difficult to even stand erect and these patients adopt a 'simian stance' (Simkin 1982), with hips and knees slightly flexed (Fig. 17.1). This can be corrected with an effort, but it quickly returns as they relax. If this posture is not present at rest, it tends to develop with walking, the patient gradually stooping further

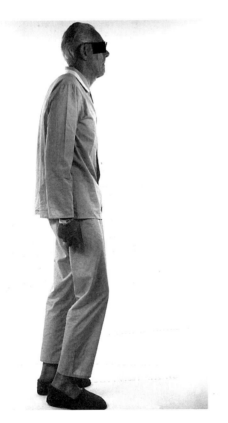

Fig. 17.1 The typical posture of a patient with neurogenic claudication, standing with flexed hips and knees in the simian stance.

Table 17.2   Signs of neurogenic claudication.

A simian stance
No spinal extension
Treadmill walking less than 500 m
Stoop forwards at the end of walking

forward until be has to stop. As claudication symptoms develop, the centre of gravity moves forwards. It recedes after each period of rest, but takes longer to return to its initial position than it takes for symptoms to settle (Hanai et al 1988). The 'stoop test' makes use of this phenomenon in diagnosing claudication of neurogenic origin, the leg symptoms being relieved by stooping forwards at the point of walking tolerance, and returning by standing upright again (Table 17.2).

The lumbar spine is often tender over several segments. Straight leg raising is generally full, the reflexes normal, the power and sensation also normal. Re-examination after exercise may alter the neurological examination. The peripheral circulation can be normal, but not infrequently arterial disease will coexist.

INVESTIGATION

A treadmill enables us to establish an objective record of walking pain, noting the speed of walking, the distance at which symptoms develop, the distribution of discomfort, the changing posture and the tolerance (Fig. 17.2). The impression gained from the patient's history can be completely different from an objective assessment of walking. When measuring a response to treatment, a treadmill is invaluable.

A plain X-ray may raise the suspicion of a shallow vertebral canal and perhaps show a degenerative spondylolisthesis, present in half the men with neurogenic claudication. When degenerative spondylolisthesis occurs with claudication, the symptoms are normally bilateral. Half of the patients with unilateral claudication have a structural lumbar scoliosis.

The lack of space in the central canal can make injection of the contrast medium very difficult, and the myelogram may have to be abandoned at the lower lumbar level (Williams 1975, Ehni 1969). Myelography alone provides insufficient

Table 17.3   Imaging of neurogenic claudication.

Plain X-ray:	degenerative change, degenerative spondylolisthesis or lumbar scoliosis
Myelogram:	'canal full of roots', multiple level stenosis
CT:	central canal less than 70 mm^2; coexistent root canal stenosis
MRI:	central canal stenosis, root canal stenosis

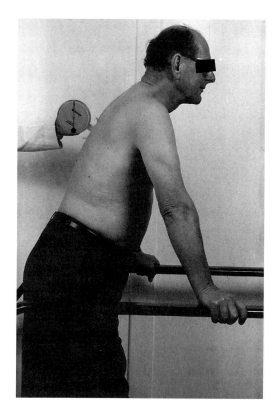

Fig. 17.2   A treadmill provides an objective method of assessing the speed, posture and walking distance.

information about the multiple nature of the stenosis and, if MRI is not available, CT should be used to image the root canals. It also demonstrates the canal's mid-sagittal diameter, cross-sectional area and shape. The CT scan must examine a longer segment of canal than the standard L4 to S1 for disc problems, increasing the radiation dose, but this is outweighed by its advantages. Bony encroachment, thickened ligamentum flavum and disc material may be evident, and the extent of undercutting facetectomy can be predicted (Table 17.3).

Ultrasound measurement can be used as a simple non-invasive method of confirming a reduced mid-sagittal diameter of the vertebral canal. Of patients with neurogenic claudication, 57% had measurement below the 10th percentile and 42% below the 5th percentile (Porter et al 1978). A narrow canal on ultrasound supports the diagnosis, but narrow canals exist without neurogenic claudication symptoms. A wide canal is incompatible with the diagnosis.

Doppler studies of the peripheral circulation are advisable. Somatosensory evoked potentials are useful if the diagnosis is in doubt.

DIFFERENTIAL DIAGNOSIS

Differential diagnosis of neurogenic claudication must include the following:

- Intermittent claudication, a phrase coined by Charcot in 1858 to describe ischaemic pain from peripheral vascular disease, is difficult to distinguish from neurogenic claudication by the history alone. It is not affected by posture, and the patient does not find himself stooping forwards the further he walks. We might expect the patient with intermittent claudication to have more difficulty climbing hills than descending them, and to find cycling the same problem as walking. However, the converse is not always true for neurogenic claudication. The bicycle test of Van Gelderen (1948), modified by Dyck and Doyle (1977), may help to differentiate between these two types of claudication. The patient is asked to cycle with the spine first extended and then flexed. The distance is the same in intermittent claudication, whilst in neurogenic claudication the flexed position allows greater exercise tolerance (Fig. 17.3). Only 30% of our patients with neurogenic claudication moderately improved their cycling distance by stooping forwards (Fig. 17.4), and this was therefore not a very sensitive discriminator between the two types of claudication (Dong & Porter 1989). Neurogenic claudication generally affects the entire leg, whilst intermittent claudication may only involve the calf or thigh. These, however, are

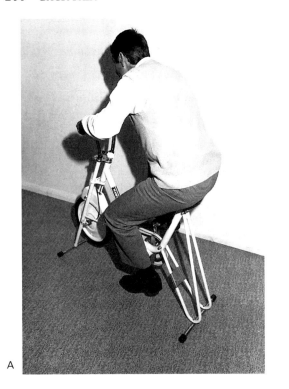

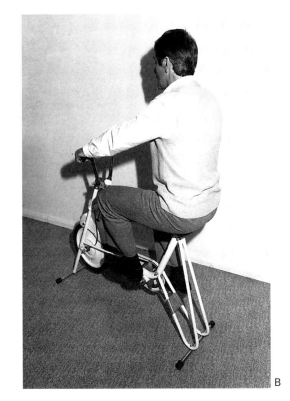

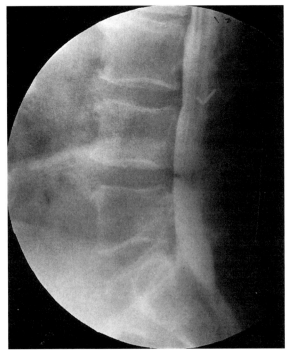

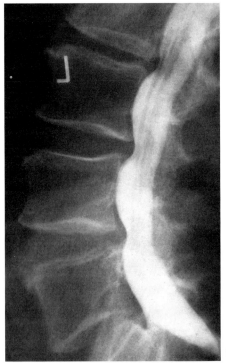

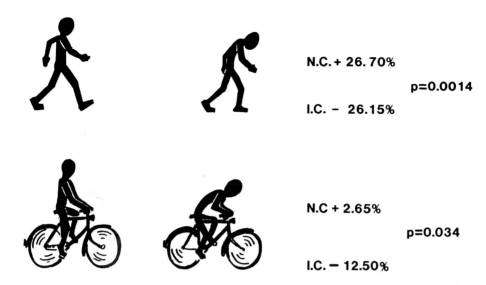

N.C. + 26.70%

p=0.0014

I.C. − 26.15%

N.C + 2.65%

p=0.034

I.C. − 12.50%

Fig. 17.4 The percentage difference of the median walking and cycling tolerance as a result of flexing forwards in 19 patients with neurogenic claudication and 11 patients with intermittent claudication. Posture significantly affected the tolerance in neurogenic claudication, but not in all patients.

generalizations, and in practice the difference between the two is not always straightforward. Impalpable peripheral pulses and femoral bruits will suggest peripheral vascular disease. It clinical examination is difficult a Doppler scan may be more objective, but an arteriogram may be necessary to be certain of the relative importance of the peripheral arterial circulation. Cerebral somatosensory evoked potentials after walking may help to differentiate neurogenic from vascular intermittent claudication (Larson & Milwaukee 1983). To confuse the issue, spinal stenosis and peripheral vascular disease often coexist (Johansson et al 1982).

- Lamberton and colleagues (1983) described sciatic claudication, an insufficiency of the inferior gluteal artery producing ischaemia of the sciatic nerve and claudication in a sciatic distribution. The claudication is in a root distribution but spinal examination and myelography are normal. It is an important condition to recognize. Endarterectomy of the aorto-iliac segments can relieve the symptoms whilst an arterial graft, by disturbing the inferior gluteal artery and its anastomoses, will be ineffective.

- Referred pain from the lower lumbar region in the buttocks and thighs, even to the upper calves can be aggravated by walking. Of Crock's patients with isolated lumbar disc resorption (Venner & Crock 1981), 18% had increasing leg pain or paraesthesia on walking distances up to 500 yards. We can recognize referred pain from its proximal distribution (not beyond the upper calves) and its presence in activities other than walking. In addition, walking long distances, though painful, may not be impossible. Normal MRI or a normal myelogram is compatible with referred pain, but not with neurogenic claudication. An unstable isthmic spondylolisthesis may give pain in the back referred into the thighs when walking, mimicking neurogenic claudication.

Fig. 17.3(A) (facing page) A patient with neurogenic claudication may be able to cycle without pain if the spine is flexed.
(B) Symptoms develop in the legs when the patient with neurogenic claudication cycles in the upright position. The symptoms of intermittent claudication are not altered by changing posture.
(C) A lateral myelogram of a claudicating patient with the spine flexed.
(D) Lateral myelogram with extended spine.

Stenosis is uncommon, however, because as the vertebra has displaced forwards the floating lamina has been left behind, widening the canal.

- Some types of root pain and multiple root pathology are made worse by walking (Jayson & Nelson 1979), probably when segmental instability is a factor in producing the root symptoms. There may be little pain at rest, but walking aggravates unilateral leg pain with a variable threshold and tolerance. The patient whose root entrapment syndrome is caused by a degenerative pars defect in isthmic spondylolisthesis, may have root pain aggravated by walking. This is not neurogenic claudication and a fusion to prevent segmental movement may relieve symptoms more effectively than decompressing the canal.
- Claudication pain is sometimes a symptom of distress. Abnormal behaviour patterns are common in patients who have a long history of back pain, and pain in the legs when walking is not infrequently a symptom inappropriate to the underlying organic problem in the spine. There are usually inappropriate signs also.

Mrs JM, a 45-year-old housewife, complained of pain in both legs when walking which had gradually developed over the past 5 years, limiting her walking distance to 30 yards. She had no previous history of back pain, but did have back pain now, interfering with housework. She found climbing stairs and going up a slope difficult. She slept fairly well. She was a little overweight. She found it difficult to get up from a chair and walked across the room slowly and awkwardly. Flexion and extension of the lumbar spine were both somewhat limited. Reflexes and motor power were normal. She had bounding peripheral pulses. There were six inappropriate signs. Axial loading and simulated rotation both gave pain in the lower lumbar region. There was widespread tenderness, discomfort to light squeezing of the lumbar skin, straight leg raising was resisted and there was non-dermatomal sensory loss. Ultrasound measurements of the vertebral canal were below the 10th percentile and, lest a genuine spinal stenosis was missed, she had a myelogram. It was normal. She was told that there was no evidence of a serious disorder causing her symptoms, that she would get better rather than worse, but she wept at the thought of not being offered an operation.

- It is difficult to accurately assess the claudicating patient who also has a litigation problem.

One can exclude a peripheral vascular lesion and, if the myelogram is normal, neurogenic claudication. An equivocal myelogram is a problem, especially as symptomless pathology is so common (Boden et al 1990). Although the diagnosis would be suspect with a number of inappropriate signs, these may mask a genuine underlying problem. Litigation can so confuse the issue that it may not be possible to decide how much of the symptoms are organic, and whether the organic element of the leg pain is neurogenic claudication, multiple root pathology or referred pain.

- There are other less common causes of claudication pain. Venous claudication can follow thrombosis before the collateral circulation takes over, the increased venous pressure affecting the perfusion pressure. The pain brought on by exercise is only relieved as the leg is elevated.
- Myxoedema claudication results from the limited potential of muscle to increase its metabolism with exercise. Pulses are normal. Symptoms are completely relieved by treating the hypothyroidism.
- Multiple sclerosis can mimic neurogenic claudication (Varty et al 1991).
- Rarely a localized deep arteriovenous fistula will present with aching and pain in the legs aggravated by exercise and standing. The muscle cannot respond to exercise by significantly increasing its arterial flow. Usually congenital or acquired fistulae demonstrate swelling, a bruit, distal venous insufficiency and hemihypertrophy in the young.
- It is not difficult to recognize degenerative changes of the weight-bearing joints as a cause of ambulatory leg pain.

PATHOLOGY

Spinal stenosis

Verbiest (1954) recognized that neurogenic claudication was associated with a shallow vertebral canal. In fact the term 'spinal stenosis' has unfortunately become synonymous with neurogenic claudication, when a shallow canal is only one factor in the pathology, and spinal stenosis can be an important factor in other back pain syndromes. Symptoms of claudication develop after middle life but there is no evidence that the vertebral canal becomes much narrower with age. There can be a little encroachment into the canal (both into the root canal and the central canal) from hypertrophy of the apophyseal joints and marginal osteophyte formation. Also, posterior vertebral bar formation on the lower and upper posterior margins of the vertebral bodies can reduce the sagittal diameter to some degree. In general, however, the central canal retains the same cross-sectional diameter throughout life.

An individual with spinal stenosis and neurogenic claudication has, therefore, had a narrow canal for many years before the development of leg symptoms (Salibi 1976, Ami Hood & Weigl 1983, Critchley 1982), and many patients with stenotic canals never have claudication pain. MRI studies of asymptomatic subjects over 60 years of age show spinal stenosis in 21% (Boden et al 1990). The canal is therefore but one factor in the pathology.

Degenerative disease

A second factor is degenerative disease of the lumbar spine associated with manual work. The majority of patients with neurogenic claudication have been involved in heavy work; few have been sedentary workers. It would seem that the cumulative effects of the mechanical stress of labouring work play a part in multiple-segment pathology, rather than the degenerative process from one disc insult in the earlier life of a sedentary worker. The high male incidence may be due to heavier manual work, or may indicate that hormonal factors are significant. Thickening of the ligamentum flavum (Schönström & Hansson 1991) or ossification (Kurihara et al 1988, Miyamoto et al 1992) may be responsible for stenosis. It can occur in vertebral hyperostosis, and in Paget's disease (Weisz 1983).

Neurogenic claudication must be very unusual in children, but Birkensfield and Kasdon (1978) described it in two adolescent boys with con-

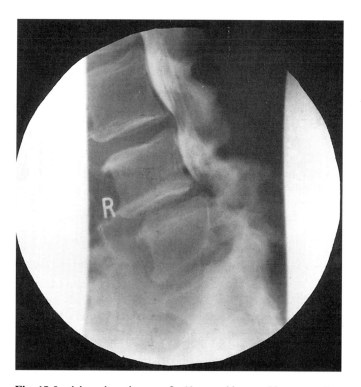

Fig. 17.5   A lateral myelogram of a 63-year-old man with neurogenic claudication showing partial occlusion at L3/4 and total occlusion at L4/5 where there is a degenerative spondylolisthesis.

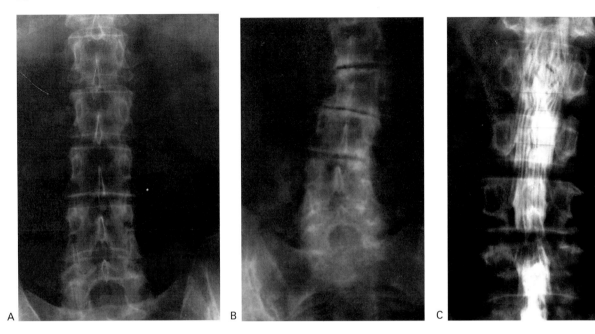

A   B   C

Fig. 17.6(A)   AP radiograph of a 47-year-old lady with back pain. **(B)**   The same patient 12 years later showing a marked degenerative lumbar scoliosis. **(C)**   A myelogram of the same patient showing spinal stenosis, a 'canal full of roots', subtotal occlusion at L3/4 and signs of venous congestion of the conus. (Fig 17.6 (A), (B) and (C) reproduced with the permission of Doncaster Royal Infirmary.)

genital lumbar ridges producing ventral defects on myelography.

Vertebral displacement

Vertebral displacement with an intact neural arch will critically narrow an already small canal (Fig. 17.5). Degenerative spondylolisthesis effectively reduces the canal size at the level of displacement (Rosenberg 1976, Wilson & Brill 1977). Although degenerative spondylolisthesis is more common in women, half of the men with neurogenic claudication in our series had a degenerative spondylolisthesis (Porter & Hibbert 1983). Women with degenerative spondylolisthesis rarely develop claudication symptoms (Fig. 17.6), but many patients with unilateral claudication and lumbar scoliosis are women. Displacement of a stenotic spine is therefore only one factor amongst many.

Abnormal nerve function

The neuropathology is probably the result of inadequate oxygenation or accumulation of me-

tabolites in the cauda equina. Nerve function is just adequate at rest, but inadequate during exercise. The effect of nerve compression has been extensively studied in animal experiments (Olmarker 1991, Rydevik et al 1991, Delmarter et al 1990), but how this is related to chronic stenosis and walking has so far been purely speculative.

Central stenosis at one level does not account for the symptoms

Although it is not possible to make the diagnosis of neurogenic claudication without central canal stenosis, there are a number of clinical reasons why central stenosis alone will not explain the mechanism. First, a steadily progressing spinal tumour can completely block the central vertebral canal without producing claudication. Second, a large central disc protrusion can block the canal without claudication. Third, a single-level central stenosis from degenerative change at L3/4 or L4/5 may almost occlude the dural sac and yet produce only back pain. Furthermore, imaging of

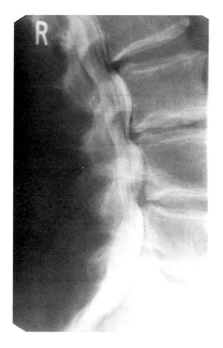 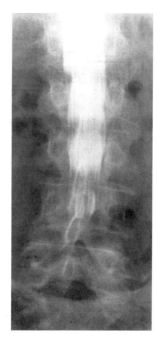 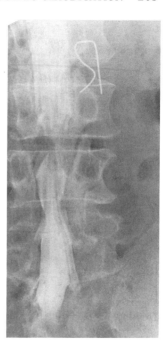

Fig. 17.7   (Left) A lateral myelogram showing the common multiple-level central canal stenosis, with partial filling defects at L2/3, L3/4 and L4/5.

Fig. 17.8   (Centre) A multiple-level occlusion, partial at L2/3, subtotal at L3/4, and total at L4/5 where there is a degenerative spondylolisthesis, in a 72-year-old man with only 3 years of back pain, and 18 months of bilateral claudication. He could walk only a few steps, and was mainly confined to a wheelchair.

Fig. 17.9   (Right) Subtotal occlusion at L3/4 and partial occlusion of the dural sac at L4/5 in a 56-year-old man. He had 18 years of low back pain, and 3 years of bilateral neurogenic claudication limiting walking to 60 m.

asymptomatic subjects confirms that stenosis is common, and patients who present with claudications must have had asymptomatic stenotic canals for many years. Again it is surprising that in canine studies, a single-level experimental stenosis constricted the cauda equina by 25% without causing neurological deficit (Delmarter et al 1990). In addition, one has to explain why claudicating patients frequently have multiple-level central stenosis and associated root canal stenosis.

Root canal stenosis

If central canal stenosis will not explain the symptoms of neurogenic claudication, can root canal stenosis be responsible? A number of authors have thought that root canal stenosis or foramina stenosis was important (Naylor 1979, Bose & Balasybramaniam 1984, Ciric et al 1980, Kirkaldy-Willis et al 1982). However, isolated stenosis of the root canal might be asymptomatic, or responsible for symptoms of root entrapment (Ch. 16). And if root canal pathology were important, why do patients with neurogenic claudication invariably have a central canal stenosis? It is now apparent that the pathophysiology of neurogenic claudication can only be explained in terms of multiple-level pathology.

Two-level low pressure stenosis — venous pooling

One of the radiological features of neurogenic claudication is the high frequency of multiple-level stenosis. We have examined the myelogram and CT studies of 50 patients with neurogenic claudication, and 47 had spinal stenosis at two or more levels (Porter & Ward 1992). There was either a two-level central stenosis (Figs 17.7, 17.8, 17.9, 17.10 and 17.11), or associated central and root canal stenosis (Fig. 17.12). Two

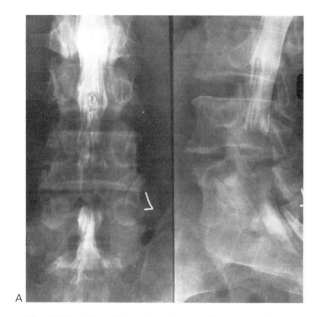
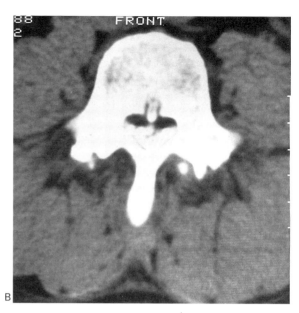

Fig. 17.19   AP and lateral myelogram of a 68-year-old man with bilateral neurogenic claudication, with a two-level stenosis (**A**). He had subtotal occlusion at L4/5 and partial occlusion at L3/4. The circular pattern at L3 is probably displaced contrast by the pressure of the extradural veins from the nutrient foramen at the back of the body of L3. This is suggested from the CT (**B**).

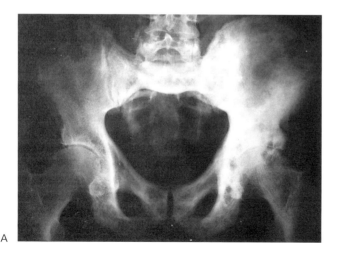
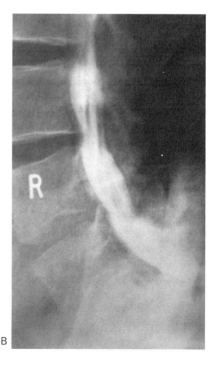

Fig. 17.20   A pelvic X-ray of a 72-year-old man with Paget's disease (**A**), reproduced with the permission of Doncaster Royal Infirmary) and coexistent spinal stenosis (**B**). Not only was back pain relieved with calcitonin, but walking distance was improved.

intramuscularly four times a week for 4 weeks. If the walking distance has not improved by the 4th week the drug is discontinued, but if there is some improvement the regimen is continued for a further 4 weeks (Fig. 17.21). Calcitonin engenders a sense of well-being, and undoubtedly some patients experience a placebo response. Some become almost euphoric at their ability to walk unlimited distances again. We do not usually continue the drug beyond 8 weeks. Some have relapsed, and others have maintained progress after cessation of the drug (Porter & Hibbert 1983).

We have found this a useful first line of treatment. The responders avoid a surgical decompression and the non-responders, although content to have had a course of injections, may decline surgery. A return of claudicating symptoms after a previous decompression is not a contraindication for calcitonin. We have observed no serious side-effects, but would withhold the drug from women of child-bearing age.

The mechanism of response to calcitonin, if not placebo, is probably vascular. Most who respond do so at about 2 weeks; this is too rapid to be due to remodelling of bone, and too slow to be an analgesic response. Canal measurements using ultrasound have not shown any increase in diameter in 16 responding patients with neurogenic claudication, nor in three patients whose Paget's paraparesis recovered with calcitonin (Douglas et al 1981). Likewise, a response in postoperative patients who have relapsed after a previous decompression is not likely to be due to bony remodelling. Calcitonin reduces skeletal blood flow (Wooton et al 1981). Venous blood drains from the vertebral bodies into Batson's extradural plexus and, if this is reduced, the neural elements will enjoy more space. Furthermore, myeloscopy shows vasodilatation of the vessels of the cauda equina 10 minutes after calcitonin injection. In patients with neurogenic

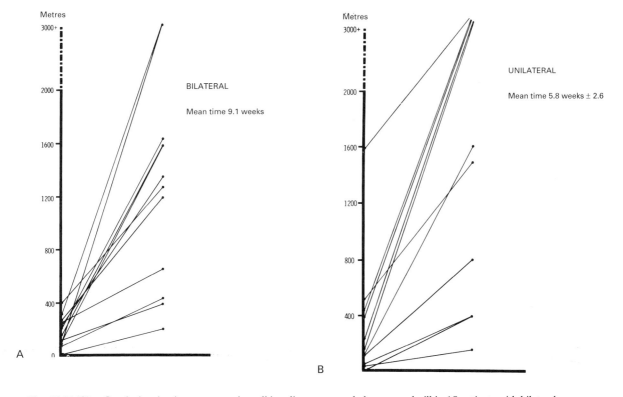

Fig. 17.21(A) Graph showing improvement in walking distance recorded on a treadmill in 15 patients with bilateral neurogenic claudication after treatment with calcitonin. **(B)** Similar results for patients with unilateral claudication.

claudication, micro-Doppler studies show a decreased blood flow when walking which improves after calcitonin injection (Ooi et al 1990b). We are not yet able to explain why only a proportion of patients respond to calcitonin.

Surgery

If symptoms of claudication are sufficiently severe they are generally relieved by surgical decompression (Verbiest 1977, Park et al 1981). Most patients are immediately impressed with the improved sensation in their legs and are soon walking long distances. However, many relapse as a laminectomy membrane of fibrous tissue develops over the posterior dura. Their walking distance again becomes reduced. Verbiest recorded that 70 out of 74 of his patients with neurogenic claudication were relieved by decompression (1977) and this probably depends on careful patient selection and adequate decompression. Russin and Sheldon (1976) likewise record excellent long-term follow-up results with decompression for stenotic symptoms, but back pain is the most common persisting problem (Getty 1980). There is evidence that the results deteriorate with time (Katz et al 1991, Johnsson et al 1991). Advanced age is no contraindication to decompression; it will often improve the quality of life for the elderly (Ami Hood & Weigl 1983). Some results are less satisfactory and in these it is claimed that decompression was less than adequate, that epidural scarring spoilt the results, or that longstanding ischaemia of the nerve roots became irreversible.

Most operative series have a hard core of failures, and there are few patient characteristics that will predict outcome (Turner et al 1992). A year after decompression, 15% of our patients were completely free of symptoms, 55% were improved but still had some walking pain, and 30% were no better. We tend to offer surgical decompression, therefore, to those patients who have not responded to calcitonin and to those most severely disabled. About half of the patients not responding to calcitonin will prefer to accept their walking limitations and live with them rather than submit to a spinal operation. The rest will accept a surgical remedy.

The spinal decompression must be adequate (Schatzker & Pennal 1968, Wiltse et al 1976). It must extend sufficiently proximal to permit a free flow of cerebrospinal fluid to the distal cauda equina and it must be sufficiently lateral to ensure that there is no occlusion of the nerve roots. It usually involves operating on three laminae, sometimes two, and occasionally four. A wide fenestration, removing only the medial parts of the inferior facets and adjoining ligamentum flavum, seems to be as effective as a total laminectomy (Nakai et al 1991). There is conflicting evidence about the extent of decompression. In one study, one- or two-level decompression for localized segmental stenosis gave better long-term results than a more extensive three-, four- or five-level decompression for multi-level disease (Grabias 1980). In another, the results of multiple-level decompression were better than one- or two-level surgery (Katz et al 1991).

The canal will have been narrow for years prior to the development of symptoms, and although there may be stenosis at multiple levels the symptomatic pathology is probably localized to two levels. The operative dilemma is to ensure that these critical segments are effectively decompressed. One tends to rely upon an intraoperative clinical impression that the tight dura and roots are given adequate space, and on the grounds of safety one may at times be more radical than is necessary. Somatosensory evoked potentials may have a place as an intraoperative diagnostic aid in determining the extent of decompression (Kiem et al 1984).

If there is degenerative spondylolithesis, it is essential not to increase the instability of that segment unnecessarily (Lin 1982). Forward postoperative displacement is unusual even with wide decompression provided there is marked degenerative change, but one should be cautious if degeneration is minimal (Grabias 1980, Shenkin & Has 1976). The integrity of the apophyseal joints should not be unduly disturbed, though the medial third of the joint must often be removed and the facet undercut. It is necessary to perform a decompression wide enough to ensure a completely free dura (Wiltse et al 1976), but not so wide as to produce either instability or such a shallow spinal gutter that a laminectomy membrane will soon compress the dura to a ribbon.

Provided there is not degenerative spondylolisthesis, it is legitimate to sacrifice the major part of the apophyseal joint on one side in order to obtain satisfactory decompression, and not jeopardize stability. When there is a degenerative spondylolisthesis and minimal degenerative change, and always in the presence of a stenosis with structural lumbar scoliosis, decompression should be accompanied by a lateral spinal fusion. Fusion is also essential when decompressing an osteoporotic patient.

If the symptoms are due to a two-level stenosis, it should be necessary to decompress only one of the levels in order to relieve the claudication. However, it would be inadequate to decompress only the central canal of the most stenotic segment if in fact root canal stenosis at this level was responsible for the distal stenosis, and there was a proximal central canal stenosis still left untreated. A double-level hypothesis, therefore has considerable surgical implications.

A fat graft applied over the decompressed dura reduces the risk of postoperative fibrous compression (Bryant et al 1983, Nussbaum et al 1990). Other materials tested both experimentally and clinically are no more effective than fat, and some produce more scar than controls (Boot & Hughes 1987). To ensure that the fat survives and is revascularized, it is applied as thin postage stamp-sized grafts rather than one large cube of fat. This is obtained from the subcutaneous layer at the operation site, but in thin men it may have to be dissected from a separate buttock incision. One should obliterate 'dead space' and secure haemostasis.

Patients are pleased to be mobilized early; they know immediately that they are better and it is difficult to restrain them. They find their own limitations and many remain highly satisfied.

REFERENCES

Ami Hood S, Weigl K 1983 Lumbar spinal stenosis: surgical intervention for the older person. Israel Journal of Medical Sciences 19: 169–171

Bergmark 1950 Intermittent spinal claudication. Acta Medica Scandinavica 246 (Suppl): 30

Birkensfield R, Kasdon D L 1978 Congenital lumbar ridge causing spinal claudication in adolescents. Journal of Neurosurgery 49: 441–444

Blau J N, Logue V 1978 The natural history of intermittent claudication of the cauda equina. Brain 101: 211–222

Blau J N, Rushworth G 1958 Observations of blood vessels of the spinal cord and their responses to motor activity. Brain 81: 354–363

Boden S D, Davis D O, Dina T S, Patronas N J, Weisel S W 1990 Abnormal magnetic resonance scans of the lumbar spine in asymptomatic subjects. A positive investigation. Journal of Bone and Joint Surgery 72-A: 403–408

Boot D A, Hughes S P F 1987 The prevention of adhesions after laminectomy: adverse results of zenoderm implantations onto laminectomy sites in rabbits. Clinical Orthopaedics 215: 296–307

Bose K, Balasybramaniam P 1984 Nerve root canals of the lumbar spine. Spine 9: 16–18

Bowen V, Shannan R, Kirkcaldy-Willis W H 1978 Lumbar spinal stenosis. Child's Brain 4: 257–277

Brish A, Lerner M B, Braham J 1964 Intermittent claudication from compression of the cauda equina by a narrowed spinal canal. Journal of Neurosurgery 21: 207–211

Bryant M S, Bomer A M, Nguyon J Q 1983 Autogenic fat transplants in the epidural space in routine lumbar spine surgery. Neurosurgery 13: 367–370

Buchtal F 1949 Problems of the pathologic physiology of poliomyelitis. American Journal of Medicine 6: 587–591

Charcot J M C 1858 Sur la claudication intermittente observee dans un cas d'obliteration complete de l'une des arteres iliaques primitives. Comptes Rendu Soc Biol 10: 225–238

Ciric L, Michael A, Mikhael M D, Tarkington J A, Vick N A 1980 The lateral recess syndrome. A variant of spinal stenosis. Journal of Neurosurgery 53: 433–443

Critchley E M R 1982 Lumbar spinal stenosis. British Medical Journal 284: 1588–1589

DeJerine J 1911 La claudication intermittente de la molle epiniere. Presse Medicale 19: 981

Delmarter R B, Bohlman H H, Dodge L D, Biro C 1990 Experimental lumbar spinal stenosis. Journal of Bone and Joint Surgery 72-A: 110–120

Dong G X, Porter R W 1989 Walking and cycling tests in neurogenic and intermittent claudication. Spine 14: 965–969

Douglas D L, Duckworth T, Kanis J A, Jefferson A A, Martin T J, Russell R G G 1981 Spinal cord dysfunction in Paget's disease of bone: has medical treatment a vascular basis? Journal of Bone and Joint Surgery 63-B: 495–503

Dyck P 1979 The stoop-test in lumbar entrapment radiculography. Spine 4: 89–92

Dyck P, Doyle J B 1977 'Bicycle test' of Van Gelderen in diagnosis of intermittent cauda equina compression syndrome. Journal of Neurosurgery 46: 667–670

Ehni G 1969 Significance of the small lumbar spinal canal cauda equina compression syndromes due to spondylosis. Journal of Neurosurgery 31: 490–494

Gathier J C 1959 A case of absolute stenosis of the lumbar vertebral canal in adults. Acta Neurochirurgica (Wein) 7: 344–349

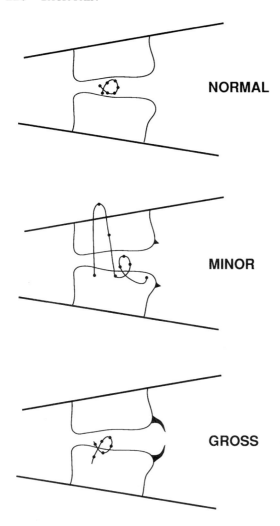

Fig. 18.2 Diagram showing that a healthy disc has a small uniform centrode (top). Early disc degeneration is associated with a long irregular centrode (middle), and further degeneration improves stability, reducing the length of the centrode (bottom).

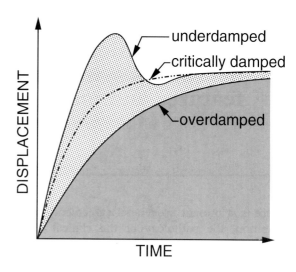

Fig. 18.3 Figure showing that a critically damped system displaces in a smooth manner, an overdamped system displaces slowly and perhaps incompletely, whilst an underdamped system displaces in a jerky manner (Hukins 1988).

tissues might be expected to contribute enough damping to produce smooth spinal motion in the three planes of rotation. Inadequate damping will produce an overswing, with irregular movement (Fig. 18.3). Instability, defined as a failure of damping, considers the spine as a whole and not necessarily excessive or erratic movement in any one motion segment.

Jerky or irregular movements of the spine as a whole can occur with healthy non-degenerate discs if, say, inadequate neuromuscular control fails to damp motion. Such jerky movements can occur in a nervous convalescing patient with healthy discs but with poor muscle control. The overswing of an extension catch may be a failure of damping, caused by a variety of soft tissue pathologies including poor neuromuscular control, fatigue (Roy et al 1989), generalized neuromuscular control, as well as early segmental degeneration. This concept of instability also explains why some patients climb up their legs when rising from the stooped position, or hold onto their knees when rising from a chair. The extra support improves the damping on an unstable spine, and hypertrophied muscle may be an attempt to compensate for inadequate damping.

PATHOLOGY

It follows from the biocmechanical definition of instability that there is uncertainty about the pathology responsible for symptoms. Even when pain is clearly associated with excessive or erratic movement of one segment, and when the disc is degenerate and the apophyseal joints hypertrophic, the source of pain still remains speculative. It may be in the pain-sensitive nerves of the outer annulus, or from abnormal nerve endings which invade the degenerate disc causing a pain-sensitive disc. Alternatively, the capsule of the apophyseal joint or the musculoligamentous structure of the segment could be a pain source. When the vertebral canal is small, the tight dura may be sensitive to segmental motion.

If the spine rather than the segment is unstable, the disc may be normal, with no degenerative change of the vertebra or facets, whilst the soft tissues are pathologically inadequate to dampen spinal motion. Soft tissues can be inadequate with an isthmic defect in the pars interarticularis; when spina bifida occulta is associated with congenitally deficient soft tissues; and when muscles are weakened through disuse. These problems are compounded by injury and in pregnancy (Svensson et al 1990, Ostgaard & Andersson 1992) from the effect of the hormone 'relaxin'.

Spina bifida occulta has too long been thought an innocuous condition unrelated to back pain, but it may be an important factor in instability. The prevalence of spina bifida occulta in patients attending a back pain clinic is no greater than in the general population, but when examining the prevalence in specific back pain syndromes, it is apparent that some syndromes have a significantly lower prevalence of spina bifida, and others a high prevalence. We have found that patients with root pathology syndromes — disc protrusion, root entrapment from lateral stenosis and neurogenic claudication — have a low incidence of spina bifida (6, 5 and 3%, respectively). The nerves may be protected because of a wider canal that is associated with spina bifida (Sand 1970, Porter et al 1991). However, patients with instability criteria and back pain without leg pain have a high prevalence of spina bifida (47%). The soft tissues are probably deficient as well as the bony neural arch, and there may be poor neuromuscular control predisposing to instability.

We have already stated that a displaced vertebra is not the same as 'instability'. A degenerative spondylolisthesis may have started with a mildly degenerative unstable L4/5 disc, but further degenerative change may restore stability. However, a lumbar scoliosis with rotatory displacement seems to remain unstable. The degenerative change is incapable of keeping pace with the increasing forces of rotatory displacement. Structural scoliosis in the elderly frequently remains unstable, progressive and painful.

Defects of the pars interarticularis are not necessarily unstable. Fibrous union across the defect and compensatory strengthening of the soft tissues can maintain stability. Marked displacement can occur in children and adolescents which is quite compatible with stability. However, the defect can weaken and the soft tissues then fail to prevent excessive or erratic movement.

SYMPTOMS OF INSTABILITY

The typical patient with instability is a middle-aged women, a little obese, with chronic back pain which first began in pregnancy. She complains of back pain but not leg pain. It is worse when she is on her feet, relieved by rest, and aggravated by certain movements. X-rays might show a spina bifida occulta at L5 or S1 and a degenerative disc at L4/5. When standing up from the stooped position, the movement is jerky and erratic.

These symptoms that are associated with excessive unnatural or erratic movement should rightly be considered symptoms of instability; That is, either when a located or displaced vertebra deforms beyond the normal restraint and yet returns again to the predeformed state, or when the spine as a whole moves in a jerky manner. These symptoms are of two types.

Symptoms of fatigue in the structures which restrain shear or maintain damping

The posterior bony elements of the vertebral arch, with coronally orientated lower lumbar apophyseal joints, are the major restraining structures. When these fail, either by deficiency in the pars interarticularis or by disorganization of the apophyseal joints, the ligamentous and muscular structures are liable to fatigue (Ferguson 1933, Wyke 1980). This probably results in backache with or without referred pain round the pelvis or into the posterior thighs. It is aggravated by walking far, especially shopping if it involves standing, walking slowly and carrying. These patients cannot stand for long. They return home from shopping and either lie down for relief or rest in an easy-chair. The pain will then settle completely. Pain is aggravated by obesity, pregnancy and by being unfit.

Symptoms of minor subluxation — jerky movement

The pain source may be in apophyseal joints, in the ligamentous structures or in the dura. It is experienced as the deformed segment returns to the predeformation position in any one of the three axes of rotation, or when the spine as a whole has an overswing from failure of efficient damping, with stretching of pain-sensitive soft tissue. Typically, the patient reports discomfort when rising from the stooped position, or pain when getting out of a low chair (Fig. 18.4). They state that when getting up from sitting they have to support themselves by taking their weight with their hands on the arms of a chair, or on their knee.

The two types of instability symptoms, fatigue and momentary subluxation, may occur independently or may coexist. Patients with isthmic spondylolisthesis tend to have fatigue symptoms but not subluxation pain.

Symptoms of neurological compromise can occur with excessive movement of an unstable segment. Dural pain, root pain and neurogenic claudication are all more probable with excessive movement if there is pre-existing stenosis. Although instability may be a factor in these syndromes, neurological compromise is not truly a symptom of instability.

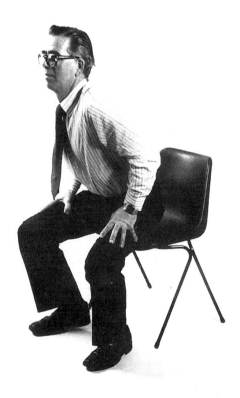 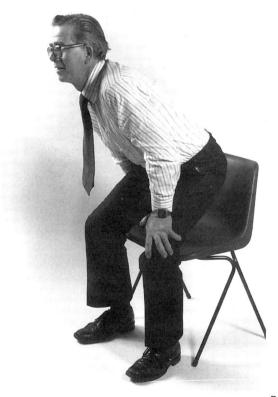

A
B

Fig. 18.4(A)   When rising from a chair, a patient with instability symptoms will flex the hips to move the centre of gravity over the feet. (**B**) He will then use his hands for support when standing upright.

SIGNS OF INSTABILITY

The paraspinal muscles may be hypertrophied, though this is certainly a very subjective sign (Fig. 9.7). Good paraspinal muscles may be present without instability, and obesity may mask muscle hypertrophy.

The patient with symptoms from an unstable lumbar spine frequently exhibits an exceptionally good range of forward flexion. Many can reach down to their toes with the knees straight, some to put their hands flat on the floor (combined straight leg raising and spinal flexion). As a group, their flexion is not better than the general population, but they are better than other patients with back pain (Table 19.2, page 236). Perhaps flexion is unimpaired because the

symptoms of instability are not related to the contents and space in the vertebral canal. Most other back pain syndromes restrict forward flexion, probably because the dura and the neural elements are involved as a factor in the symptomatology.

A patient with symptoms of momentary subluxation will have a classical pattern of spinal motion when standing up again from the stooped position. The normal smooth motion of the spine is broken by a sudden jerky movement, the extension catch. To prevent this, some patients will use their hands to support the spine as they stand up straight from the stooped posture, by 'climbing up their legs' (Fig. 18.5), or as they rise from a chair.

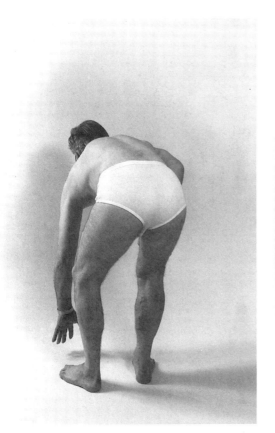
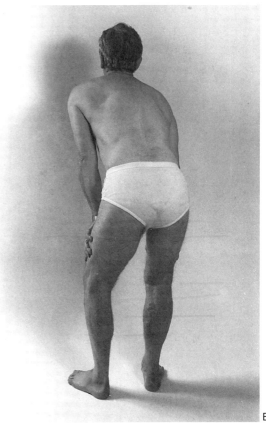

A

B

Fig. 18.5(A)   A patient with instability symptoms often has discomfort rising from the stooped position. (**B**) He will use his hands to 'climb up his legs' when rising from the stooped position.

RADIOLOGICAL FEATURES OF INSTABILITY

Instability symptoms are often associated with radiological changes. Disc space narrowing with traction spurs of the two adjacent vertebrae indicates that the segment is, or has been, unstable with excessive or erratic movement (Fig. 18.6) (Macnab 1971). A lytic pars is potentially unstable, but there may be fibrous union and not instability.

There is really no uniform agreement about the value of flexion and extension radiographs, partly because even good quality radiographs do not ensure accuracy of measurement (Fig. 18.7) (Schaffer et al 1990), and partly because the degree of segmental movement does not correlate with symptoms. Using conventional radiography, Mensor and Duvall (1959) and Hayes and colleagues (1989) found increased motion in a

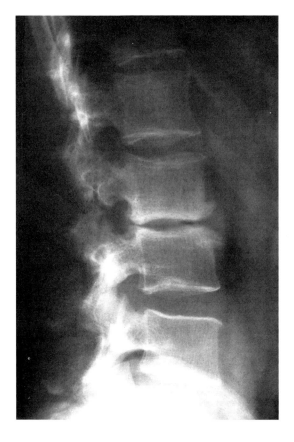

Fig. 18.6 A lateral radiograph showing marked disc degeneration at L2/3, with a reduced disc space, large traction spurs and posterior vertebral bars.

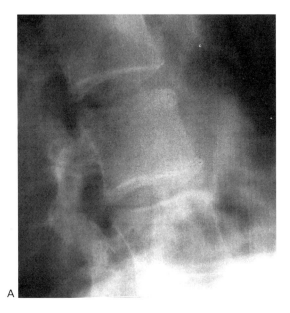

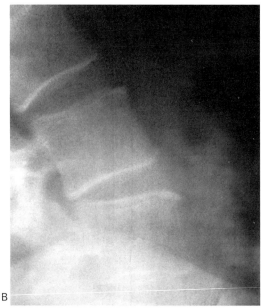

Fig. 18.7(A) Lateral radiograph of L3/4 disc space in flexion showing small traction spurs. (**B**) In extension there is the impression (difficult to quantify) of irregular segmental movement with some displacement of L3. Probably more unstable than patient in Fig. 18.6.

similar number of patients with and without back pain. Video radiographs are no more helpful. Stereoscopic radiography provides interesting information about segmental movement in health and disease but has yet to be applied to the clinically unstable back (Pearcy et al 1984). We need a measurement of dynamic motion rather than static vertebral positions (Boden & Wiesel 1990). Compression–traction radiography may have a place in assessing younger patients with instability symptoms (Friberg 1987, Kalebo et al 1990), but traction radiography might be hazardous for the older disabled patient.

Although the symptoms are not necessarily related to space within the vertebral canal, if space is restricted then unnatural segmental movement can compromise the canal's contents (Fig. 18.8). Neurological symptoms then coexist with instability, and flexion and extension views are helpful (Liyang et al 1989).

Segmental motion can be assessed in vivo by computer analysis of flexion radiographs of isolated segments, measuring transitional and angular components of motion. Patients with symptomatic degenerative disc disease have significantly more

segmental translation relative to angulation than do asymptomatic age-matched controls (Weiler et al 1990).

The divorce between biomechanical instability and symptoms results in a clinical dilemma. Excessive segmental movement may be symptomless, and mild instability troublesome. Typical symptoms may not be associated with any abnormal radiological changes at all, perhaps because in these patients the pathology is not in the discs or vertebrae, but in the soft tissues which fail to damp motion. Frequently, however, there are radiological features that match the symptoms and make 'instability' a recognizable back pain syndrome.

TREATMENT OF INSTABILITY

The severity of the symptoms, the degree of disturbance they produce in family and working life, the expectations of the patient — these will dictate the way in which the problem is managed.

Symptoms of fatigue which develop after standing, walking about and shopping may be either a mild intermittent nuisance or a severe

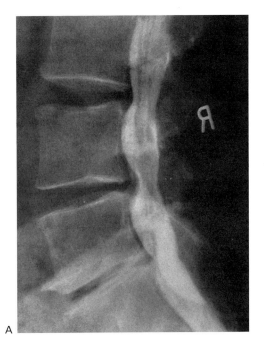
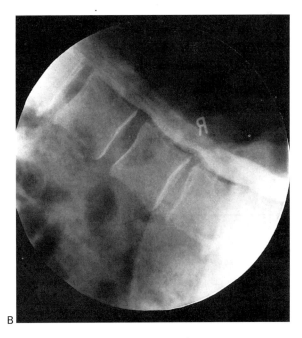

A

B

Fig. 18.8(A)   Lateral radiograph showing posterior dural displacement from a bulging L4/5 disc in extension.
(B) The same spine in flexion showing the dural bulge is largely abolished.

disability. Most patients are seeking a diagnosis and advice about their future prospects, and ways of making the discomfort manageable without resorting to surgery. The mechanism of the pain is easily described to the patient. Even though they cannot be promised a cure with the passage of time, it is usually possible to say that with care, the symptoms will probably not get worse. If the patient is obese, it is worth taking weight reduction seriously. Simple techniques like using a shopping trolley, not walking further than necessary, using a stick for longer distances, not standing too long and getting a high stool to perch on in the kitchen can be recommended; these are all ways to reduce the shear forces on the spine. The advice can be reinforced in a 'Back School' situation, reducing the level of apprehension about backache. The patient is advised to avoid stooping forward more than necessary and to avoid lifting in the stooped position. They may need to modify their working environment, and even change their job if that is practical. The 'Back School' situation is an ideal way to spend time with the patient, looking at their activities through a normal day. Many will be helped by wearing a lumbosacral corset intermittently, say at work or when shopping.

A more rigid jacket should be prescribed with caution. Although it can provide temporary relief of back pain, the muscular weakness which develops with such a support makes it counterproductive. A functional rehabilitation programme to improve fitness, strengthen muscles and soft tissues can be more productive.

Apart from the obese woman with degenerative spondylolisthesis and some patients with isthmic spondylolisthesis, the prognosis can be good. Many a subluxating unstable spine becomes stable as the spine stiffens with the years. Patients learn to avoid the movement that produces pain, and that arc of movement is eventually lost. The fact that instability symptoms peak in the fifth decade suggests that the problem lessens with time.

INDICATIONS FOR SURGERY

For a few, however, this reassurance is inadequate; occasionally the fatigue pain is of such intensity and duration that it interferes with normal life and surgery must be considered. If the segmental level of the pain source can be confidently identified, if movement causes pain and if a spinal fusion of that segment can be guaranteed, it should be possible to promise a cure. Surgical failure results from either making the wrong diagnosis, or from not obtaining a satisfactory fusion.

Fusion is the most popular operation for an unstable segment, but poor results have caused surgeons to seek other methods of surgical treatment. Ligamentous reinforcement with loops of Dacron (Graf 1991) attempts to provide temporary stabilization of the facet joints in lordosis permitting a measure of repair. The Dacron is secured under tension on pedicular screws. The maximum follow-up is limited at present, and we must await the long-term results.

Disc replacement (Fig. 18.9) also stems from a dissatisfaction with the late results of fusion (Brock et al 1991). Many prosthetic devices are under experimental development. Unjust comparisons are made with the success of hip and knee arthroplasty (Fairbank 1992), and a flexible disc neglects other pathologies in the three-joint complex (Deburge 1992). There is concern also about the long-term outcome of disc replacement, and fusion remains the operation of choice for a single abnormal symptomatic motion segment.

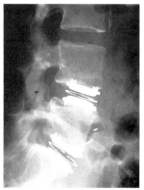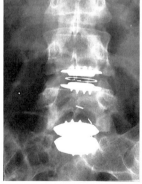

Fig. 18.9 Lateral and AP radiographs of disc replacements at L4/5 and L5/S1, which successfully relieved back pain in the short term for a patient who had previously had an unsuccessful discectomy.

Surgical assessment follows a logical sequence:

- *Is the diagnosis of segmental instability correct?* The patient may have an unstable spine rather than an unstable segment. They may be obese, with spina bifida occulta and poor neuromuscular control of the lower spine, without a single segment pathology.
- *Can the symptomatic segment be identified?* If the symptoms suggest that the back pain and referred pain originate from an unstable segment, and if this is supported by abnormal signs, further investigations may help. MRI will confirm disc degeneration but will not guarantee that it is the painful segment. Neither does an abnormal discogram mean this is the level of the nociception. Provocative discography simulating the distribution of pain does not guarantee that this is the pain source (Fig. 18.10).

One of the main problems with regard to fusing a spine for symptoms of instability is that one has presumptive evidence only about the pain source. Pain relief after applying an external fixator does not mean that fusion at that segment will be effective, and fixators are not without the complications of pin tract infection and nerve root damage. It is difficult to be sure of the painful segment, and a policy of random fusion for severe backache will only result in a hard core of failures.

- *Is the disability sufficiently severe, and has it persisted sufficiently long to make surgery worthwhile?* The majority of patients with instability who do not respond to conservative management have an isthmic spondylolisthesis and even these, if observed for a period of time, may respond to reducing spinal stress and a period in a corset.
- *Is there a possibility of exaggeration of the symptoms?* The surgeon is generally persuaded to operate because of the degree and persistence of the patient's symptoms, and therefore objective assessment of the disability is essential. Are there many inappropriate symptoms in addition to the back and referred pain? Are there inappropriate signs? What is the psychological profile? The results of surgery can be less than successful if there is evidence of exaggeration of the symptoms.
- *What is the state of the segment proximal to the proposed fusion segment?* A fusion should not be attempted unless the disc above the proposed

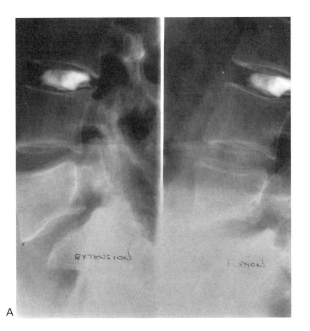
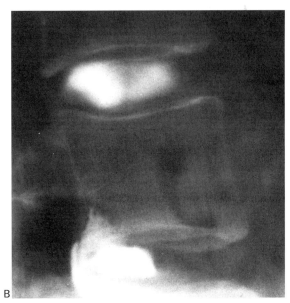

Fig. 18.10(A)   Lateral radiograph of a patient with an isthmic spondylolisthesis at L5 and excessive segmental motion at L4/5 on flexion and extension views. **(B)** A discogram of the same patient, showing an annular tear with painful posterior extravasation. This may be the symptomatic segment.

fusion can be shown to be normal by MRI, CT or discography. If degenerate, it could be the pain source or become a source of pain after the surgery. A more distal fusion will then add to the patient's problem, increasing that instability. The vertebral canal at the proximal end of the proposed fusion should also be of adequate dimensions. Even a normal segment proximal to the fusion could become unstable from the added stresses that will be applied to it (Kim et al 1991, Deburge 1992), and if the canal is already narrow, it could eventually cause stenosis symptoms.

Instability is a major cause of chronic low back pain. Fortunately only a minority fulfil the criteria for spinal fusion, which is discussed in Chapter 24.

REFERENCES

Boden S D, Wiesel W 1990 Lumbo sacral segmental motion in named individuals: have we been measuring instability properly. Spine 15(6): 571–576

Brock M, Mayer H M, Weigl K 1991 The artificial disc. Springer-Verlag

Deburge A 1992 Modern trends in spinal surgery. Journal of Bone and Joint Surgery 74-B: 6–8

Fairbank J 1992 The artificial disc. Review. Journal of Bone and Joint Surgery 74-B: 167

Farfan H G 1973 The mechanical disorders of the lower back. Lea and Febiger, Philadelphia

Ferguson A B 1933 The clinical and roentgenographic interpretation of lumbo-sacral anomalies. Radiology 22: 548–558

Friberg O 1987 Lumbar instability. A dynamic approach by traction–compression radiography. Spine 12: 119–129

Gertzbein S D, Seligman J V, Holtby R, Chen K H, Kapasouri A, Tile M, Cruickshank B 1985 Centrode patterns and segmental instability in degenerate disc disease. Spine 10: 256–261

Graf H 1991 Instabilite vertebrale. Traitment a l'aide d'un system souple. Rachis (in press)

Hayes M A, Harvard J C, Cruel C R, Kopta J A 1989 Roentgenographic evaluation of lumbar spine flexion–extension in asymptomatic individuals. Spine 14(3): 327–331

Hukins D W L 1990 Clinical signs and dynamics of segmental instability. In: Fairbank C T, Pynsent P B (eds) Back pain, classification of symptoms. Manchester University Press, Manchester, p 139–144

Kalebo P, Kadziolka R, Sward L 1990 Compression–traction radiography of lumbar segmental instability. Spine 15: 351–355

Kim Y E, Weinstein J N, Lim T 1991 Effect of disc degeneration on one level on the adjacent level in axial mode. Spine 16: 331–335

Liyang D, Yinkan X, Wenming Z, Zihua Z 1989 The effect of flexion–extension motion of the lumbar spine on the capacity of the spinal canal: an experimental study. Spine 14(5): 523–525

Macnab I 1971 The traction spur. Journal of Bone and Joint Surgery 53-A: 663–670

Mensor M C, Duvall G 1959 Absence of motion at the fourth and fifth lumbar interspaces in patients with and without low back pain. Journal of Bone and Joint Surgery 41-A: 1047–1054

Ostgaard H C, Andersson G B J 1992 Post partum low-back pain. Spine 17: 53–55

Pearcy M, Portek I, Shepherd J E 1984 Three dimension x-ray analysis of normal movement in the lumbar spine. Spine 9: 294–297

Pope N H, Panjabim M 1985 Biomechanical definitions of spinal instability. Spine 10: 255–256

Porter R W, Powers R, Pavitt D 1991 Vertebral changes proximal to spinal bifida occulta. An archaeological study with clinical significance. European Journal of Physiology, Medicine and Rehabilitation 4: 97–100

Roy S H, DeLuca C J, Casavant D A 1989 Lumbar muscle fatigue and chronic low back pain. Spine 14: 992–1001

Sand P G 1970 The human lumbo-sacral vertebral column: an osteometric study. Thesis, University of Oslo

Schaffer W O, Spratt K F, Weinstein J, Lehmann T R, Goel V 1990 The consistency and accuracy of roentgenograms for measuring sagittal translation in the lumbar vertebral motion segment: an experimental model. Spine 15: 741–750

Svensson H, Anderssen G J, Hegstal A, Janssen P 1990 The relationship of low back pain to pregnancy and gynaecological factors. Spine 15: 371–375

Weiler P J, King G T, Gertzbein S D 1990 Analysis of sagittal plane instability of the lumbar spine in vivo. Spine 15: 1300–1306

Wyke B D 1980 The neurology of low back pain. In: Jayson M I V (ed) The lumbar spine and back pain, 2nd edn. Pitman Medical, London, ch 11, p 265–339

19. Lysis of the pars interarticularis — pathology, identification of the defect, clinical significance and management

Lysis of the pars interarticularis is of great interest to clinicians treating back pain because it is assumed that such an obvious anatomical anomaly must have symptomatic significance. It is, however, a relatively common condition, frequently symptomless, with a variable prevalence amongst selected groups. Roche and Rowe (1951) carried out a large study of white skeletons and found an overall prevalence of bilateral lysis in 4.2% of 2300 skeletons, there being a male to female ratio of almost three to one. Studies in vivo have shown a greater prevalence in selected athletic groups, from 5 to 54% (Kono et al 1975, Troup 1975, Jackson et al 1976, Murray-Leslie et al 1977, Bird et al 1980, Hitoshi 1980, Hardcastle et al 1992).

CLASSIFICATION

Spondylolisthesis means the forward displacement of a proximal vertebra on a distal vertebra. There is much confusion about classification, but the most common cause is lysis of the pars interarticularis, with varying degrees of displacement. The pars may, however, be attenuated with no lysis. Displacement may result from acute fracture of the pars or fracture of any part of the neural arch. In degeneration spondylolisthesis, forward displacement occurs with an intact neural arch (Table 19.1). In this chapter we shall be discussing type I, lysis of the pars interarticularis.

PATHOLOGY OF LYSIS OF PARS INTERARTICULARIS

Lysis of the pars is more common at L5 than at L4 (Fig. 19.1). It is generally accepted that when lysis occurs it has a traumatic origin (Wiltse et al 1976, Cyron et al 1976), but some individuals may be constitutionally predisposed to develop a defect (Newman 1963, Farfan 1973, Fredrickson et al 1984). The existence of unilateral spondylolysis suggests that not all lytic defects result from trauma, though probably most of them do. The high incidence amongst the Eskimo races led Roche and Rowe (1951) to suspect that it was a congenital condition but they later modified their

Table 19.1 Classification of spondylolisthesis.

Classification	Spinal level	Aetiology
I Lysis of the isthmus of the pars interarticularis		
a. No vertebral displacement — spondylolysis	L5 (occasionally L4 or 3)	stress fracture
b. Moderate displacement — spondylolisthesis	L5 (occasionally L4 or 3)	stress fracture
c. Gross displacement — spondylolisthesis	L5	congenital defect
d. Unilateral spondylolysis (Ch. 20)	L5	congenital defect
II Attenuation of pars interarticularis — dysplastic	L5	dysplasia
III Acute fracture of the posterior elements		
a. Traumatic spondylolisthesis	any level	acute fracture
b. Pathological spondylolisthesis	any level	bone disease
IV Degenerative displacement, with intact neural arch, no dysplasia		
a. Degenerative spondylolisthesis (Ch. 21)	usually L4/5	inadequate restraint
b. Degenerative scoliosis (Ch. 22)	L2–5	not known

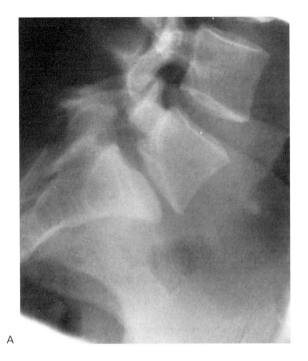 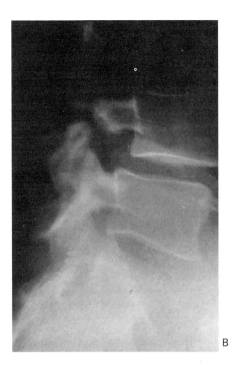

Fig. 19.1(A)   Lateral radiograph of a patient with lysis of the pars articularis at L5. **(B)** Lysis at L4.

views (1953) suggesting that certain postures adopted by the Eskimo may generate unacceptable high stresses in the pars interarticularis, causing a stress fracture. Troup (1975) has shown that the shearing forces across the pars are particularly high in forced spinal extension, and such repetitive forces may produce stress fracture in gymnasts and other athletes accounting for their high incidence of lysis. It could equally be argued, however, that an athletic career is often chosen by subjects with lysis because they are in some respects hypermobile. We are ignorant about both the aetiology of spondylolysis and also the factors responsible for the variable degree of displacement.

Vertebral displacement

Lysis can occur with no vertebral displacement at all (spondylolysis). Commonly there is moderate forward displacement (spondylolisthesis), or there may be gross forward displacement with complete dislocation of the proximal vertebra. The degree of displacement is expressed as a percentage of the forward displacement of the posterior margin of the proximal vertebral body over the antero-posterior diameter of the vertebra below (Fig.

19.2) (Blackburne & Velikas 1977, Wiltse & Winter 1983). The mean displacement of 162 patients attending out clinic with lysis was 17% and only four patients has a slip ratio greater than

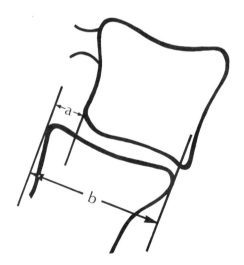

$$\frac{a}{b} \times 100 = \text{Slip ratio}$$

Fig. 19.2   Method of measuring the slip ratio. (Reproduced with the permission of Doncaster Royal Infirmary.)

40%. Gross displacement is usually associated with congenital anomalies of the posterior vertebral arch, a wide spina bifida and attenuation of the pars with or without lysis — 'dysplastic spondylolisthesis'. Wiltse and colleagues (1976) in their classification distinguished this from the more common 'isthmic spondylolisthesis', in which there is a lytic defect of the pars without dysplasia. Sometimes the difference is more apparent than real, and the two may be but extremes of one condition.

The term 'slip' is a misnomer. The degree of displacement has not been shown to suddenly increase with a forward slip. Displacement can be shown to progress gradually during childhood but after maturity, displacement, at least at L5/S1, does not increase significantly (Danielson et al 1991) (Figs 19.3 and 19.4). The displacement should rather be considered a growth phenomenon, with gradual remodelling of the posterior vertebral elements in response to the forces of shear. The degree of displacement that exists at maturity probably changes little thereafter. This growth concept is supported by the asymmetrical development of vertebrae with unilateral spondylolysis (Ch. 20).

Injury

Lysis of the pars undoubtedly follows stress fracture in some athletes whose spines are subject to high torque, e.g. fast bowlers. Fast bowlers can sequentially fracture one vertebra after another. This may occur at L4, then L3 and L2. It is possible, however, that the common L5 lysis which is present from an early age has a different aetiology.

About one patient in four with a lysis will clearly recollect an acute childhood injury to the spine. They remember a fall downstairs, from a wall or tree. If such an injury were to cause an acute fracture or to damage a pre-existing lytic defect of the pars and result in instability, the posterior elements would not then be able to adequately restrain the shear forces. Growth remodelling would allow progressive displacement until maturity. The age at which such an injury occurred would affect the degree of displacement. Hitchcock (1940) has suggested that the hyperflexion and torsion of a traumatic birth delivery could fracture the pars. He produced neural arch fractures by cadaveric experiments, but this was not supported by the work of Rowe and Roche

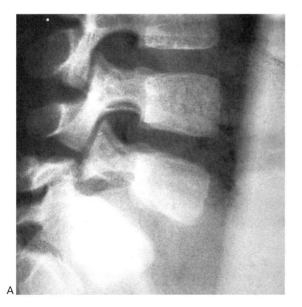 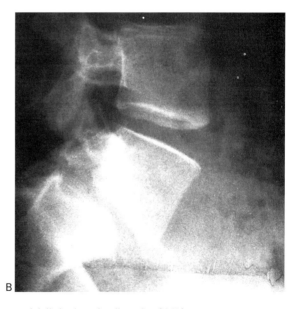

Fig. 19.3(A)   Lateral radiograph of a 7-year-old girl with isthmic spondylolisthesis and a slip ratio of 34%.
(B) At 18 years of age the slip ratio was measured at 40% (not significantly different from the slip at 7 years of age).

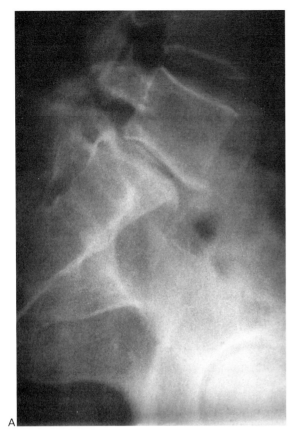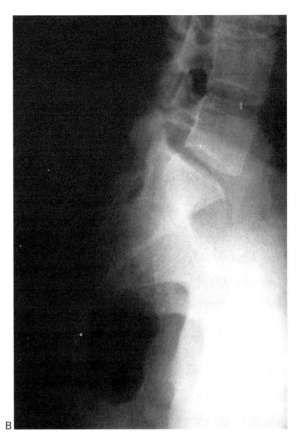

A

B

Fig. 19.4(A)   Lateral radiograph of a 63-year-old woman with isthmic spondylolisthesis at L5/S1 and a slip ratio of 17%. **(B)** Radiograph of the same patient at 34 years of age when the slip ratio was measured at 13% (not significantly different from (**A**)).

(1953). If birth injury were a significant factor in the development of a lysis, one would expect spondylolysis to be uncommon in children born by Caesarean section. Only one of our 162 patients with lysis of the pars had been born by Caesarean section, far less than the 5% section rate in the 1940s. Perhaps birth injury is significant.

Although the aetiology of isthmic spondylolisthesis is unresolved, it is a good working hypothesis to accept that some individuals are predisposed to develop a lysis of the pars; that it probably occurs very early in life; and that it is usually stable, being adequately supported by soft tissues which restrain the shear forces and prevent forward displacement, leaving only a spondylolysis. Others may injure the site of the existing defect causing instability; and the unrestrained shear forces then result in a growth remodelling process

with forward displacement of the proximal segment. The degree of that displacement will depend on two factors: the age at which the instability occurs, and the degree to which the soft tissues are able to withstand shear.

Tensile forces develop across the pars from the downward pull of the muscles attached to the laminae and spinous processes, and from the shear forces across the disc (Fig. 19.5) (Stott et al 1981). These forces are acceptable in an intact pars, and are presumably adequately restrained in many a spondylolytic defect. The intact disc itself is a powerful restrainer of shear, with the disc at the level of spondylolisthesis having characteristic histology (Roberts et al 1982). The anterior lip of the first sacral body develops a prominence to match the proximal vertebra, also resisting displacement. Stability may become absolute by a spontaneous bony fusion.

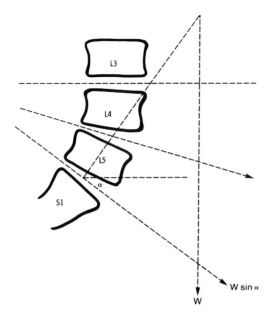

Fig. 19.5   Diagram to show shear through the lumbosacral disc, where W is the body weight above the disc, and α is the lumbosacral angle.

Dysplastic neural arch

Should unacceptable bending movement cause an isthmic defect of the pars to become unstable in infancy, and should the soft tissues prove unable to restrain shear, there will be a long period of growth available for these forces to elongate the pars and for considerable displacement to occur. Displacement by growth would have less time to develop from a similar injury in later childhood. Wiltse and Jackson (1976) noted that displacement increases most rapidly if spondylolisthesis is detected at the start of the growth spurt.

A defect that remains stable throughout growth may produce no displacement provided the soft tissues maintain that stability. The ability of the soft tissues to restrain the forces of shear will affect the degree of displacement. The greatest displacement occurs in 'dysplastic spondylolisthesis', where hypoplastic posterior vertebral elements are also associated with anomalies of the attachments of multifidus and the lumbar fascia. In 'isthmic spondylolisthesis' there is a high incidence of spina bifida occulta (Fredrickson et al 1984); 32% of our patients had spina bifida at

L5 or S1 but these did not have a greater degree of displacement than those without a spina bifida.

Ossification of the spinous process proceeds in a cranio-caudal direction, sometimes being delayed at L5 and the sacrum. There is a high incidence of incomplete ossification of the neural arch in young children and a decreasing incidence with age, until about 10% of the adult population have spina bifida occulta. Complete ossification of the neural arch probably depends on tensile forces mediated through the soft tissues and if there is a pars defect, these tensile forces will be deficient. This is turn will inhibit complete ossification of the neural arch, with resultant spina bifida occulta. Thus the high incidence of spina bifida occulta in patients with spondylolisthesis may be the result of the defect and not part of the original dysplastic pathology.

Joint laxity

The elastic properties of the spinal ligamentous structures may be a factor in vertebral displacement (Bird et al 1980). This is difficult to measure, but probably the Leeds hyperextensiometer (Jobbins et al 1979) is the most useful index of generalized joint mobility (Fig. 19.6). We found a correlation of 0.26 ($p < 0.05$) between the slip ratio of the 162 patients with lysis and the hyperextensiometer measurement of the second left metacarpal.

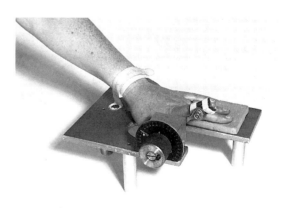

Fig. 19.6   The Leeds hyperextensiometer measures mobility of the second metocarpophalangeal joint.

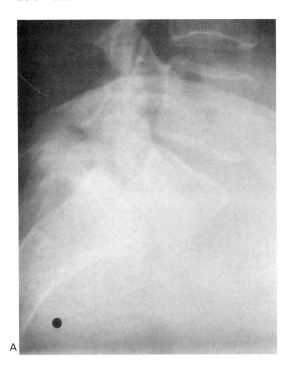

A

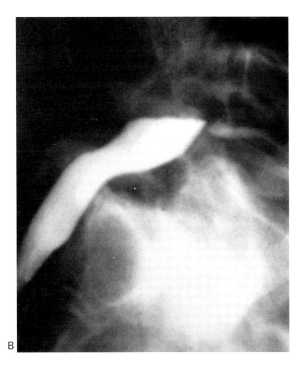

B

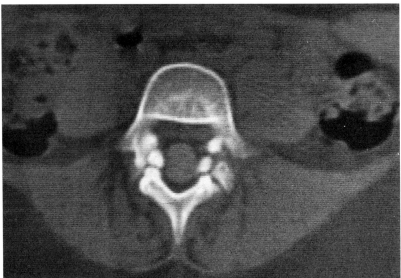

C

Fig. 19.7(A)   A lateral radiograph of a patient with an isthmic spondylolisthesis and 40% slip ratio. (**B**) A myelogram showing that the displacement has produced a capacious canal. (**C**) CT scan showing the lysis in the pars, and a large dome-shaped vertebral canal.

Lumbosacral angle

There is a positive correlation between the lumbosacral angle and the degree of displacement (Blackburne & Velikas 1977). The lumbosacral angle is best measured between the L3/4 and L5/S1 disc spaces (Farfan 1973), and in our series this showed a correlation of 0.39 ($p < 0.01$) with the degree of displacement. It does not follow that an initial steep angle of inclination is related to the speed of displacement. Rather, it is probable that, as displacement occurs slowly during growth, the body of L5 becomes gradually wedged (Porter & Park 1982), and the lumbosacral angle in adult life merely reflects the growth change of the vertebral body. However, once established, this increasing angle will produce greater shear forces tending to accelerate the displacement.

The vertebral canal

Vertebral displacement with elongation of the pars has the advantage of widening the sagittal diameter of the central vertebral canal (Fig. 19.7) and thus protecting the patient to some degree from back pain syndromes that are related to a narrow central canal. The powerful epigenetic influence of the neurological tissue ensures that in the growth remodelling displacement process, the root canal remains adequate for the nerve root, even with gross displacement. In a dysplastic spondylolisthesis 'crisis', however, there is a relatively sudden final displacement, with neurological compromise.

IDENTIFICATION OF A PARS DEFECT

From the history

One may suspect a defect from certain features in the history and examination. The patient who has a long history of pain in the back, sometimes referred to the thighs and perhaps with some childhood injury, would make the clinician think of a lysis, more so if they stated that they were previously of good athletic ability and that they could feel a 'click' in the back. Some patients will give a history of an industrial accident with some heavy weight falling on the back, or symptoms dating from pregnancy, which may have made a previously symptomless defect painful.

By examination

Many patients with a lysis seem to be highly flexible. They can bend forwards with straight legs and place the flat of the hands on the floor (Jackson et al 1976) (Fig. 19.8). However, it is not the lumbar spine that is hypermobile, but this manoeuvre is possible because straight leg raising is so good, often well above 90°. Most patients with back pain are not able to put their hands flat on

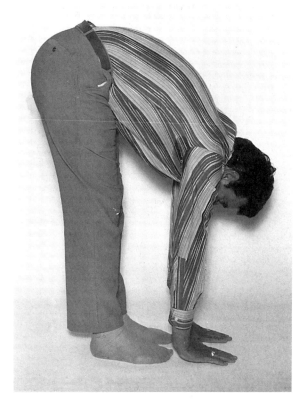

Fig. 19.8 Patient with isthmic spondylolisthesis and chronic low back pain, able to place the hands flat on the floor (a reflection of good straight leg raising rather than spinal flexion).

the floor because spinal flexion and/or straight leg raising are limited. Patients with lysis are in distinct contrast to others with back pain because in spite of their pain, they are often sufficiently flexible to touch the floor. Their flexibility is little different to non-back pain subjects, however (Table 19.2).

A careful examiner may be able to detect an unstable lysis by palpating the lower lumbar spinous processes first in the neutral position, and then in maximum rotation. The patient lies on their side and a finger tip is placed on the lower three spinous processes. The patient is then rotated and in an intact spine the processes move in step. The process of L5 will not move with L4 if there is an unstable lysis at L5 (Fig. 9.8 page 93).

The mid-line hollow created by a forward displaced vertebra is often obvious, both to

Table 19.2 Ability of patients with isthmic and degenerative spondylolisthesis to flex forwards with straight knees, compared with other patients and volunteer subjects.

	Isthmic spondylolisthesis (*n* = 98)	Degenerative spondylolisthesis (*n* = 53)	Patients with back pain but no spondylolisthesis (*n* = 115)	Volunteer subjects without back pain (*n* = 61)
Able to place flat of hands on floor	18%	21%	9%	23%
Able to touch floor with finger tips	35%	36%	22%	62%
Unable to touch the floor	47%	43%	69%	15%

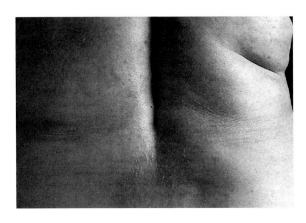

Fig. 19.9 Photograph of the mid-line hollow created by a spondylolisthesis.

inspection (Fig. 19.9) and to palpation of the back.

By ultrasound

A displaced vertebra can easily be recognized by ultrasound examination (Fig. 19.10) when, by virtue of the forward rotational element of the displacement, it is more obviously out of line than in radiographic examination. Ultrasound is therefore a useful non-invasive investigation for epidemiological studies of spondylolisthesis.

Radiography

If the lysis is not obvious on a lateral X-ray, oblique 45° projections will usually demonstrate the defect, with the typical 'scottie dog collar effect' (Fig. 19.11). This may be enhanced by cranial projections (Porter & Park 1982, Lisbon & Bloom 1983).

Scintigraphy

Increased vascularity of the pars interarticularis can be demonstrated by scintigraphy after spinal trauma. It is not possible to say whether this is evidence of a stress fracture in an inherently weakened pars, or disruption of a pre-existing pars defect.

CLINICAL SIGNIFICANCE

We are tempted to assume that lysis of the pars is in some way the cause of a patient's backache because it is such an obvious anomaly, but both backache and lysis are common and they may at times be unrelated (Supik & Broom 1991) (Fig. 19.12). Studies of gymnasts' spines, in spite of the many series being dissimilar in age, sex and nationality, agree on two counts: spondylolysis and spondylolisthesis are common (5–21%); and many of the subjects with a defect have no symptoms.

The lysis was symptomless in 33% of Bird's series (1980), and in 45% of Jackson's (1976). In Hitoshi's series (1980), 76% of subjects with lysis were symptomless, there being no significant difference in back pain incidence between those athletes with lysis and those without. Semon and Spengler (1981) reached the same conclusion, finding that 27% of 507 college football players had back pain, but only 2.4% had pain and a spondylolisthesis. In the short term, the lysis did not appear to have clinical significance. What then is the relevance of lysis of the pars in a patient complaining of back pain?

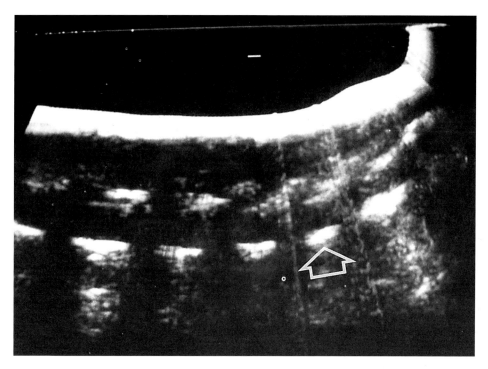

Fig. 19.10   Ultrasound B-scan of five lumbar vertebrae and sacrum, showing forward displacement of the body of L5 and a wide vertebral canal.

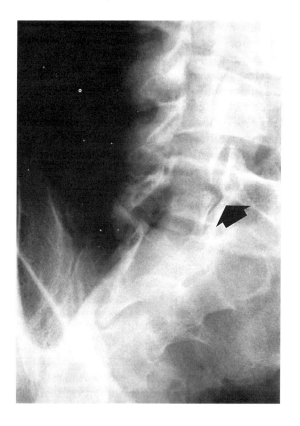

Fig. 19.11   45° oblique radiograph showing a pars defect at L5, the 'scottie dog collar'.

Back and referred pain

This is the most common problem for a patient with lysis of the pars interarticularis (Table 19.3). One in three attending hospital with a defect will have pain across the back and round the pelvis into the buttocks, and when on their feet for long it will affect the thighs and even the upper calves. It has the characteristics of the fatigue pain of instability, being worse standing, walking far, and especially when shopping. It is relieved by lying down. The patient may add an interesting symptom: they hear or feel a 'click' in the lower back.

There is often a long history with intermittent pain from childhood, and one in four can remember some violent accident in early life. Others may have a more recent history of an industrial accident when a weight fell on their back. One woman out of five complaining of these

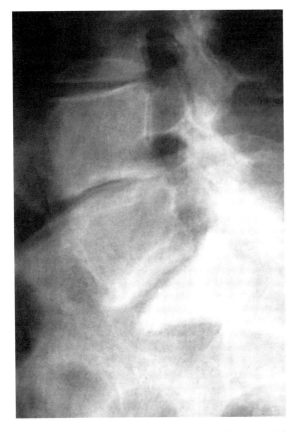

Fig. 19.15   Lateral radiograph of a 74-year-old woman with isthmic spondylolisthesis at L5/S1 and disc degeneration at L4/5. She recollected back pain in her youth, and that she had been told a vertebra was displaced, but she had had no back pain for 40 years.

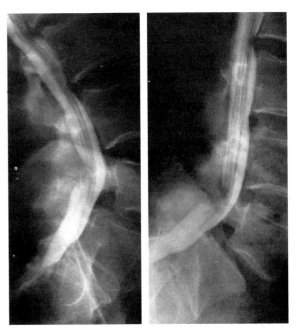

Fig. 19.16   Lateral myelography of a 54-year-old woman with neurogenic claudication. She could only walk 100 yards. She had an isthmic spondylolisthesis at L5/S1. The first sacral vertebra is lumbarized. Note the two-level stenosis — at L2/3, and at the cranial aspect of L5. She was cured by decompressing only L5, and an associated fusion.

proximal stenotic lesion (Fig. 19.16). Many patients with lysis do have discomfort in the legs which increases with walking and limits the walking distance, but this is not neurogenic claudication. Instability back pain can give referred pain into the buttock or thigh, and root entrapment can become more painful when walking because of movement at the lysis.

Spondylolisthesis crisis

The adolescent who has marked displacement of L5 on S1 may develop fairly sudden severe symptoms in the back and legs. The crisis is probably due to a relatively acute increase in the forces of shear at S1. The marked degree of displacement is associated both with wedging of the body of L5 and increased lumbosacral angle. With the increased weight associated with a growth spurt, instability at the lysis becomes a problem. The vertebral canal which is widened in spondylolisthesis can be distorted by the relatively sudden accelerating displacement. The neural contents have not been able to keep pace with the bony changes, and excessive movement at the lysis is the final insult to the cauda equina. There is pain in the back and legs with restricted movements of the spine, spasm and restricted straight leg raising.

Is the defect of any significance at all? In a series of 2360 patients attending a back pain clinic, we recorded 5.6% of patients with bilateral lysis of the pars, which is probably no greater than the incidence of the defect in the general population. It could be suggested reasonably that the demonstration of lysis is an incidental finding, unrelated to the cause of back pain. Two facts, however, indicate that the defect can be clinically significant. The first is the considerable difference in the incidence of two back pain syndromes (the symptomatic disc lesion, and back and referred pain) when comparing patients with and without a lysis (Porter & Hibbert 1984) (Table 19.3). The second observation is that proportionally more women than men who have lytic defects attend the hospital with back pain. Roche and Rowe (1951) recorded a spondylolisthesis sex ratio of three men to one woman. Comparing our population to this finding, we have twice as many women attending with lysis as would be expected (a sex ratio to 1.7 to 1). Perhaps the effects of pregnancy are important in initiating instability symptoms.

MANAGEMENT OF BACK PAIN AND SPONDYLOLISTHESIS

Conservative management

A spondylolisthesis which is recognized in early life should not give rise to undue concern. Pain of course can be severe and ultimately require surgical treatment, but in general, patients with a spondylolysis or spondylolisthesis manage as well as patients without a defect. They are no more likely to visit the hospital with back pain than the rest of the population. They are more likely than the rest of us to develop back and referred pain, but this is often a manageable problem, and they are better protected against the disabling symptoms of the acute disc lesion.

It would probably be wise for a young man with a known lysis to avoid those occupations which are stressful to the spine, but in other respects he is at no greater risk than his peers. However, the young person with a painful spondylolysis or low-grade spondylolisthesis who cannot enjoy sports and recreation is greatly helped by bone grafting and internal fixation at the site of the defect (Nicol & Scott 1985, Bradford & Iza 1985, Pederson & Hagen 1988, Johnson & Thompson 1992).

A young woman with a known lysis should receive precautionary advice in pregnancy, as she is at risk of developing instability. She should not be overweight, and should avoid unnecessary lifting and carrying. Frequent periods of rest are advisable, especially in the third trimester. She should be doubly cautious not to fall, and postural advice about pelvic rotation to reduce the lumbosacral angle may be useful (Maring-Klug 1982). Unfortunately, many women progress through pregnancy oblivious of a hidden spondylolisthesis, only to learn of the lesion when they later develop back pain. An earlier diagnosis is possible if the ultrasonographer performing the first fetal scan will look at every mother's spine for a displaced vertebra.

It is important to spend time describing to a patient what is meant by a spondylolisthesis or they will imagine a slipping vertebra which will eventually dislocate altogether. A few words to explain that the displacement has probably been present from early life and that it will not materially alter can allay many fears. Each syndrome is then treated on its own merits.

The common problem of pain in the back referred to the thighs is usually managed satisfactorily by an understanding of the instability fatigue pain mechanism and advice about limiting the mechanical stress on the spine. The load carried, its duration and the strength of the spine are topics for discussion. How can the patient reduce the amount and frequency of lifting and carrying? Can they improve on their fitness? Are they too heavy? Here is the role of the 'back school'. A good car seat makes a difference and, for those over middle age, there is a place for a lumbosacral corset. If there has been a sudden increase in symptoms it might be useful to support the spine in a jacket for 3 months. Most patients with back and referred pain can be effectively managed by conservative means and, although they will probably never be entirely free of symptoms, they can usually cope with the problem.

Children and adolescents with spondylolysis or spondylolisthesis fare as well with conservative treatment as with surgery (Seitsalo et al 1991). There is no general agreement about the management of the young athlete with acute low back pain who has a demonstrable pars defect and a positive scintiscan. If this represents a stress fracture, immobilization may allow bony union. Some would advocate a spica for 3 months. The 'hot spot' may only indicate that a pre-existing lysis has become unstable, and immobilization is then likely to be unproductive. Some would recommend simply withdrawal from sporting activities. The need for surgical fusion is open to debate, but if symptoms persist which affect an athletic career, it is certainly worthwhile.

Surgery

Instability symptoms

Patients with continuing back pain unrelieved by conservative treatment need surgery. With careful assessment and a sound fusion (Ch. 24), these are amongst the most grateful of patients (Attenborough & Reynolds 1975), especially the younger patients with disabling instability pain (Haraldsson & Willner 1983). Scott's wire fixation and fusion of the defect is generally successful in the adolescent and young adult, especially at L4. A posterior laminar fusion also produces excellent results. A severe dysplastic fusion may also do well with a posterior fusion in situ, but some favour anterior fusion with or without reduction.

Disc symptoms

A patient with classical disc symptoms may have a lytic defect of the pars which is incidental to the back pain problem. Admittedly these disc symptoms are rare in the presence of a lysis, but the defect may be stable and symptomless and a protruding disc proximal to the lysis responsible for the root lesion. Management is no different from that offered to other patients with a disc lesion.

Root entrapment

Root entrapment occurs in the presence of a lysis with much the same frequency as in patients without a lysis. The defect, however, is usually a factor in the causation of the symptoms, either from degenerative changes around the lysis or from more proximal or distal involvement. Conservative management for root entrapment is the same as for patients without a defect, though an epidural injection is not likely to influence the 'far out syndrome'. Those few patients requiring surgical help may need both adequate decompression of the nerve root and a fusion; fusion alone may relieve the pain, but this cannot be guaranteed (Haraldsson & Willner 1983). Adequate exposure of L5 and S1 is imperative

because either root can be responsible for the symptoms at several possible sites: L5 at the region of the lysis, or at the L4/5 disc level in the central canal; and S1 from involvement under the cranial lip of the first sacral lamina. If the lesion is in the root canal, then instability forms part of the pathological process and a fusion in necessary; it is also worthwhile if backache accompanies the root pain. A lateral fusion is the procedure of choice when performing a synchronous decompression.

Claudication

When the major complaint is painful legs when walking, with limited walking distance, a careful assessment is necessary to find the cause. It is unlikely to be neurogenic claudication because lysis and displacement tend to widen the vertebral canal. MR, CT or myelography will exclude or confirm a more proximal spinal stenosis. More often the walking pain is spinal instability pain referred into the thighs, and it is usually managed by conservative means, reducing weight, strengthening the back and living within the limitations of pain. Only when this is not possible is surgery considered. A fusion will help, provided the canal is wide enough and the proximal disc intact.

Crisis

The rare complication of spondylolisthesis crisis in the adolescent spine requires fusion. A good fusion will relieve the symptoms, and most surgeons would fuse the spine in situ (Zindrick & Lorenz 1989, Frennered et al 1991). Johnson and Kirwan (1983) reviewed the long-term results of fusion in situ for severe spondylolisthesis, and most had excellent ratings 20 years after surgery. McPhee and O'Brien (1979) recommend reduction of a severely displaced adolescent spondylolisthesis prior to fusion to improve the cosmetic appearance, though cauda equina lesions are a feared complication. A serious attempt to reduce the displacement is probably not logical if we believe that slow vertebral displacement is accompanied by growth remodelling. The epigenetic influence of the nerves will have shaped the central and root canals, and attempts to reduce a so-called slip, which is really a growth phenomenon, are likely to cause neurological damage. However, cauda equina lesions are not unknown even when the spine is fused in situ (Maurice & Morley 1989).

Fortunately, although spondylolysis affects about 5% of the population the majority have no symptoms at all, and those who do can be managed without major surgery.

REFERENCES

Attenborough C G, Reynolds M T 1975 Lumbo-sacral fusion with spring fixation. Journal of Bone and Joint Surgery 57-B: 283–288

Bird H A, Eastmond C J, Hudson A, Wright V 1980 Is generalised joint laxity a factor in spondylolisthesis? Scandinavian Journal of Rheumatology 9: 203–205

Blackburne J S, Velikas E P 1977 Spondylolisthesis in children and adolescents. Journal of Bone and Joint Surgery 59-B: 490–494

Bradford D S, Iza J 1985 Repair of the defect in spondylolysis or minimal degrees of spondylolisthesis by segmental wire fixation and bone grafting. Spine 10: 673–679

Cyron B M, Hutton W C, Troup J D G 1976 Spondylolytic fractures. Journal of Bone and Joint Surgery 58-B: 462–466

Danielson B I, Frennered A K, Irstam L K H 1991 Radiologic progression of isthmic lumbar spondylolisthesis in young people. Spine 16: 422–425

Farfan H F 1973 The mechanical disorders of the lower back. Lea and Febiger, Philadelphia

Fredrickson B E, Baker D, McHolick W J, Juan H A, Lubicky J P 1984 The natural history of spondylolysis and spondylolisthesis. Journal of Bone and Joint Surgery 66-A: 699–707

Frennered A K, Danielson B I, Nachemson A L, Nordwall A B 1991 Mid-term follow-up of young patients fused in situ for spondylolisthesis. Spine 16: 409–416

Haraldsson S, Willner S 1983 A comparative study of spondylolisthesis in operations on adolescents and adults. Archives of Orthopedic Trauma Surgery 101 (2): 101–105

Hardcastle P, Annear P, Foster D H, Chakera T M, McCormick C, Khangure M, Burnett A 1992 Spinal abnormalities in young fast bowlers. Journal of Bone and Joint Surgery 74-B: 421–425

Hitchcock H H 1940 Spondylolisthesis. Journal of Bone and Joint Surgery 22: 1–16

Hitoshi H 1980 Spondylolysis in athletes. Physician Sports Medicine 8: 75–79

Jackson D W, Wiltse L L, Cirincone R J 1976 Spondylolysis in the female gymnast. Clinical Orthopaedics 117: 68–73

Jobbins B, Bird H A, Wright V 1979 A joint hyperextensiometer for the quantification of joint laxity. Engineering in Medicine 8: 103–105

Johnson G V, Thompson H G 1992 The Scott wiring technique for direct repair of lumbar spondylolisthesis. Journal of Bone and Joint Surgery 74-B: 426–430

Johnson J R, Kirwan E O'G 1983 The long term results of fusion in situ for severe spondylolisthesis. Journal of Bone and Joint Surgery 65-B: 43–46

Kono S, Hayashi N, Kashahara G, Akimoto T, Keneko F, Sugiura Y, Harada A 1975 A study of the aetiology of spondylolysis with reference to athletic activities. Journal of Japanese Orthopaedic Association 49: 125–131

Lisbon E, Bloom R A 1983 Anteroposterior and angulated view: a new radiographic technique for the evaluation of spondylolysis. Radiology 149: 315–316

McCulloch J A 1977 Chemonucleolysis. Journal of Bone and Joint Surgery 59-B: 45–52

McPhee I B, O'Brien J P 1979 Reduction of severe spondylolisthesis. Spine 4: 430–434

Maring-Klug R 1982 Reducing low back pain during pregnancy. Nurse Practitioner 7: 18–24

Maurice H D, Morley T R 1989 Cauda equina lesions following fusion in-situ and decompressive laminectomy for severe spondylolisthesis. Four case reports. Spine 14: 214–216

Murray-Leslie C F, Lintott D J, Wright V 1977 The spine in sport and veteran military parachutists. Annals of Rheumatic Diseases 36: 332–342

Newman P H 1963 The etiology of spondylolisthesis. Journal of Bone and Joint Surgery 45-B: 39–59

Nicol R O, Scott J A S 1985 Lytic spondylolisthesis: repair by wiring. Journal of Bone and Joint Surgery 67B: 673–674

Pederson A K, Hagen R 1988 Spondylolysis and spondylolisthesis. Treatment by internal fixation and bone-grafting of the defect. Journal of Bone and Joint Surgery 70-A: 15–24

Porter R W, Hibbert C S 1984 Symptoms associated with lysis of the pars interarticularis. Spine 7: 755–758

Porter R W, Miller C G 1986 Back pain and the trunk list. Spine 11: 596–600

Porter R W, Park W 1982 Unilateral spondylolysis. Journal of Bone and Joint Surgery 64-B: 344–348

Roberts S, Beard H K, O'Brien J P 1982 Biochemical changes of intervertebral discs in patients with spondylolisthesis or with tears of the posterior annulus. Annals of the Rheumatic Diseases 41: 78–85

Roche M B, Rowe G G 1951 The incidence of separated neural arch and coincident bone variation: a survey of 4200 skeletons. Anatomical Records 109: 233–252

Rowe G G, Roche M B 1953 The aetiology of separate neural arch. Journal of Bone and Joint Surgery 35-A: 102–110

Seitsalo S, Osterman K, Hyväinen H, Tallroth K, Schlenzka D, Poussa M 1991 Progression of spondylolisthesis in children and adolescents: a long-term follow-up of 272 patients. Spine 16: 417–421

Semon R L, Spengler D 1981 Significance of lumbar spondylolysis in college football players. Spine 6: 172–174

Stott J R R, Cyron B M, Hutton W C, Wall J C 1981 The mechanics of spondylolysis. Orthopaedic mechanics, procedures and devices, Academic Press, London, p 65–93

Supik L F, Broom M J 1991 Epidural lipoma causing a myelographic block in a patient who had sciatica and lumbosacral spondylolisthesis. Journal of Bone and Joint Surgery 73-A: 1104–1107

Troup J D G 1975 Mechanical factors in spondylolisthesis. Clinical Orthopaedics and Related Research 117: 59–67

Wiltse L L, Jackson D W 1976 Treatment of spondylolisthesis and spondylolysis in children. Clinical Orthopaedics and Related Research 117: 92–100

Wiltse L L, Winter R B 1983 Terminology and measurement of spondylolisthesis. Journal of Bone and Joint Surgery 65-B: 768–772

Wiltse L L, Newman P H, Macnab I 1976 Classification of spondylolysis and spondylolisthesis. Clinical Orthopaedics and Related Research 117: 23–29

Wiltse L L, Guyer R, Spencer C, Glen W, Porter I 1984 Alar transverse process impingement of the L5 spinal nerve: the far out syndrome. Spine 9: 31–41

Zindrick M R, Lorenz M A 1989 The non-reactive treatment of spondylolisthesis. Seminars in Spine Surgery 1: 116–123

20. Unilateral spondylolysis — pathology, diagnosis and clinical significance

PREVALENCE

Bilateral spondylolisthesis probably occurs in approximately 5% of the population. In contrast, unilateral spondylolysis is rather rare. The classification of spondylolysis and spondylolisthesis by Wiltse and colleagues (1976) refers to bilateral lesions only and not to the unilateral defect. It has been reported by Stewart (1953) and was present in one-sixth of the spondylitic specimens of Roche and Rowe (1951), one in four of those of Willis (1923), and one in three of Einstein's specimens (1978). We described the vertebral morphology of five specimens of unilateral spondylolysis (1982), each showing developmental asymmetry (Porter & Park 1982).

PATHOLOGY

The defect is more common on the right side (Willis 1931). The pedicles and the superior apophyseal joints are in normal symmetrical relationship with the vertebral body (Fig. 20.1). There is, however, marked asymmetry of the neural arch, the inferior apophyseal joints and the posterior elements (Figs 20.2 and 20.3). The combination of these effects produces a rotation of the spinous process away from the side of the lesion (Maldagne & Malghem 1976), the inferior apophyseal joint on that side being placed more dorsally than the superior. When viewed from behind, the neural arch is rotated in an anti-clockwise direction in the vertebra with a right-sided defect, and clockwise in a left-sided defect. The combined deformity results in horizontal orientation of the lamina on the affected side. There is usually quite marked asymmetrical pos-

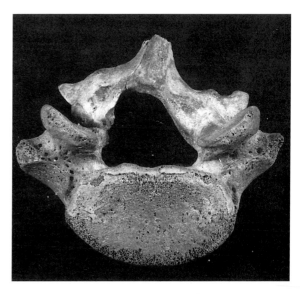

Fig. 20.1 L5 lumbar vertebra with a right-sided unilateral spondylolysis, photographed from above. The superior facets are symmetrical, but the spinous process is deviated to the left.

terior wedging of the vertebral bodies, with reduction in the vertical height at the posterior angle of 2–4 mm.

Radiographs show that the areas of asymmetry are accompanied not only by a reduction in size of the lamina, apophyseal joint and transverse process, but also by thinner cortices and fewer trabeculae in these locations (Fig. 20.4). There is usually a reactive stenosis in the contralateral pedicle (Maldagne & Malghem 1985). Posterior asymmetrical wedging of the vertebral body is shown in Figure 20.5 and this is accompanied by a tendency to horizontal orientation of the pars interarticularis and the inferior apophyseal joint

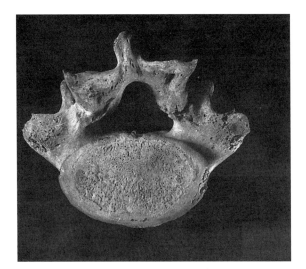

Fig. 20.2   L5 lumbar vertebra photographed from below, with a right-sided unilateral spondylolysis. The inferior facets and laminae are asymmetrical, with the spinous process deviated to the left.

on the affected side. The spondylolytic defects vary in width, which determines the facility with which they can be demonstrated radiologically. A defect of 1 mm cannot be demonstrated by an axial projection, even when using thin section computerized tomography.

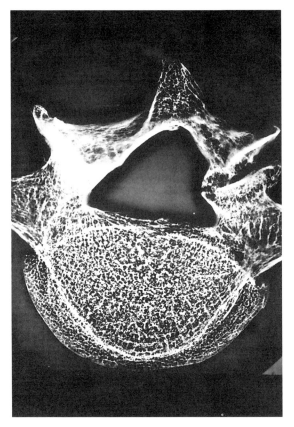

Fig. 20.4   Radiograph of unilateral spondylolysis.

Sometimes a stress fracture will occur in the opposite pedicle (Aland et al 1986, Garber & Wright 1986, Gunzburg & Fraser 1991), or in the opposite lamina (O'Beirne & Horgan 1988). An associated spina bifida occulta is not uncommon (Burkus 1990).

DIAGNOSIS

Although unilateral spondylolysis may well occur in a little less than 1% of the population, its detection is extremely difficult. We seldom make the diagnosis of unilateral spondylolysis in clinical practice. This may be because it rarely produces symptoms. The wide dome-shaped vertebral canal produced by elongation of the pars, albeit asymmetrical, does protect the neural elements from compression in the presence of disc pathology, degenerative change and segmental movement. In addition, the intact, thickened unilateral pars

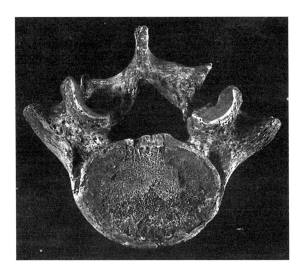

Fig. 20.3   A left-sided unilateral spondylolysis again showing symmetrical inferior facets, but laminar and canal asymmetry.

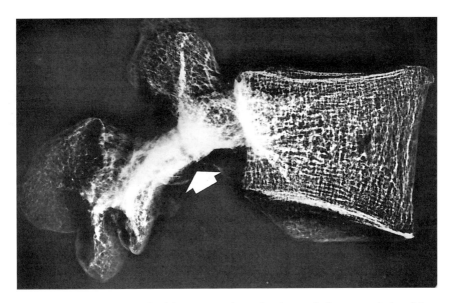

Fig. 20.5   Lateral radiograph of the same specimen showing marked asymmetrical wedging of the vertebral body and pars defect.

does resist shear and avoids the instability that can accompany bilateral defects. Furthermore, we may fail to recognize unilateral defects because we do not suspect them and, even if suspected, they are difficult to demonstrate radiologically. Such a defect may be suspected when there is asymmetrical posterolateral wedging of the vertebral body, horizontal orientation of the lamina, hypoplasia of one inferior apophyseal facet or sclerosis of the contralateral pedicle. Computerized

tomography may not always reveal the defect. Radiographs taken at a 45° oblique angle, with the tube inclined 20° cranially, may be of help (Fig. 20.6) and may give some additional information about hypertrophic bone indenting the root canal. Because of these difficulties in visualization, it is possible that symptomatic unilateral spondylolysis is more frequent than is generally acknowledged.

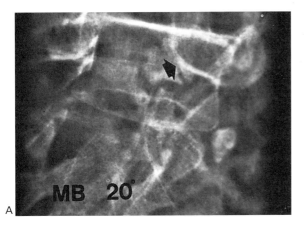

Fig. 20.6(A)   An oblique radiograph with a 20° incline showing the unilateral defect on the left side.

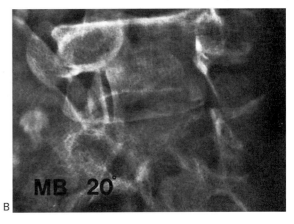

Fig. 20.6(B)   A 20° inclined plane on the unaffected side shows no abnormality.

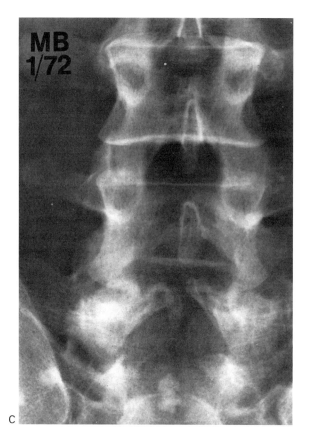

C

Fig. 20.6(C) An AP film shows spina bifida occulta at L5, not uncommon with a unilateral defect.

AETIOLOGICAL SIGNIFICANCE

It is difficult to reconcile the morphological finding of unilateral spondylolysis with the various theories on the aetiology of bilateral spondylolysis. Opinions vary on the cause of the lytic defect in the pars interarticularis. The major controversy centres on whether the defects are congenital or traumatic. A number of authors (Newman 1963, Farfan 1973, Troup 1975, 1977) have felt that the two are not mutually incompatible, and that an individual may be congenitally predisposed to a stress fracture of the pars. Undoubtedly, fractures of the pars may be seen to heal (Devas 1963, Murray & Colwill 1968, Krenz & Troup 1973, Jackson et al 1976). Specimens of unilateral

spondylolysis, however, do not show any evidence of a healed fracture in the pars opposite to the defect, nor of attempted healing of the unilateral lysis. It would be unlikely for a single fracture to occur in a ring of bone like the neural arch, and if a double fracture occurred, it would be unusual for one of the fractures alone to heal. The very existence of the unilateral spondylolysis questions the concept that lysis of the pars is always the result of a stress fracture.

The morphological changes in unilateral spondylolysis with unilateral asymmetry and hypoplasia also provide some understanding of the changes that are observed in bilateral spondylolysis. At least some features are common to both unilateral and bilateral conditions. Wedging of the vertebral body occurs with bilateral lysis, and unilateral wedging of the body with unilateral lysis. Both laminae are orientated horizontally with the bilateral defect, and one lamina is asymmetrically orientated in the horizontal plane with the unilateral defect. In an isolated vertebra there is an obvious deformity with asymmetry of the neural arch, with deviation of the spinous process away from the side having the hypoplastic elements. In the articulated spine, however, the spinous process may maintain a mid-line position. This could only occur with forward rotation of the vertebra on the affected side, resulting in a hemilisthesis. It is probable that these asymmetrical morphological changes occur before skeletal maturity is complete and that they are a growth phenomenon. If we extrapolate to the bilateral situation, all the characteristics of bilateral spondylolisthesis are present, with elongation of the pars, horizontal orientation of the laminae, and olisthesis and wedging of the vertebral body. Thus the changes recorded in unilateral spondylolysis suggest that many of the changes in bilateral spondylolisthesis are a growth phenomenon. In degenerative spondylolisthesis it is reasonable to describe displacement as a 'slip', but in isthmic spondylolisthesis displacement is not a 'slip', but a growth change.

There is histological evidence that growth remodelling occurs in the posterior elements. Park and colleagues (1980) have studied the changes in grossly displaced adolescent spondylolisthesis. This revealed pronounced elongation of the pars interarticularis as a result of remodelling secondarily to the stress loading. It was accompanied by underdevelopment of the posterior elements, notably of the inferior facets.

CLINICAL SIGNIFICANCE

The clinical implications of unilateral spondylolysis must remain speculative. Possible factors could include the effects of unilateral rotation with torsional damage to the intervertebral disc and disturbance of the nerve root (Farfan et al 1970), which could then be aggravated by hypertrophic bone projecting into the nerve root canal (Fig. 20.7). A significant factor is likely to be the presence of spina bifida which will produce a free-floating fragment (Miki et al 1991) (Figs 20.8 and 20.9), or a stress fracture of the opposite pedicle or lamina, contributing to segmental instability. Increased facet degenerative change has been noted on the side opposite to the defect, which may result from or contribute to instability (Kornberg 1988). The opposite pedicle has been known to fracture (Weatherley et al 1991). The fifth lumbar roots can be at risk in the root canal at either side. Burkus (1990) treated three patients whose sciatic pain was associated with unilateral spondylolysis, by hemilaminectomy, excision of the pseudoarthrosis and

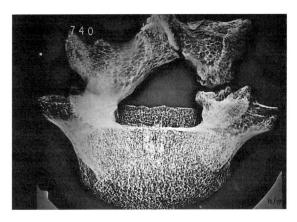

Fig. 20.8 Radiograph of a unilateral spondylolysis with a spina bifida and free-floating fragment. (Reproduced with the permission of Doncaster Royal Infirmary.)

bilateral posterolateral fusion.

As with bilateral spondylolisthesis, however, the absence of the trefoil configuration ensures that even with a compromising lesion, the neural contents in the central canal are protected. We should be aware of its presence, and it should be specifically sought in patients with asymmetrical vertebral wedging and associated hypoplasia of the neural arch. As we become more proficient in its diagnosis, the full clinical implications will be revealed.

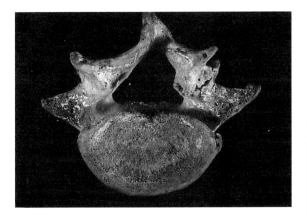

Fig. 20.7 A right-sided unilateral spondylolysis at L5 with hypertrophic bone encroaching into the central canal producing a lateral recess, which with soft tissue could compromise the L5 root. Note the absence of a lateral recess on the left. (Reproduced with the permission of Doncaster Royal Infirmary.)

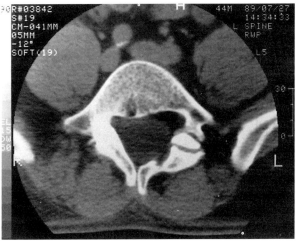

Fig. 20.9 CT scan of a unilateral defect with spina bifida occulta.

REFERENCES

Aland C, Rineberg B A, Malberg M, Fired S H 1986 Fracture of the pedicle of the fourth lumbar vertebra associated with contralateral spondylolysis. Journal of Bone and Joint Surgery 68-A: 1454–1455

Burkus J K 1990 Unilateral spondylolysis associated with spinal bifida occulta and nerve root compression. Spine 15: 555–559

Devas M B 1963 Stress fractures in children. Journal of Bone and Joint Surgery 45-B: 528–541

Einstein S M C 1978 Spondylolysis. A skeletal investigation of two population groups. Journal of Bone and Joint Surgery 60-B: 488–494

Farfan H F 1973 The mechanical disorders of the lower back. Lea and Febiger, Philadelphia

Farfan H F, Cossette J W, Robertson G H, Wells R V, Kraus H 1970 The effects of torsion in the production of disc degeneration. Journal of Bone and Joint Surgery 52-A: 468–497

Garber J E, Wright A M 1986 Unilateral spondylolysis and contralateral pedicle fracture. Spine 11: 63–66

Gunzburg R, Fraser R D 1991 Stress fracture of the lumbar pedicle: case reports on 'pediculolysis' and review of the literature. Spine 16: 185–189

Jackson D W, Wiltse L L, Cirincone R J 1976 Spondylolysis in the female gymnast. Clinical Orthopaedics 117: 68–73

Kornberg M 1988 Spondylolisthesis with unilateral pars interarticularis defect and contralateral facet joint degeneration: a case report. Spine 13: 712–713

Krenz J, Troup J D G 1973 The structure of the pars interarticularis of the lower lumbar vertebrae and its relation to the aetiology of spondylolysis with a report of the healing fracture in the neural arch of a fourth lumbar vertebrae. Journal of Bone and Joint Surgery 55-B: 735–741

Maldagne B F, Malghem J J 1976 Unilateral arch hypertrophy with spinous process tilt: a sign of arch deficiency. Radiology 121: 567–574

Maldagne B, Malghem J 1985 La spondylolyse en activite. Journal of Radiology 55: 263–274

Miki T, Tamura T, Senzoku F, Kotani H, Hara T, Masuda T 1991 Congenital laminar defect of the upper lumbar spine associated with pars defect. Spine 16: 353–355

Murray R O, Colwill M R 1968 Stress fractures of the pars interarticularis. Proceedings of the Royal Society of Medicine 61: 555–557

Newman P H 1963 The etiology of spondylolisthesis. Journal of Bone and Joint Surgery 45-B: 39–59

O'Beirne J G, Horgan J G 1988 Stress fracture of the lamina associated with unilateral spondylolysis. Spine 13: 220–222

Park W M, Webb J K, O'Brien J P, McCall I W 1980 The microstructure of the neural arch complex in adolescence: a histological and radiological correlation in spondylolisthesis. Proceedings of the Institute of Mechanical Engineering 35–36

Porter R W, Park W 1982 Unilateral spondylolysis. Journal of Bone and Joint Surgery 45-B: 39–59

Roche M B, Rowe G G 1951 The incidence of separated neural arch and coincident bone variations: a survey of 4200 skeletons. Anatomical Records 109: 233–252

Stewart T D 1953 The age-incidence of neural arch defects in Alaskan natives, considering the standpoint of aetiology. Journal of Bone and Joint Surgery 35-A: 937–950

Troup J D G 1975 Mechanical factors in spondylolisthesis and spondylolysis. Clinical Orthopaedics and Related Research 117: 59–67

Troup J D G 1977 The etiology of spondylosis. Orthopaedic Clinics of North America 81: 57–64

Weatherley C R, Mehdian H, Vanden Burghe L 1991 Low back pain with fracture of the pedicle and contra lateral spondylolysis. Journal of Bone and Joint Surgery 73-B: 990–993

Willis T A 1923 The lumbo-sacral column in man, its stability of form and function. American Journal of Anatomy 32: 95–123

Willis T A 1931 The separate neural arch. Journal of Bone and Joint Surgery 13: 709–721

Wiltse L L, Newman P H, Macnab I 1976 Classification of spondylolysis and spondylolisthesis. Clinical Orthopaedics and Related Research 117: 23–29

21. Degenerative spondylolisthesis — pathology, symptoms and management

PATHOLOGY

Forward displacement of a proximal vertebra in relation to its adjacent vertebra when associated with an intact neural arch, no congenital anomaly and in the presence of degenerative change is known as 'degenerative spondylolisthesis'. It was described by Junghanns (1930) and Schmorl and Junghanns (1932) who noted that it was more common in women, and often occurred between the fourth and fifth lumbar vertebrae. This contrasts with isthmic spondylolisthesis (Table 21.1).

The displacement, when it occurs, begins in the sixth decade and patients generally attend with symptoms around 60 years of age (Newman & Stone 1963). The displacement is limited and a slip ratio of more than 15% is unusual (Fig. 21.1) (Junghanns 1930, Macnab 1950).

Causes of displacement

Many factors have been blamed for this failure, but most without much foundation:

1. Constitutional variation in the orientation of the apophyseal joints. Forward displacement

results partly from a failure of the apophyseal joints to restrain shear. They are orientated in the sagittal plane in the upper lumbar spine, and become progressively more coronally orientated towards to lower lumbar spine (Table 7.1, page 73). The increasing shear forces in the lower lumbar lordotic spine are balanced by the progressively efficient restraint of the coronally orientated lower lumbar facets. L4/5 appears to be the level where the joints may fail to restrain shear (Fig. 21.2).

The inclination of the superior articular process may be significant (Newman and Stone 1963). Facetectomy in vitro certainly affects the stability of the segment (Abumi et al 1990). Those individuals whose L4/5 facets are more sagittally orientated than the rest of the population will be more prone to displacement (though see Fig. 21.3).

Table 21.1 Comparison between the segmental level and sex ratio in degenerative and isthmic spondylolisthesis.

	Degenerative Spondylolisthesis ($n = 53$)	Isthmic spondylolisthesis ($n = 107$)
Percentage male	22%	57%
L3/4	12%	2%
L4/5	78%	15%
L5/S1	12%	85%

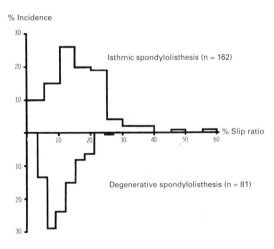

Fig. 21.1 Histogram to show the limited slip ratio of patients with degenerative spondylolisthesis compared with isthmic spondylolisthesis.

251

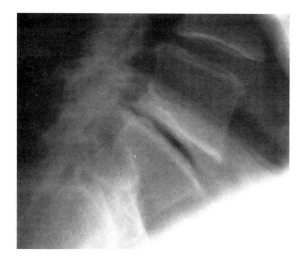

Fig. 21.2 Lateral radiograph of a transitional sixth lumbar vertebra, disc degeneration at L5/S1 and a vacuum disc but no displacement, and degenerative spondylolisthesis at L4/5 where the coronally placed facets fail to restrain shear. (Reproduced with the permission of Doncaster Royal Infirmary.)

Table 21.2   Mean lumbosacral angle for patients with degenerative spondylolisthesis, isthmic spondylolisthesis and other patients with back pain.

	Mean LS angle (degrees)
Degenerative spondylolisthesis (n = 58)	30.8 (±7.1)
Isthmic spondylolisthesis (n = 107)	37.3 (±8.3)
Other patients with back pain (n = 60)	30.3 (±6.4)

soft tissues (1963), and they thought the high incidence of spina bifida occulta important. There is no evidence that these patients have generalized ligamentous or joint laxity.

6. Obesity disproportionate to muscle strength increases the shear.

Several of these factors in combination may explain the higher incidence of degenerative spondylolisthesis in women, but none are proved.

Neurological compromise

The proximal vertebra steadily displaces forwards deforming the vertebral canal, the root canal and the intervertebral foramina (Figs 21.4 and 21.5). If the central canal is already constitutionally narrow, then vertebral displacement with an intact neural arch will deform the dura and its contents. The root canal can also become critically narrow, especially at the foraminal exit. When a dynamic element is superimposed on the reduction of space for the neural contents, pathological changes develop in the dura and nerve roots, producing symptoms.

Instability problems

The proximal vertebra may be displaced and yet theoretically be in a neutral equilibrium; that is, segmental movement may not cause further displacement beyond the limits of normal restraint. Alternatively, it may be displaced and be unstable, being further displaced by movement beyond the normal limits of restraint. This is a theoretical distinction, but it does have practical implications. A vertebra which has displaced but has reached a position of neutral equilibrium is unlikely to produce symptoms of fatigue in the soft tissues which restrain shear, nor momentary subluxation

2. The mechanical strength of the subchondral bone. The osteoporotic spine will be vulnerable to microfractures, with deformity of the facets. It had been suggested that an increased angle between the pedicle and inferior articular facet would allow forward subluxation of the upper vertebra (Junghanns 1930, Macnab 1950, Tsunoda et al 1980). However, Newman and Stone (1963) found no increase of this angle in the slipping vertebra and suspected that progressive widening of the angle may accompany the progressive slip from remodelling in response to microscopic stress fractures.

3. A degenerate disc will less effectively restrain Shear (Larson 1983, Fitzgerald & Newman 1976, Matsunaga et al 1990).

4. An increased lumbar lordosis will increase the force of shear (Fitzgerald & Newman 1976). There is no evidence that these patients have an increased lumbosacral angle (Table 21.2), but posture, especially in pregnancy when the ligamentous restraint is less effective, is probably significant.

5. Poor spinal and abdominal muscles place proportionally greater strain on the apophyseal joints. Newman and Stone believed that the facets give way from an acquired instability of the

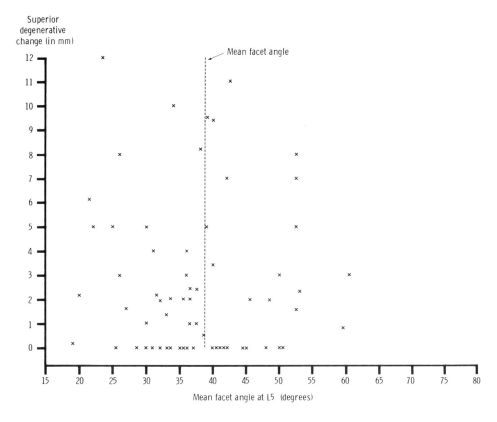

Fig. 21.3   Graph showing the degree of degenerative change of the upper facet of L5 compared with the sagittal orientation of the facets. There does not appear to be a correlation. (Reproduced with the permission of Doncaster Royal Infirmary.)

pain in the apophyseal joints or dura. A displaced vertebra with a degree of associated unnatural segmental movement may produce either of these symptoms.

Degenerative change

Degenerative changes develop in the apophyseal joints and at the margins of the vertebral bodies, until a degree of stability occurs (Fig. 21.6). These osteophytic changes can encroach into the root canal. It is interesting that the vertebral body of degenerative spondylolisthesis does not become wedge-shaped as in the displaced body of an isthmic spondylolisthesis, the former displacing in adult life, the latter during growth.

SYMPTOMS ASSOCIATED WITH DEGENERATIVE SPONDYLOLISTHESIS

The anatomical displacement of one vertebra upon another does not necessarily cause symptoms. If symptoms do occur they are generally either symptoms of instability or symptoms of compromise with embarrassment of the dura and nerve roots within a small deformed central canal or root canal.

Symptoms of instability

Momentary jerky movement is a common symptom and sign, with discomfort rising from the stooped position or getting up out of a chair. To avoid this patients will support the trunk with the

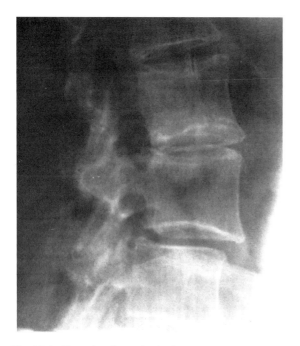

Fig. 21.4   Lateral radiograph of a degenerative spondylolisthesis at L4/5 with deformation of the root canal.

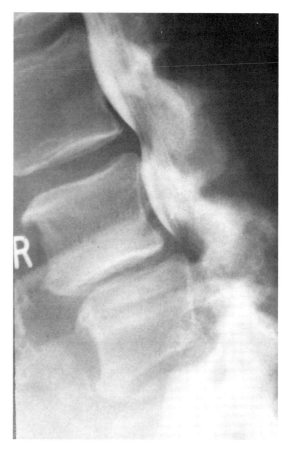

Fig. 21.5   Myelogram of a man with neurogenic claudication, where a degenerative spondylolisthesis at L4/5 completely blocks the flow of contrast. (Reproduced with the permission of Doncaster Royal Infirmary.)

hands on their thighs as they stand up after stooping. Sudden movements and turning in bed can be painful. Standing and walking also cause fatigue pain, with aching in the back and thighs. It is relieved by rest. Flexion is not limited, and they can frequently place the flat of the hands on the floor. They may have an extension catch and no lumbar extension. Tenderness is localized to the level of the displacement. There are no abnormal neurological signs unless there is another associated lesion.

The mechanism of these instability symptoms is speculative. Some believe that the apophyseal joints are probably the pain source, but this does not explain why some patients with degenerative spondylolisthesis are quite symptom-free. Our ultrasound measurement of the vertebral canal in 81 patients with back pain and degenerative spondylolisthesis suggests that some have narrow central canals, the mean measurement at L5 being 1.39 cm (SD 0.08 cm). If the canal size is a relevant factor, then the momentary pain with jerky movement may be dural in origin (Fig. 21.7).

Root entrapment pain

The L4 root within its root canal is at risk in an L4/5 degenerative spondylolisthesis. It can produce the classical symptoms of root entrapment, but the pain is particularly influenced by posture and spinal rotation. The L5 root is also vulnerable as it crosses a rolled rim of L4/5 disc (Fig. 21.8), especially if the L5 central canal is trefoil in shape.

Neurogenic claudication

This can be precipitated by a degenerative spondylolisthesis, especially in men. Although degenerative spondylolisthesis is more common in

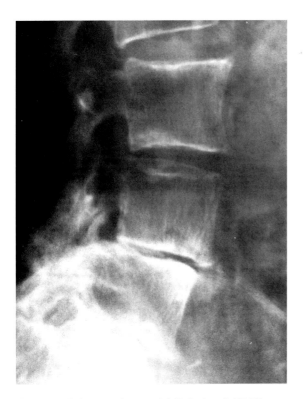

Fig. 21.6 A degenerative spondylolisthesis at L4/5. The marked disc degeneration and hypertrophied superior facet at L5 probably restored stability.

women than in men, when neurogenic claudication occurs with degenerative spondylolisthesis, the patients are usually male. About half the male patients with bilateral neurogenic claudication have some vertebral displacement with an intact neural arch. A pre-existing narrow canal with some forward vertebral displacement is an unpleasant combination, but a single-level stenosis is not likely to result in neurogenic claudication. A single-level central stenosis at L4/5 will give back pain aggravated by movement, but not neurogenic claudication. The high male incidence of degenerative spondylolisthesis and neurogenic claudication is probably because neurogenic claudication is a two-level lesion, and men are more likely than women to have a second level of degenerative pathology.

MANAGEMENT OF SYMPTOMS ASSOCIATED WITH DEGENERATIVE SPONDYLOLISTHESIS

Instability pain is effectively managed with an explanation of the pain mechanism and appropriate advice. Pain in the back, perhaps referred to the buttocks and thighs, is seldom so severe that the patient cannot be managed by a conservative approach. They are helped by the 'back school' programme, when fitness and obesity may be discussed. Lifting is demonstrated and practised, avoiding stooping and twisting, and using the legs and not the back. They are reassured that with time and the inevitable stiffness of age, their unstable spinal segment should become more stable and less troublesome. If instability symptoms are the only problem, the natural history is good.

Root entrapment syndrome can usually be managed conservatively, though occasionally the severity, disability and duration of the pain make surgical intervention necessary. It may not be possible to recognize preoperatively which nerve root is involved, whether L5 in the central canal or L4 in the root canal. The clinical examination may help with support from electromyographic (EMG) studies, nerve root infiltration and a CT scan or MRI, but it may only be at the time of operation after adequate decompression and exposure that the correct root is identified.

Removal of the lamina usually reveals an hour-glass constriction of the dura, compressed from either side by osteophytic outgrowths of the apophyseal joint. The L4 root can be involved in the deformed root canal, and it needs complete decompression while laterally removing much of the inferior and superior facets of the apophyseal joints on the affected side. The decision to fuse the spine as well as decompress depends on the degree of degenerative change at L4/5, and on the amount of bone to be removed. Provided the joint is not completely removed and the contra-lateral joint is undisturbed, if the disc space is degenerative then there is no real risk of subsequent increase in the vertebral displacement (Epstein et al 1983). However, concomitant fusion seems to give superior results to decompression alone (Herkowitz & Kurz 1991). Some advocate anterior decompression and interbody fusion

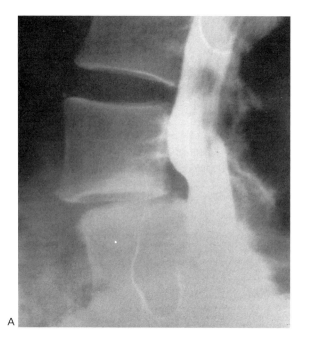
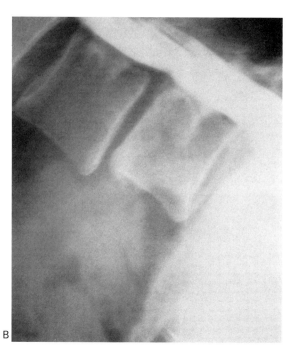

Fig. 21.7(A) Radiculogram of a patient with degenerative spondylolisthesis at L4/5 where the contrast is distorted in extension. **(B)** The anterior dural deformation is largely corrected in flexion. The anterior dura and anterior longitudinal ligament are richly innervated, and could be a nociceptive source if the canal is narrow.

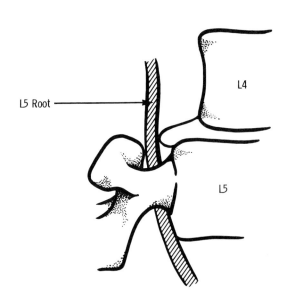

Fig. 21.8 Diagram demonstrating that the L5 root can be affected in the central canal between the rolled edge of the L4/5 disc and the cranial edge of the lamina of L5, especially if the canal is trefoil in shape.

(Takahashi et al 1990), and others would attempt to reduce the displacement prior to fusion (Chang 1990).

The L5 root can be involved in the central canal as it passes over the ridged L4/5 disc. There is counter-compression dorsally from the cranial edge of the lamina of L5. Attempts to remove the thickened rim of L4/5 disc are not usually very successful and removal of the posterior vertebral bar of L5 is likewise difficult, but the bone can be surgically impacted. Decompression of the central canal by removal of the L5 lamina does, however, provide more space for the L5 root. The L5 root is often kinked in the lateral recess of a trefoil-shaped central canal, under the overlapping superior facet. The medial edge of the facet must be excised and the facet undercut to effectively decompress the root.

The treatment of neurogenic claudication is discussed in Chapter 17. It is a two-level pathology, and the surgeon must decide which are the two significant levels. If surgical decompression is attempted at the level of the degenerative spondylolisthesis, it is important to leave a remnant of the inferior facets to prevent further subluxation of the displaced vertebra, and to fuse the segment to avoid further displacement (Fujiya et al 1990). Radical decompression without fusion risks only temporary benefit.

REFERENCES

Abumi K, Panjabi M M, Kramer K M, Duranccau J, Oxland T, Crisco J J 1990 Biomechanical evaluation of lumbar spinal stability after graded facetectomies. Spine 15: 1142–1147

Chang K W 1990 Degenerative spondylolisthesis treated with reduction fixation system. Journal of Surgical Association, Republic of China 23: 120–127

Epstein N E, Epstein J A, Carras R, Lavine S 1983 Degenerative spondylolisthesis with an intact neural arch; a review of 60 cases with analysis of clinical findings and the development of surgical management. Neurosurgery 13: 555–561

Fitzgerald J A, Newman P A 1976 Degenerative spondylolisthesis. Journal of Bone and Joint Surgery 58-B: 184–192

Fujiya M, Saita M, Kaneda K, Abumi K 1990 Clinical study on stability of combined distraction and compression rod instrumentation with posterolateral fusion for unstable degenerative spondylolisthesis. Spine 15: 1216–1222

Herkowitz H N, Kurz L T 1991 Degenerative lumbar spondylolisthesis with spinal stenosis. Journal of Bone and Joint Surgery 73-A: 802–808

Junghanns H 1930 Spondylolisthesen ohne Spalt im zwischengelenkstuck. Archiv fur Orthopaedische und Unfall Chirurgie 29: 118

Larson S J 1983 Degenerative spondylolisthesis. Neurosurgery 13: 560–561

Macnab I 1950 Spondylolisthesis with an intact neural arch: so-called pseudospondylolisthesis. Journal of Bone and Joint Surgery 32-B: 325

Matsunaga S, Sakou J, Morizono Y, Masuda A, Demirtas A M 1990 Natural history of degenerative spondylolisthesis: pathologies and natural course of the slippage. Spine 15: 1204–1210

Newman P H, Stone K H 1963 The etiology of spondylolisthesis. Journal of Bone and Joint Surgery 45-B: 39–59

Schmorl G, Junghanns H 1932 Die gesunde und krande wirbelsaule. George Thieme, Leipzig

Takahashi K, Kitahara H, Yamagata M, Murakami M 1990 Long-term results of anterior interbody fusion for treatment of degenerative spondylolisthesis. Spine 15: 1211–1215

Tsunoda N, Kurace S, Sakaki K 1980 Radiological study of degenerative spondylolisthesis. Rinsho Seikei Geka 15: 1216–1222

22. Retrolisthesis and degenerative lumbar scoliosis — pathology, clinical significance and treatment

PATHOLOGY

Coupled displacement

Vertebral displacement can occur in any one of the three axes of rotation: sagittal, coronal or transverse (Fig. 22.1). Retrolisthesis implies a posterior displacement of the proximal vertebral body in the sagittal plane, but in practice it is more often coupled in two or even three planes (Farfan 1973). A single radiograph in the lateral projection may show what appears to be a posterior displacement (Fig. 22.2) and this may indeed be confirmed by the absence of lateral and rotational displacement in the anteroposterior view.

The lateral radiograph, however, often gives a hint of a combined rotational displacement by the double shadow of the posterior vertebral body margin (Fig. 22.3). The asymmetrical facets in the anteroposterior film suggest a rotational element in the displacement. If the facets are constitutionally symmetrical the vertebra will displace posteriorly, but one spine in three will have facets with more than 5° of asymmetry (page 74), and this will encourage rotational displacement (Cyron & Hutton 1980). Unequal facet degeneration may produce asymmetry, with remodelling from stress and microfracture and subsequent rotational displacement. Malalignment of the spinous processes also suggests a rotational element to the vertebral displacement (Fig. 22.4).

Retrolisthesis with posterior and/or rotational displacement is the result of disc degeneration, loss of disc height and the shingling effect of the apophyseal joints (Chandnani & Chabria 1978). It usually occurs at the L4/5 or L3/4 level, or at the segment adjacent to a fusion or congenital block vertebra (Fig. 22.5). Rotational displacement can progress quickly in a few years, particularly in postmenopausal women, to produce a marked degenerative lumbar scoliosis (Fig. 22.6). The causative mechanism may be similar to that of degenerative spondylolisthesis, with a single factor deciding whether the displacement is forwards, backwards or rotational.

The vertebral canal

When the displacement is in any of the three planes of rotation, the vertebral canal and its contents may be compromised. If the canal is small, the dura is vulnerable from changes in spinal posture (Fig. 22.7). The nerve root is also at risk in the root canal or at the foramen.

The effects of the displacement are compounded by bony and soft tissue degenerative change around the apophyseal joints, and by the formation of a

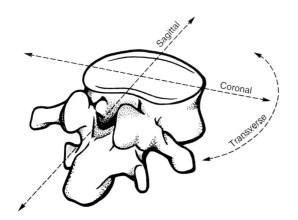

Fig. 22.1 Diagram to show axes of rotation.

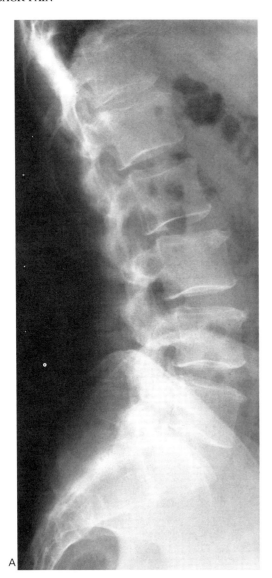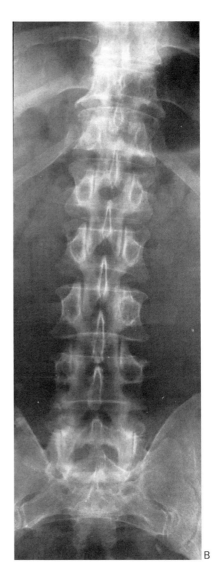

Fig. 22.2(A)   Lateral radiograph showing posterior displacement of L2 and L3, and L3 on L4 with traction spurs. **(B)**   An AP radiograph suggests that the displacement is mainly in the sagittal plane, with symmetrical sagitally orientated apophyseal joints, mid-line spinous processes, and no rotation.

posterior vertebral bar and ridging of the disc annulus. Then a rotatory movement or lateral flexion at the level of displacement further reduces the cross-sectional area of the foramen.

When space is critically limited by vertebral displacement, it is the combination of change of posture and nerve root excursion that produces pathological changes in the root, with symptoms of root entrapment.

Retrolisthesis rarely causes symptoms in the upper lumbar spine, where the canal and foramina are more spacious. It is lower lumbar displacement, with associated pathological changes, that affects the neural elements.

Because posterior and rotational displacement often affect more than one segmental level, it is not uncommon to find a multiple-level central canal stenosis, with associated root canal stenosis

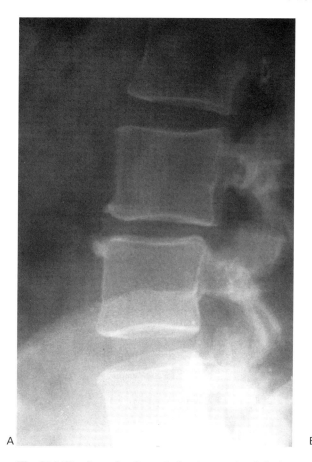
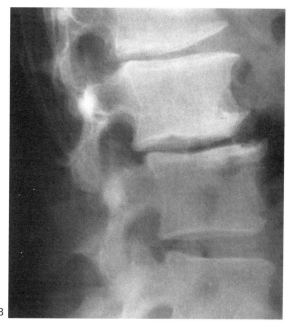

Fig. 22.3(A) Lateral radiograph showing rotational displacement at L3/4, confirmed by the double shadow of the posterior aspect of L3. **(B)** Similar coupled displacement, with marked disc degeneration at L3/4.

at a more distal level (Fig. 22.8). A two-level venous occlusion with pooling and venous stasis may then be responsible for symptoms of neurogenic claudication. The claudication symptoms of a patient with lumbar scoliosis are usually unilateral, probably because the root is affected in a distal root canal from asymmetrical degenerative changes with a second proximal occlusion from central stenosis (Fig. 17.17 p. 211).

CLINICAL SIGNIFICANCE

Root entrapment

Of our 177 patients attending with a retro- (or rotational) listhesis, 42% had root pain below the knee incriminating a single nerve. Displacement

at L4 can affect the fourth root in the root canal, or the fifth root in the central canal, over a posterior vertebral bar or beneath a superior facet. L3 displacement can similarly affect the third or fourth root. The root pain is affected by spinal posture. It is not the major cause of root entrapment, but when displacement does occur, the root is at risk.

Posture-related back pain

Retrolisthesis is an important factor in posture-related back pain in the middle-aged and elderly, either from dural irritation or apophyseal joint pain. In both of these syndromes limited spinal flexion is not a feature of the examination but, probably because extension decreases the space in

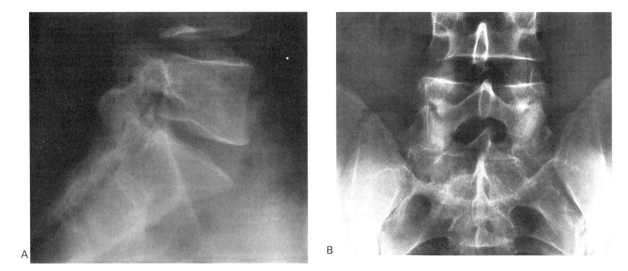

Fig. 22.4(A)   Retrolisthesis at L4/5. **(B)**   AP film of the same patient suggests a rotational component to the displacement, with asymmetrical facets at L4/5 and malalignment of the spinous process of L4.

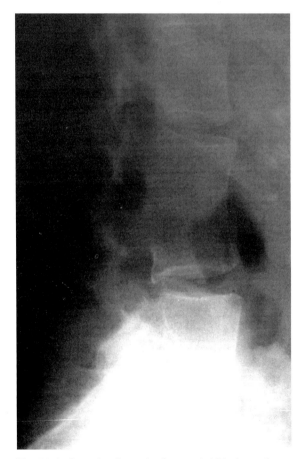

Fig. 22.5   Lateral radiograph of congenital block vertebrae at L3/4 with retrolisthesis at L4/5.

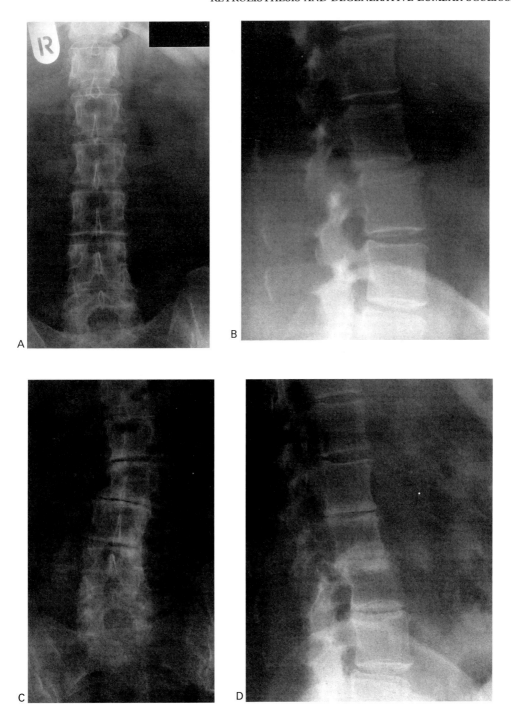

Fig. 22.6   AP (**A**) and lateral (**B**) radiographs of a 45-year-old woman with early signs of coupled retrolisthesis at L2/3. AP (**C**) and lateral (**D**) radiograph of the same patient 6 years later showing a structural lumbar scoliosis. She now had symptoms of unilateral neurogenic claudication.

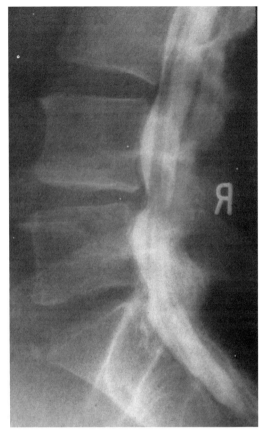

Fig. 22.7 Lateral radiograph of a myelogram showing posterior displacement of L4 on L5, and a posterior bulge of the annulus. This is not a disc protrusion, and excision of the disc will not cure the patient. Excessive or erratic segmental movement associated with chronic disc degeneration is probably responsible for back pain, and surgery must address the problem of both stenosis and instability.

the central and root canal, spinal extension is reduced or absent. Space seems to be highly significant in the causation of symptoms. Nearly half of our 177 patients with retrolisthesis had ultrasound measurement of the central canal below the 10th percentile for asymptomatic subjects.

Unilateral (root) claudication

Of our patients with claudication symptoms in one leg, 50% had rotational vertebral displacement with a two-level stenosis — a central canal stenosis proximally, and a more distal unilateral root canal stenosis. One-third of these patients were women past the menopause.

TREATMENT

Conservative

If the patient has learnt that symptoms are related to certain movements and to posture, a change of posture when pain develops and avoidance of movements that cause pain is obvious advice which can be reinforced in a back school with an explanation of ways of reducing spinal stress in everyday life. A corset with a frame rather than parallel steels will restrict rotation and lateral flexion. It should be accompanied by advice about maintaining good muscle and bone strength by swimming and walking. Severe root pain may require epidural injections.

Surgery

A few patients need surgical help. With root entrapment every effort should be made to identify the affected root before surgery. The lesion may be too distal for identification by myelography and, although CT scan and MR may show bony encroachment, this is not necessarily the side of the lesion. The root may be recognized at operation from its size, its colour, its consistency and more significantly from its tension.

If the root is affected in the central canal the cranial lip of the lamina is excised, perhaps with part of the rolled ridge of annulus and impaction of the posterior vertebral bar at the level of displacement. Involvement in the root canal requires adequate decompression with undercutting of the superior facet on the affected side and a major part of the apophyseal joint.

If back pain is the problem and the central canal is stenosed with posterior displacement, bilateral decompression by excision of the cranial part of the lamina can help. Radical decompression, however, may increase the instability. When it can be shown that the dura is significantly affected by posture (Fig. 17.3), distraction fusion is useful (Fujiya et al 1990).

The patient with degenerative lumbar scoliosis and unilateral claudication requires not only a two-level decompression of the affected root, but also a fusion to prevent further postoperative displacement.

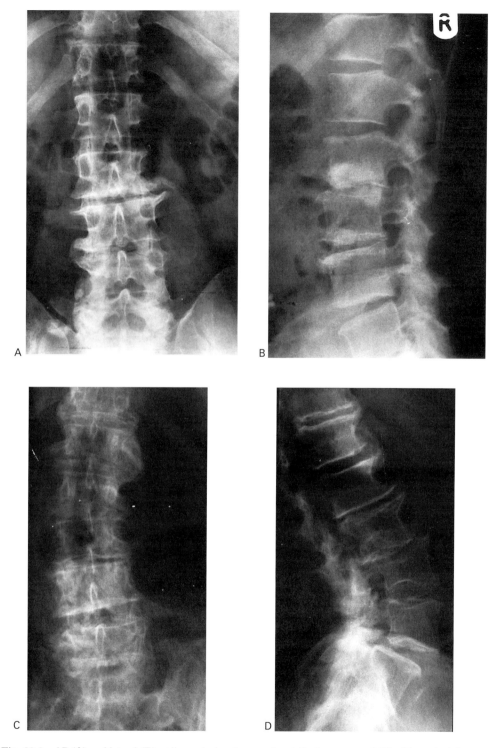

Fig. 22.8 AP (**A**) and lateral (**B**) radiograph showing rotational displacement at L2/3 with marked degenerative change at that level and at L3/4, 4/5 and L5/S1, on the right. The patient had right root claudication with central stenosis at L2/3 and root canal stenosis at L4 and L5. AP (**C** and lateral **D**) radiograph of a patient with root claudication. There is an isthmic spondylolisthesis at L5/S1 with root compromise at that level, and a structural mid-lumbar scoliosis causing central stenosis at L3/4.

REFERENCES

Chandnani P G, Chabria P B 1978 Posterior spinal compression by the cephalad edge of the laminae and its role in the etiology of backache. Neurology India 26: 7–9

Cyron B M, Hutton W C 1980 Articular trophism and stability of the lumbar spine. Spine 5: 168–172

Farfan H F 1973 The mechanical disorders of the lower back. Lea and Febiger, Philadelphia

Fujiya M, Saita M, Kaneda K, Abumi K 1990 Clinical study of combined distraction and compression and instrumentation with posterolateral fusion for unstable degenerative spondylolisthesis. Spine 15: 1216–1222

23. Fractures of the vertebrae — spinal injury, pathology, symptoms, management, natural history — and osteoporotic fractures

FRACTURES OF HEALTHY BONE

Pathology

The commonest fractures of the thoracic and lumbar spines occur as a result of a vertical compression force, sometimes combined with flexion, lateral flexion, rotation or extension. T12, L1 and L2 are the vertebrae most often affected, with decreasing incidence proximally and distally (Nicoll 1949, Young 1973). Two or more vertebrae, not necessarily adjacent to each other, may be fractured.

It is helpful to classify vertebral fractures in relation to the three columns: first, the anterior and middle parts of the vertebral body and anterior annulus; second, the posterior cortex and posterior annulus; and third, the posterior elements (Denis 1983, McAfee et al 1983). In addition there are two clinical questions related to the pathology which are important in planning management: is the spine stable?, and is there neurological impairment? (Bohlman 1985).

Wedge compression fracture

This is the most common vertebral fracture, resulting from an isolated failure of the anterior column following axial loading and flexion. It is stable. The vertebrae become wedged-shaped, varying in degree. There is usually no neurological deficit but nerve damage can occasionally occur, depending on the size of the vertebral canal, the severity of the initial injury and the degree of kyphosis initially or in later years.

Stable burst fracture

Both the anterior and middle columns fail as a result of a compressive load, but with integrity of the posterior elements the spine is stable. Displacement of bony fragments or disc material can, however, compromise the vertebral canal with neural compression. Holdsworth suggested that, provided the posterior elements were undamaged, there was usually no neurological deficit (Holdsworth 1963); however, CT imaging has shown how much more extensive is the fracture of the posterior column than was originally appreciated from conventional radiographs (Figs 23.1 and 23.2). Neurological deficit can develop some years after the injury (Fig. 23.3). In a study by Ballock and colleagues (1992), one-quarter of fractures diagnosed as wedge compression fractures on plain radiographs were, when examined by CT, really burst fractures affecting the middle and sometimes the posterior columns.

Unstable burst fracture

In this type of fracture, all three columns have failed. There is a tendency to kyphosis, with progressive neurological symptoms.

Chance fracture

A chance fracture (Chance 1948) is a horizontal avulsion injury of the vertebral body following tensile flexion around an axis anterior to the anterior longitudinal ligament.

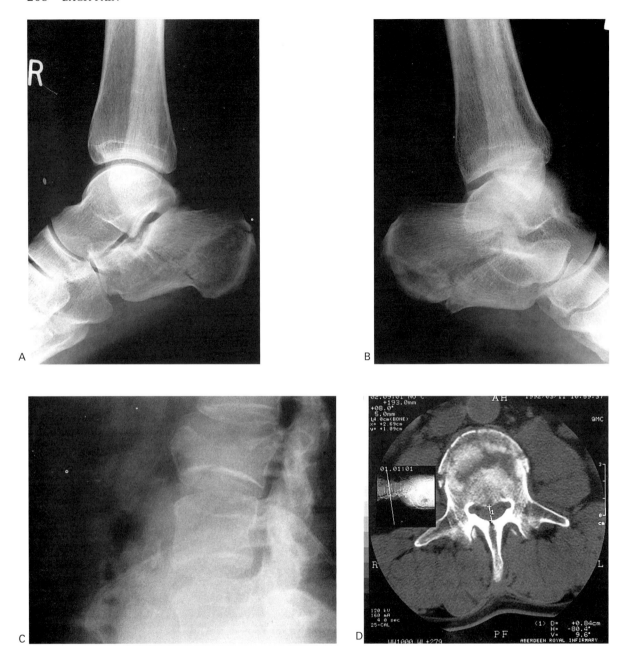

Fig. 23.1   Fractures of both os calces (**A**) and (**B**) in a man who fell 18 feet from a ladder. In addition he had an anterior and middle column fracture of the body of L1 (**C**). The CT scan (**D**) shows bony encroachment into the vertebral canal, but he had no abnormal neurological signs.

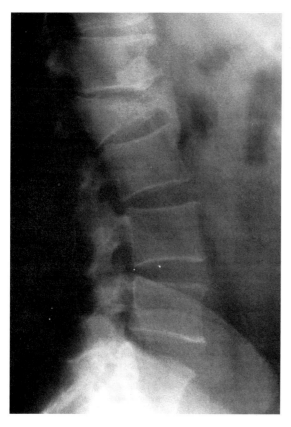

Fig. 23.2 Lateral radiograph of a burst fracture with failure of the anterior and middle columns. Integrity of the posterior column ensures stability. There was no neurological compromise, but this could subsequently develop.

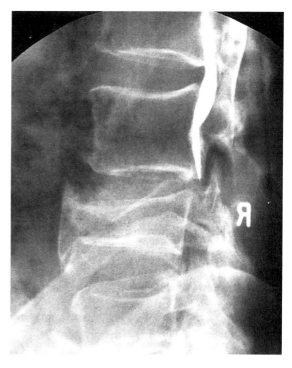

Fig. 23.3 Lateral myelogram (some contrast is extradural) of a 73-year-old man who sustained a stable burst fracture 16 years previously. He now presents with 5 years of neurogenic claudication, and has a complete block at L3/4.

Flexion–distraction fracture

A flexion–distraction fracture affects all three columns, following compression of the anterior column and tension of the middle and posterior columns (Fig. 23.4).

Translational injuries

Translational injuries are those in which the spine is displaced in the transverse plane at the fracture site.

Hyperextension injuries

These constitute less than 3% of all spinal injuries. Disruption usually occurs through the disc with no bony damage to the anterior or middle column.

The posterior elements are usually comminuted with gross neurological damage (Denis & Burkus 1992).

Fractures of the limbus

Fractures of the posterior superior or posterior and inferior margins of the mid- and lower lumbar vertebral bodies are not uncommon. These fractures tend to occur in adolescents and young adults. They can be avulsion fractures of the posterior cortical rim of the vertebra; they may involve some cancellous bone; they may be only a chip fracture, or a fracture of the whole length of the vertebral margin (Epstein & Epstein 1991).

Disc injury

In addition to the bony injury, flexion and compression can affect a lower lumbar disc (Pratt et al 1990). This is frequently missed clinically, being overshadowed by the more obvious fracture,

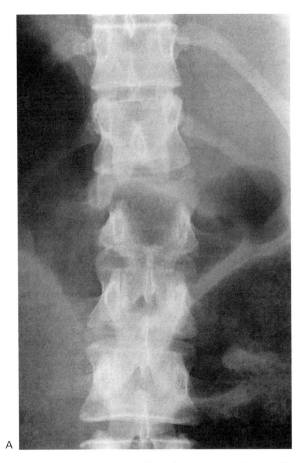 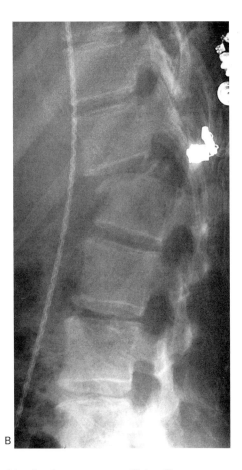

Fig. 23.4 AP (**A**) and lateral (**B**) radiographs of a 23-year-old woman involved in a head-on motor car collision. She was wearing a lap belt, sustained a flexion distraction fracture at D12/L1 and was paraplegic below that level. She also had major visceral injuries.

but persisting lower lumbar symptoms make one suspect this associated injury. A painful tear of the posterior annulus is probably not uncommon. Adams and Hutton (1982) showed that experimental disc compression in flexion can injure the annulus. It may be more significant if the annulus is already pathological.

Our studies of 71 patients with compression fractures of the spine recorded a correlation between the persistence of symptoms and the size of the vertebral canal (Table 23.1). Whether the pain source was at the fracture site or from a more distal lesion is uncertain.

Damaged viscus

Rear seat passengers of motor vehicles involved in accidents may suffer unrecognized intra-abdominal injuries as well as the spinal flexion injury. The isolated use of the lap belt is probably responsible. They need careful observation for 48 h to exclude a ruptured viscus, and early laparotomy if injury is suspected (Legay et al 1990).

Symptoms

Symptoms at the time of fracture are variable in degree and do not appear to be related to the severity of the compression (Nicoll 1949, Young 1973). A few patients with wedge compression fracture are able to remain on their feet, but most have quite severe back pain and tenderness at the site of injury. Retroperitoneal or mediastinal bleeding can be copious and this adds to the

Table 23.1 Relationship between ultrasound measurements (cm) of the vertebral canal and persistent back pain symptoms in 71 patients following compression fracture (mean time after fracture 4.4 years). Significance between groups 1 and 2 at L5 is $p < 0.02$.

	Back pain		
Level	None or very mild* ($n = 28$)	Intermittent[†] ($n = 26$)	Severe or constant ($n = 17$)
L1	1.50	1.48	1.47
L2	1.46	1.45	1.44
L3	1.45	1.42	1.41
L4	1.42	1.40	1.39
L5	1.43	1.39	1.38

*Occasional symptoms not limiting activities; [†] limiting activities.

discomfort. Such bleeding can simulate rupture of a major vessel and may need CT or MR for diagnosis.

Abnormal neurological signs may be absent, incomplete or complete at the level of the lesion. Holdsworth (1970) observed that a complete spinal cord or cauda equina injury that had not recovered at 48 h would be permanent. In the thoracic spine, incomplete lesions can cause anterior cord syndrome with sparing of some distal motor function and sparing of posterior column modalities of position and vibratory sense. Less common is the central cord syndrome, with greater proximal than distal paralysis and varying degrees of sensory sparing. Rarely, a Brown-Séquard syndrome will give hemiparesis. Incomplete lesions have potential for some recovery (Bohlman 1985).

Management

CT or MR scanning is advisable for all patients with vertebral body fractures, because the severity of the injury is rarely appreciated from conventional radiographs alone (Kerslake et al 1991). However, CT can cause apprehension when the clinician sees large bony fragments distorting the vertebral canal. In the absence of immediate neurological damage, there is the fear that narrowing will inevitably cause stenotic symptoms later but this is unfounded (McEvoy & Bradford 1985). In fact, substantial remodelling of the vertebral canal is possible (Fidler 1988, Johnsson et al 1991). It is not necessary to remove even large bony fragments

from the vertebral canal if there is normal neurology, or only slight impairment, but a significant neurological lesion requires early operative decompression and stabilization. A complete lesion for more than 48 h will not respond to decompression, and even early decompression for complete lesions has poor results. However, patients with incomplete lesions have significant potential for recovery with decompression; one can not say how many would have recovered without surgery. Decompression is often best accomplished by an anterior approach with stabilization.

When the spine is deemed unstable and there is no neurological damage, the decision must be made whether to treat the patient conservatively and await fracture union and stability, or to recommend surgical fusion. The latter assists early return to optimal function, avoids the traumatic effect that an unstable segment might have on the neurological structures, and obviates the need for later fusion if it does not occur naturally.

In a stable spine without neurological damage, bed rest is advisable until a reduction in pain allows mobilization in reasonable comfort. This may take a few days or a couple of weeks. Graded mobilization is encouraged. There is no evidence that either long periods of bed rest or even energetic exercises influence recovery. What is probably more important is a careful explanation of the significance of the fractured vertebra. It is reassuring for the patient with a stable fracture to know that eventually they should become symptom-free and, should some pain persist, it is likely to be only intermittent and not disabling. A temporary corset can help a mid- or lower lumbar fracture, but otherwise is to be avoided. Plenty of walking and swimming helps in the recovery period.

Natural history

If patients with litigation problems are excluded, then the majority of patients with stable vertebral fractures become free of symptoms within a few months of injury. Litigation influences the natural history considerably. This may be because these injuries result from industrial and road accidents, often with more violence than domestic accidents.

Alternatively, the financial implications associated with litigation may generate genuine distress and abnormal pain behaviour.

The severity of kyphosis with compression fractures may be a factor affecting the natural history (Legay et al 1990), and it is suggested that a kyphosis of more than 40° is likely to increase further in the first 3 months (Bohlman 1985). However, in our study of 71 patients up to 10 years after a stable spine fracture, pain, when it did persist, tended to become less troublesome with time. This agrees with the observation that relatively few patients with a previous wedge compression fracture seek help with back pain later in life.

OSTEOPOROTIC COMPRESSION FRACTURE OF THE SPINE FROM SKELETAL FAILURE

Although there is no precise information about the prevalence of vertebral compression fractures due to skeletal failure, population surveys suggest that 15.1 new fractures per 1000 person years occur in white American women over 50 years of age. This is twice the incidence of hip fracture (Cooper & Melton 1992) though they have a lesser morbidity, with only 8% being admitted to hospital. Such fractures are much less common in men.

Low bone mineral density is the most important determinant in osteoporotic compression fractures, with a deficiency in bone mass per unit volume. The bone present is essentially normal, but the mass reduced.

Age, sex and especially the menopause are important in the development of osteoporosis, but bone mass may be reduced by immobilization, corticosteroid drugs, hyperparathyroidism, Cushing's syndrome, hypogonadism and by bone replacement by metastases myelomatosis and reticuloendothelial disorders. These need to be excluded before one can assume that a compression fracture in the elderly is the result of the more common age-related (senile) osteoporosis.

Osteomalacia, in which the bone mass is reduced with decreased mineralization of the osteoid, may coexist with osteoporosis and also needs to be excluded. It is probably frequently unrecognized.

The degree of osteoporosis is related to bone stock developed in earlier life and the rate of bone loss thereafter. The rate of cortical bone loss is comparable in males and females (0.5–1% per annum) but because men have a greater initial bone mass, the amount of bone remaining in men is greater than in women. Trabecular bone loss is probably related to lack of ovarian function and thus, after the menopause, the superimposition of increased trabecular loss increases the risk of skeletal failure in the vertebral bodies. There is unequivocal deficiency of trabecular bone if assessed by iliac crest bone biopsy (Nordin 1983).

We know little about abnormality of the matrix, and when added to osteoporosis this may hold the key to skeletal failure.

Clinically

One or several vertebral bodies may collapse suddenly or slowly. Sudden failure of one vertebral body results in spontaneous severe back pain. It becomes less severe, settling over several weeks, unless another vertebra collapses. Gradual failure of several vertebrae is often associated with chronic back pain, sometimes with episodic increase in the pain with development of a kyphosis (the 'dowager's hump') and loss of height (Fig. 23.5). Many patients have persistent back pain 6 months after the fracture (Ringe 1987). Abdominal skin folds appear and with gross collapse, the ribs can rest on the iliac crest. The cosmetic embarrassment of this appearance is often more troublesome than the symptoms of pain.

After a recent fracture there is localized tenderness to pressure over the spinous process, muscle spasm and restricted movement.

A patient may present with cervical symptoms from a compensatory cervical lordosis rather than with a painful thoracic spine, or alternatively with low back pain from a compensatory exaggerated lumbar lordosis. The centre of gravity is thrown forwards by the upper thoracic kyphosis and, in attempting to compensate for this, the lumbar spine extends. This can disturb the apophyseal joints, cause impingement of the spinous process and, if there is a spinal stenosis, the neural elements can be embarrassed. There is some

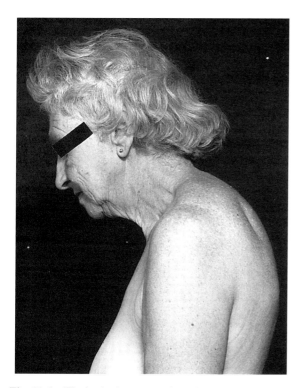

Fig. 23.5 The kyphotic posture of vertebral osteoporosis.

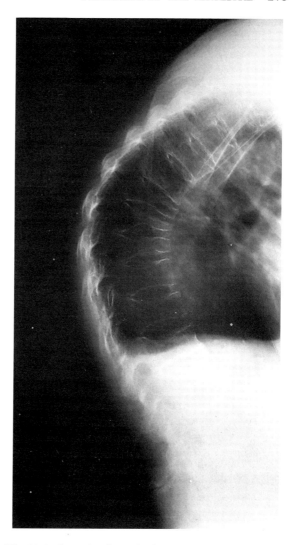

Fig. 23.6 Lateral radiograph of an osteoporotic thoracic spine with several compression fractures, and biconcave intervertebral discs where there have been subchondral microfractures beneath the end-plates.

evidence that, in contrast to men whose peak incidence of back pain is at 40 years of age, there is a steadily increasing incidence of back pain in women with advancing age (Fin Biering-Sorensen 1982), and we can speculate that menopausal osteoporosis is partly responsible.

Investigations

The clinical diagnosis is confirmed radiologically. One or more vertebrae are collapsed, with a loss of mineral content appearing as decreased density. The trabecular bone may become almost radio-lucent and the cortical shell give the appearance of a 'ghost vertebra'. In the thoracic spine, collapse of the vertebral body is mainly at the anterior aspect, producing the kyphus. There are three types of fracture pattern — wedge, crush and biconcave end-plate fracture. The intervertebral discs develop a biconcave appearance as subcortical microfractures permit the disc to encroach into the adjacent vertebrae, described as 'cod fish vertebrae' (Resnick 1982) (Fig. 23.6). The radio-logical signs of demineralization are not always so apparent because one-third of the skeletal mass is lost before there is bone rarefaction on the plain radiograph (Stevenson & Whitehead 1982).

Most patients with collapsed vertebral bodies have age-related osteoporosis and, because active treatment is of doubtful value, too much investigation for an elderly patient is not justified. Investigations are necessary, however, if there is a suspicion that the demineralization can be treated, or if there are signs of osteomalacia. Is there a past history of gastric surgery, with the possibility of deficient dietary intake and poor absorption? Is there evidence of renal disease or biliary cirrhosis? Is she receiving corticosteroids? Is there evidence of hyperparathyroidism? Is there a blood dyscrasia, or a suggestion of skeletal metastases? Are there radiological loozer zones? The patient whose initial severe pain is now settling down is more likely to have age-related skeletal failure than the patient whose back is steadily getting worse. The latter needs thorough investigation.

Biochemical assays have proved of little value in the diagnosis of osteoporosis, apart from excluding other conditions. In osteomalacia, blood tests may show low to normal calcium and phosphorus and raised alkaline phosphatase but a bone biopsy is necessary for confirmation. Bone density can be quantified by Dual Energy X-ray Absorptiometry (DXA, Fig. 23.7), but is seldom required for a diagnosis. The spinal readings will be artificially raised from spinal compression fractures. Ultrasound has the potential to measure bone density and is affected by architecture and elasticity (Fig. 23.8) (Langton et al 1984, Porter et al 1990, 1991, Massie et al 1993), and is probably a more useful discriminator than DXA for osteoporotic fractures (Massie et al 1992).

Management

The sudden severe pain of a collapsed vertebra does require a few days' rest in bed, but because of increased bone loss associated with recumbency (Leblanc et al 1990, Van der Wiel et al 1991),

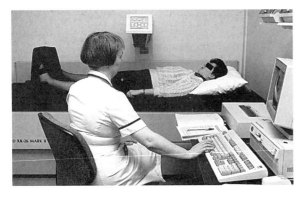

Fig. 23.7 Dual energy X-ray absorptiomery (DXA).

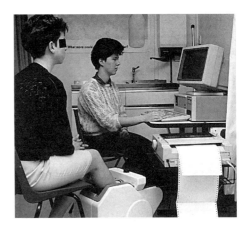

Fig. 23.8 The measurement of broad-band ultrasound attenuation (BUA) across the heel. The patient's foot is placed in a water bath, a transmitting transducer at one side and a receiver at the other. Attenuation of sound is measured.

this should be for a minimum of time. Early mobilization and activity are encouraged. In fact, exercise is the only known way of naturally reducing the rate of demineralization (Beverly et al 1989). A word of encouragement that the pain will slowly settle is appreciated. Corsets are unhelpful and tend to be more cumbersome than useful.

The slowly developing kyphus of several collapsing vertebrae cannot be prevented by a support, though a brace is often requested. Mobilization techniques should be avoided, lest they precipitate further injury.

Impingement of the twelfth rib on the iliac crest can be a troublesome source of back pain and girdle pain; in this situation it is difficult to palpate between the rib and the pelvis in the seated patient. The offending rib is tender and its excision can produce welcome relief (Fig. 23.9). An unstable spinal fracture secondary to metastatic carcinoma is best treated by segmental spinal stabilization (Galasko 1991), with postoperative radiotherapy treatment of the primary tumour where possible.

At present there is no sure way of reducing the rate of demineralization in osteoporosis, let alone replacing bone. A moderate exercise programme is probably beneficial for osteoporotic bone (Jones et al 1991, Dargie & Grant 1991), and smoking is unhelpful. It is worth ensuring that there is an

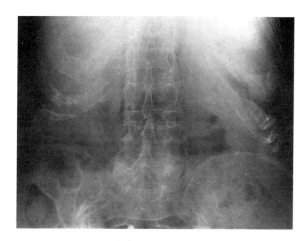

Fig. 23.9 An AP radiograph of a 74-year-old woman with osteoporosis and pain beneath the left 12th rib. Excision of the rib which was impinging on the iliac crest relieved her pain.

adequate dietary intake of calcium and vitamin D but supplements are unnecessary if the diet is adequate. There is no good evidence that oral calcium supplement can prevent postmenopausal and senile osteoporosis (Law et al 1991). Several therapeutic regimens have been shown to reduce demineralization, some even to increase total body calcium, including hormone replacement therapy (Munk-Jensen et al 1988), calcium, vitamin D, anabolic steroids, fluoride (Riggs et al 1990) and calcitonin and bisphosphonates (Fleisch 1989), but it has yet to be proved that they can reduce the incidence of subsequent fractures. Perhaps as we improve our techniques of quantitating osteoporosis, we shall be better able to monitor the methods of its prevention and eventually reduce this troublesome cause of back pain in the elderly.

REFERENCES

Adams M A, Hutton W C 1982 Prolapsed intervertebral disc, a hyperflexion injury. Spine 7: 184–191

Ballock R T, Mackersie R, Abitbol J J, Cervilla V, Resnick D, Garfin S R 1992 Can burst fractures be predicted from plain radiographs? Journal of Bone and Joint Surgery 74-B: 147–150

Beverly M C, Rider T A, Evans M J, Smith R 1989 Local bone mineral response to brief exercise that stresses the skeleton. British Medical Journal 299: 233–235

Bohlman H H 1985 Current concepts review: treatment of fractures and dislocations of the thoracic and lumbar spine. Journal of Bone and Joint Surgery 67A: 165–169

Chance G O 1948 Note on type of flexion fractures of the spine. British Journal of Radiology 21:453–453

Cooper C, Melton L J 1992 Vertebral fractures (letter). British Medical Journal 304: 793–794

Dargie H J, Grant S 1991 Exercise. British Medical Journal 303: 910–911

Denis F 1983 The three column spine and its significance in the classification of acute thoracolumbar spinal injuries. Spine 8: 817–831

Denis F, Burkus J K 1992 Shear fractures — dislocations of the thoracolumbar spine associated with forceful hyperextension (lumberjack paraplegia). Spine 17: 156–161

Epstein N E, Epstein J A 1991 Limbus lumbar vertebral fractures in 27 adolescents and adults. Spine 16: 962–966

Fidler M W 1988 Remodelling of the spinal canal after burst fracture: a prospective study of two cases. Journal of Bone and Joint Surgery 70B: 730–732

Fin Biering-Sorensen 1982 Low back trouble in a general population of 30-, 40-, 50- and 60-year-old men and women. Danish Medical Bulletin 29: 289–299

Fleisch H 1989 Bisphophonates: a new class of drugs in diseases of bone and calcium metabolism. Recent Results Cancer Research 116: 1–28

Galasko C J B 1991 Spinal instability secondary to the metastatic cancer. Journal of Bone and Joint Surgery 73B: 104–108

Holdsworth F W 1963 Fractures, dislocations and fracture dislocations of the spine. Journal of Bone and Joint Surgery 45-B: 6–20

Holdsworth F W 1970 Dislocations, and fracture dislocations of the spine. Journal of Bone and Joint Surgery 52A: 1534–1551

Johnsson R, Herrlin K, Hagglund G, Stromqvist B 1991 Spinal canal remodelling after thoracolumbar fractures with intraspinal bone fragments. 17 cases followed 1–4 years. Acta Orthopedica Scandinavica 62: 125–127

Jones P R M, Hardman A E, Hudson A, Morgan N G 1991 Influence of brisk walking on broadband ultrasound attenuation of the calcaneus in primarily sedentary women aged 30–61. Calcified Tissue International 49: 112–115

Kerslake R W, Jaspan T, Worthington B S 1991 Magnetic resonance imaging of spinal trauma. British Journal of Radiology 64: 386–402

Langton C McD, Palmer S B, Porter R W 1984 Measurement of broad band ultrasonic attenuation in cancellous bone. Engineering in Medicine 13: 89–91

Law M R, Wald N J, Meade T W 1991 Strategies for prevention of osteoporosis and hip fracture. British Medical Journal 303: 453–459

Leblanc A D, Schneider V S, Evans H J, Engelbretson D A, Krebs J M 1990 Bone mineral loss and recovery after 17 weeks of bed rest. Journal of Bone and Mineral Research 5: 843–850

Legay D A, Petrie D P, Alexander D I 1990 Flexion and distraction injuries of the lumbar spine and associated abdominal trauma. Journal of Trauma 30: 436–441

McAfee P C, Yuan H A, Fredrickson B F, Lubicky J P 1983 The value of computed tomography in thoraco lumbar fractures. Journal of Bone and Joint Surgery 65-A: 451–473

McEvoy R D, Bradford D S 1985 The management of burst fractures of the thoracic lumbar spine: experience in 53 patients. Spine 10: 631–637

Massie A, Porter R W, Reid D M 1992 Broadband ultrasound attenuation and dual energy x-ray absorptiometry in women with hip fracture: a comparison. Journal of Bone and Joint Surgery 74B (Suppl iii): 318

Massie A, Reid D M, Porter R W 1993 Screening for osteoporosis: comparison between Dual Energy X-ray absorptionometry and broadband ultrasound attenuation in 1000 perimenopausal women. Osteoporosis International 3: 107–110

Munk-Jensen N, Nielson S P, Obel F B, Erikson P B 1988 Reversal of postmenopausal vertebral bone loss by oestrogen and progesterone: a double blind placebo controlled study. British Medical Journal 296: 1150–1152

Nicoll E A 1949 Fractures of the dorso-lumbar spine. Journal of Bone and Joint Surgery 31-B: 376–394

Nordin B E C 1983 In: Wright V (ed) Osteoporosis. Bone and joint disease in the elderly. Churchill Livingstone, Edinburgh, 167–180

Porter R W, Johnson K, McCutcheon J D S 1990 Wrist fracture, heel bone density and thoracic kyphosis: a case control study. Bone 11: 211–214

Porter R W, Miller C G, Grainger D, Palmer S B 1991 Prediction of hip fracture in elderly women: a prospective study. British Medical Journal 301: 638–641

Pratt E S, Green D A, Spengler D M 1990 Herniated intervertebral discs associated with unstable spine injuries. Spine 15: 662–666

Resnick D L 1982 Fish vertebrae. Arthritis and Rheumatism 25: 322–325

Riggs B L, Hodgson S F, O'Fallon M, Chao E Y S, Wahner H W, Muhs J M, Cedel S L, Melton L J 1990 Effect of fluoride treatment on the fracture rate in postmenopausal women with osteoporosis. New England Journal of Medicine 322: 802–809

Ringe J D 1987 Clinical evaluation of salmon calcitonin in bone pain. In: Christiansen C (ed) Osteoporosis 1987. Proceedings of the International Symposium on Osteoporosis, vol 2, p 662–666

Stevenson J L, Whitehead M I 1982 Calcitonin secretion and postmenopausal osteoporosis (letter). Lancet 1(8275): 804

Van der Wiel H E, Lips P, Netelsnbos J C, Hazenberg G C 1991 Biochemical parameters of bone turnover during ten days of bed rest and subsequent mobilisation. Bone Mineral 13: 123–129

Young M H 1973 Long term consequences of stable fractures of the thoracic and lumbar vertebral bodies. Journal of Bone and Joint Surgery 55-B: 295–300

24. Spinal fusion — indications and methods

R. Porter — J. Dove

Spinal fusion for conditions other than spondylolisthesis has had a poor reputation, partly because of the high rate of pseudoarthrosis (Shaw & Taylor 1956, Prothero et al 1966, Nelson 1968). A recent long-term follow-up study of fusion found that 53% of patients were taking analgesics for back pain, and 15% had undergone recent surgery (Lehmann et al 1987). A short-term review of fusions with pedicle screw fixation considered that 28% were a clinical failure (West et al 1991).

Dissatisfaction with the late results of fusion have spawned new procedures to stabilize the spine and replace discs (Deburge 1992). However, fusion still remains a popular operation amongst surgeons and with better assessment and improved quality and range of investigations, and with new methods of fixation reducing the pseudoarthrosis rate, good results might be expected. There is a small group of patients for whom spinal fusion is rewarding, and preferable to other techniques. Who are they, and how should the operation be done?

INDICATIONS FOR SPINAL FUSION

Spinal fusion aims to reduce segmental movement and/or segmental loading. The surgeon therefore attempts to establish whether segmental movement or segmental loading is responsible for the pain and disability.

Patient selection

It is probably unreasonable to fuse a spine when root pain is the main complaint, unless there is an obvious dynamic component to the root lesion. Segmental pain can, however, be referred even into the upper calf, which is no contra-indication to fusion. Spinal fusion, however, aims to relieve back pain, and if the source can be localized to one or two segments, fusion can be remarkably successful. The symptoms need to be sufficiently severe and protracted and it must be established that abnormal pain behaviour is not a major component to the disability. Nowhere is a careful appraisal of inappropriate symptoms and signs more important than in assessment for spinal fusion. Painstaking assessment is essential because a failed fusion is a disaster. The presence of abnormal pain behaviour does not exclude a segmental back pain problem, but inappropriate symptoms and signs and the presence of litigation increases the risk of a poor response.

A detailed history and examination of a patient with a complex back problem is laborious but essential. It may involve an extensive protocol sometimes with computerized interview (Gardner et al 1986, Thomas et al 1989), a back pain disability questionnaire and a pain drawing (Ransford et al 1976). Assessment over several days is possible if the patient is admitted. They can then be observed by the ward staff with a functional assessment from experienced physiotherapists. Only when it is decided that the patient has a significant chronic organic disability is an attempt made to identify the painful segment.

The painful segment

It is rarely possible to identify the painful segment from a clinical examination alone or from plain radiographs (Fig. 24.1). Degenerative

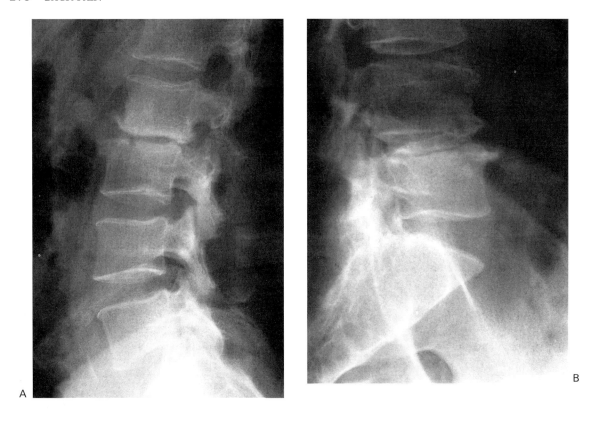

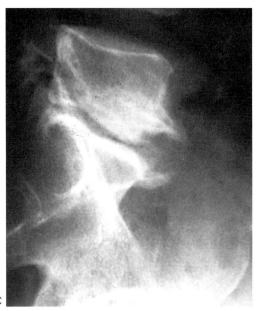

Fig. 24.1(A)   When disc degeneration is localized to a single upper lumbar segment this is probably the nociceptive source. However, a single level floating fusion will not guarantee relief of pain. **(B)** Fusion of a degenerate L4/5 disc, when pain has been reproduced by provocating injection or probing, is likely to be successful. The fusion should probably extend to S1. **(C)** A lateral radiograph showing gross degeneration at L5/S1. This may be relatively stable and is not necessarily the nociceptive source.

changes are so often symptomless that even when located to a single segment they are no guarantees that that level is the pain source.

Some features in the history might suggest whether the pain arises from the posterior joints or from the anterior column. Pain in extension and pain at night and in the early morning might suggest facet joint pain (Eisenstein & Parry 1987), while pain brought on by sitting and worse later in the day might suggest discogenic pain, but it would be unwise to rely on these features alone.

Anterior pain source

Magnetic resonance imaging will identify a loss of disc signal, and whether this is generalized or located to one or two discs. If it is restricted to no more than two levels then a pain provocation discogram will help to establish whether or not the relevant levels constitute a pain source.

Posterior pain source

A diagnostic facet joint injection under X-ray control can help identify joints responsible for pain. However, both these and provocative discograms are not totally reliable, and they require cautious interpretation.

The segment proximal to the fusion

The initial good results of fusion often deteriorate with time (Cauchoxi & David 1985). Hypermobility and retrolisthesis frequently occur at the level above the fusion, and it is therefore important to be sure before surgery that this segment is not degenerate also. Fusion is the preferred method of treatment for a single painful segment, but multiple-level pathology does less well.

Provided one or two levels are recognized as the source of pain, the proximal disc is normal on MRI, and the vertebral canal is not stenotic, then a fusion is appropriate. However, the patient should be warned that in spite of apparently identifying a painful segment and in spite of expecting a sound fusion there is no guarantee of success. There is no method which will con-

fidently predict successful fusion. An attempt to assess the effect of segmental movement by recording pain relief with a plaster spica including one thigh, or relief using an external fixator (North et al 1989), still does not ensure a good result from fusion.

The planning of assessment, investigations and counselling of a patient for spinal fusion is laborious. However, because fusion is a major procedure, failure a disaster and the late results of even a good fusion are so uncertain, there is no alternative to this careful approach, and therefore relatively few patients proceed to surgery.

THE METHOD OF SPINAL FUSION

The choices of fusion methods are numerous: anterior or posterior, intra- or intertransverse, with or without fixation, screws, wires or springs, plates, rods or rectangles. It is logical that the presumed pain source should influence whether the spine is fused from behind or in front. If the degenerative change is primarily in the anterior column, and the vertebral canal and facet joints are essentially normal, then anterior disc excision and fusion is reasonable. If, however, the primary problem is posterior with degenerative changes in the facets and less disc pathology, a posterior fusion is preferable, incorporating some decompression and undercutting of facets if the canal is also stenosed. Advanced pathology of the whole motion segment may require a combined anterior and posterior approach (O'Brien & Speck 1987).

SURGERY OF THE ANTERIOR COLUMN

The preferred approach for a two-level fusion is anterolateral by a retroperitoneal approach. However, for a single-level L5/S1 fusion, a transperitoneal approach through a Pfannenstiel incision is sometimes easier (Freebody et al 1971). The disc is thoroughly excised with curettage of the endplates down to cancellous bone, and large blocks of cortico-cancellous graft from the iliac crest are inserted across the disc space (Sacks 1965).

Tricortical grafts leave a defect in the iliac crest which can cause significant morbidity (Summers & Eisenstein 1989). This can be avoided with a dowel system (Crock 1982) or by a proplast graft filling (Hochschuler et al 1988). Because of donor site morbidity, allograft from a bone bank is an acceptable substitute. Calcium phosphate ceramic is useful only if it is in close contact with the host bone (Passuti et al 1989). However, its use as an osteoconductive material with bone morphogenic protein or growth hormone as an osteoinductive factor may prove useful.

A disc excision and interbody fusion can be carried out through a posterior approach by placing blocks of bone graft across the disc space. This Cloward interbody fusion (1963), is a difficult technique but biomechanically it places the graft at the ideal site.

A two-level anterior disc excision and fusion carries a risk of pseudoarthrosis, particularly at the upper level. The surgeon may therefore prefer to supplement the anterior fusion with internal fixation, using for example a standard AO fracture plate, or a system specifically developed for anterior fusion (Ryan et al 1986, Kostuick & Thomas 1986). Without internal fixation, even when a solid fusion occurs, there may be collapse of the graft with loss of disc height which can result in important secondary changes in the posterior column. The Hartshill horseshoe incorporating a central bone graft or bone graft substitute attempts to avoid this complication. It is screwed into place in the disc space and acts as a spacer (Valentine et al 1989).

SURGERY OF THE POSTERIOR COLUMN

Posterior surgery is normally carried out through a mid-line approach, though bilateral L5/S1 intertransverse fusion can be approached transversely (Wiltse & Bateman 1965). The facet joints can be fixed with a screw (Andrew et al 1986), but it is not very substantial and leaves the problem of the narrow lateral recess unresolved. Hypertrophic degenerative change of the lumbar facet joints which causes narrowing of the lateral recess with bony nerve root compression requires undercutting facetectomy (Getty et al 1981). This allows bony decompression of the nerve root without destabilizing the spine. It addresses the problem of leg pain, but this alone does not solve the problem of back pain if pain arises from the degenerative facet joints.

If significant degenerative changes in the lumbar facet joints is believed to be the source of pain, then surgery should consist of wide excision of the relevant facets supplemented by a fusion with internal fixation. For one-level stabilization at L5/S1, it is probably reasonable to perform a bony intertransverse fusion alone without internal fixation, but if more than one level is involved or if the single-level fusion is above L5, then internal fixation should normally be used.

Nicol and Scott (1986) introduced a wiring technique to stabilize the repaired defect in a spondylolysis or low-grade spondylolisthesis in a young patient, particularly at L4. The method is admirable in its simplicity. The defects are cleared of fibrous and cartilaginous tissue and the sclerotic margins curetted. A 2-mm diameter hole is drilled at the base of the transverse process and braided wire passed first through this hole and then through a similar hole at the base of the spinous process. Cancellous bone is packed into the defects. Results are good for those under 25 years of age (Johnson & Thompson 1992).

There is a wide choice of systems for internal fixation to supplement a posterior lumbosacral fusion (Attenborough & Reynolds 1975, Cotrel & Dubousset 1984, Dove 1986, Kaneda et al 1986, Krag et al 1986, Louis 1986, Luque 1986, Selby 1986, Steffee et al 1986, Zielke & Stempel 1986, Dick 1987, Roy-Camille et al 1987, Horowitch et al 1989). Each system has both merits and disadvantages. Most provide adequate stabilization of the lumbar spine, but the common unresolved problem is adequate fixation to the sacrum. Any internal fixation device should provide secure fixation and it should not be too bulky. It should allow preservation of the normal lumbar lordosis. It should be inexpensive, adaptable to incorporate sublamina wiring and pedicle screw fixation, and in order to provide torsional stability, there should be cross-links. Each surgeon selects his method of choice but the technique should be learned either from the originator or from another surgeon with practical experience of the device.

HARVESTING BONE

Any fixation system will be loose within 6 months, by which time a successful fusion depends on sound bony union. It is, therefore, imperative that as much care be taken with the bone graft and the cancellous bed as with the fixation device. The recipient site and the amount of cortex to be removed depend on personal preferences, but it is imperative that the bone graft lies on a good vascular bed of cancellous bone. The posterior ilium is the best source of autogenous bone in a posterior fusion; abundant cancellous bone can be harvested from the posterior ileum without transgressing the inner table.

A posterior defect of the iliac crest can cause a troublesome lumbar hernia (Fig. 24.2). In addition, the cutaneous nerves deserve respect, not straying more than 8 cm lateral to the posterior superior iliac spine. The sacroiliac joint is not to be transected, and the sciatic notch is avoided to spare the superior gluteal artery (Catinella et al 1990).

COMBINED ANTERIOR AND POSTERIOR SURGERY

Advanced degenerative change of the whole motion segment may require stabilization of both anterior and posterior columns, because a solid

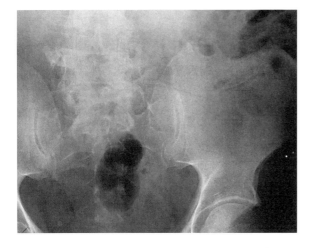

Fig. 24.2   AP radiograph of a patient with a large lumbar hernia after a posterior fusion and bone graft from the iliac crest. The donor site was unnecessarily lateral, and included both tables of the ileum. The ideal site is lateral to the sacroiliac joint preserving the inner table of the pelvis.

posterior fusion with internal fixation will not exclude all movement of the anterior column. This can be responsible for subsequent discogenic pain (Weatherley et al 1986).

In dysplastic spondylolisthesis with marked displacement there is a place for anterior disc excision and fusion, followed under the same anaesthetic by posterior fusion and internal fixation (O'Brien & Speck 1987, Kozak & O'Brien 1990). Fusion of isthmic spondylolisthesis with a lesser displacement is satisfactorily accomplished through the posterior approach. One method is to expose the relevant disc space on each side, retracting the dura medially and removing a dowel of disc and bone from each side. Dowels or bone graft or bone graft substitute are hammered into place across the disc space from behind to form a modified posterior lumbar interbody fusion. This is combined with facet joint excision and fusion with internal fixation, which gives a very secure fixation of both columns.

The problems of spinal fusion are still unresolved. In spite of improved imaging techniques the pain source remains elusive. Interpedicular screws provide rigid fixation, but the pedicle is often inadvertently transgressed with risk of neurological damage. The cortex is probably penetrated if saline injected into the screw track fails to return (An et al 1992). Pedicle screws also cause considerable damage to the intricate blood supply of the vertebral body with possible effects on disc nutrition. What is the long-term effect of this on the disc proximal to the fusion? And is it safe to use diagnostic fixators, with their risk to disc nutrition, to nerve root and the potential of pin-track infection? Does surgical exposure lateral to the facets cause significant neuromuscular damage? Should we be encouraging percutaneous fusion (Shepperd 1989)?

In the postoperative period, fusions without rigid internal fixation do better in an orthosis for 5 months than for 3 months (Johnsson et al 1992), though most surgeons favour rigid internal fixation and an orthosis for 3 months. Good results can be expected from fusion, with very grateful patients, provided they are carefully selected and surgery is expeditious. That means a good cancellous bed, adequate bone graft and secure fixation. However, the long-term benefits await a comparative randomized trial between surgery and the natural history of segmental spinal pain.

REFERENCES

An H, Benoit P, Nguyen C 1992 A new saline injection technique to confirm pedicle screw path: a cadaveric study. Presented to the International Society for the Study of the Lumbar Spine, Chicago, May 1992

Andrew T A, Brooks S, Piggott H 1986 Long term follow up evaluation of screw and graft fusion of the lumbar spine, 1986 Clinical Orthopaedics and Related Research 203: 113–119

Attenborough C G, Reynolds M T 1975 Lumbosacral fusion with spring fixation. Journal of Bone and Joint Surgery 57B: 283–288

Catinella F P, DeLaria G A, DeWald R Z 1990 False aneurysm of the superior gluteal artery. Spine 15: 1360–1362

Cauchoxi J, David T 1985 Arthrodeses lombaires resultats apres plus de dix ans. Revue de Chirurgie Orthopedique 71: 263–268

Cloward R B 1963 Lesions of the intervertebral discs and their treatment by interbody fusion methods. Clinical Orthopaedics 27: 51

Cotrel Y, Dubousset J 1984 Nouvelle technique d'osteosynthese rachidienne segmentaire par voie posterieure, 1984. Revue de Chirurgie Orthopedique 70: 489–495

Crock H V 1982 Anterior inter body fusion. Clinical Orthopaedics and Related Research 165: 157

Deburge 1992 Modern trends in spinal surgery. Journal of Bone and Joint Surgery 74-B: 6–8

Dick W 1987 The 'fixateur interne' as a versatile implant for spine surgery. Spine 12: 882–900

Dove J 1986 Internal fixation of the lumbar spine: the Hartshill rectangle. Clinical Orthopaedics and Related Research 203: 135–140

Eisenstein S M, Parry C R 1987 The lumbar facet arthrosis syndrome: clinical presentation and articular surface changes. Journal of Bone and Joint Surgery 69 B: 3–7

Freebody D, Bendall R, Taylor R D 1971 Anterior transperitoneal lumbar fusion. Journal of Bone and Joint Surgery 53 B: 617

Gardner A D, Pursell L M, Murty K, Smith D G 1986 The management of the clinical problem of spinal pain with the assistance of a micro-computer. In: Hukins D W L, Mulholland R C (eds) Back pain. Manchester University Press, p 24–41

Getty C J M, Johnson J R, Kirward E O'G, Sullivan M F 1981 Partial undercutting facetectomy for bony entrapment of the lumbar nerve root. Journal of Bone and Joint Surgery 63B: 330–335

Hochschuler S H, Guyer R D, Stith W J, Ohnmeiss D D, Rashbaum R F 1988 Proplast reconstruction of iliac crest defects. Spine 13: 378–379

Horowitch A, Peek R D, Thomas J C, Widell E H, Dimartino P P, Spencer C W, Weinstein J, Wiltse L L 1989 The Wiltse pedicle screw fixation system. Spine 14: 461–467

Johnson G V, Thompson A G 1992 The Scott wiring technique for direct repair of lumbar spondylolysis. Journal of Bone and Joint Surgery. 74-B: 426–430

Johnsson R, Stromqvist B, Axelsson P, Selvik G 1992 Influence of spinal immobilisation on consolidation of posterolateral lumbosacral fusion. Spine 17: 16–21

Kaneda K, Kazama H, Satoh S, Fujiya M 1986 Follow-up study of medial facetectomies and posterolateral fusion with instrumentation in unstable degenerative spondylolisthesis. Clinical Orthopaedics and Related Research 203: 159–167

Kostuik J P, Thomas J E 1986 Techniques of internal fixation for degenerative conditions of the lumbar spine. Clinical Orthopaedics and Related Research 203: 219–231

Kozak J A, O'Brien J P 1990 Simultaneous combined anterior and posterior fusion. An independent analysis of a treatment for the disabled low back patient. Spine 15: 322–328

Krag M H, Beynnon B D, Pope M H, Frymoyer J W, Haugh L D, Weaver D L 1986 An internal fixator for posterior application to short segments of the thoracic, lumbar or lumbosacral spine. Clinical Othopaedics and Related Research 203: 75–98

Lane J M, Muschler G F 1992 Principles of bone fusion. In Rothman Simeone (eds) The spine. W B Saunders, Philadelphia, p 1739–1755

Lehmann T R, Spratt K F, Tozzi J E 1987 Long term follow up of lower lumbar fusion patients. Spine 12: 97–104

Louis R 1986 Fusion of the lumbar and sacral spine by internal fixation with screw plates. Clinical Orthopaedics and Related Research 203: 18–23

Luque E R 1986 Interpedicular segmental fixation. Clinical Orthopaedics and Related Research 203: 54–57

Nelson M A 1968 A longterm review of posterior spinal fusion. Proceedings of the Royal Society of Medicine 611: 558–559

Nicol R O, Scott J H 1986 Lytic spondylolysis: repair by wiring. Spine 11: 1027–1030

North A D, Roberts A P, Wilde G P, Pembleton C J, Mulholland R C, Webb J K 1989 The Harlow Wood external fixator. Proceedings of the Institute of Mechanical Engineers, London 2: 53–66 ISBN 0 85298 688

O'Brien J P, Speck G R 1987 Simultaneous combined anterior and posterior fusion of the lumbar spine. Journal of Bone and Joint Surgery 69B: 164

Passuti N, Daculsi G, Rogez J M 1989 Macroporous calcium phosphate ceramic performance in human spine fusion. Clinical Orthopaedics 248: 169–176

Prothero S R, Parkes J C, Stinchfield F E 1966 Complications after low back pain fusion in 1,000 patients: a comparison of two series one decade apart. Journal of Bone and Joint Surgery 48A: 57–65

Ransford A O, Cairns O, Mooney V 1976 The pain drawing as an aid to the psychologic evaluation of patients with low-back pain. Spine 1: 127–134

Roy-Camille R, Saillant G, Christian M 1987 Internal fixation of the lumbar spine with pedicle screw plating. Clinical Orthopaedics and Related Research 203: 7–17

Ryan M D, Taylor T F K, Phil D, Sherwood A A 1986 Bolt-plate fixation for anterior spinal fusion. Clinical Orthopaedics and Related Research 203: 196–202

Sacks S 1965 Anterior interbody fusion of the lumbar spine. Journal of Bone and Joint Surgery 47B: 211

Selby D 1986 Internal fixation with Knodt's rods. Clinical Orthopaedics and Related Research 203: 179–184

Shaw E G, Taylor J G 1956 The results of lumbosacral fusion for low back pain. Journal of Bone and Joint Surgery 38B: 485

Shepperd J 1989 Current possibilities of percutaneous disc surgery. Percutaneous lumbar discectomy. Shepperd, Hastings, p 185–187

Steffee A D, Biscup R S, Sitkowski D J 1986 Segmental spine plates with pedicle screw fixation. Clinical Orthopaedics and Related Research 203: 45–53

Summers B N, Eisenstein S M 1989 Donor site pain from the ilium. Journal of Bone and Joint Surgery 71B: 677–680

Thomas A M C, Fairbank J C T, Pynsent P B, Baker D J 1989 A computer based interview system for patients with back pain. Spine 14: 844–846

Valentine N W, Aziz R, Sell P J, Dove J 1989 A pedicle screw bridge modification of the Hartshill system. Presented at the Combined Meeting of the Scoliosis Research Society and European Spinal Deformity Society, Amsterdam

Weatherley C R, Prickett C F, O'Brien J P 1986 Discogenic pain persisting despite solid posterior fusion. Journal of Bone and Joint Surgery 68B: 142–143

West J L, Bradford D S, Ogilvie J W 1991 Results of spinal arthrodesis with pedicular screw-plate fixation. Journal of Bone and Joint Surgery 73-A: 1179–1184

Wiltse L L, Bateman J G 1965 Experience with transverse process fusion of the lumbar spine. Journal of Bone and Joint Surgery 47A: 848–849

Zielke K, Stempel A V 1986 Posterior lateral distraction spondylodesis using the twofold sacral bar. Clinical Orthopaedics and Related Research 203: 151–158

25. Soft tissue injury

Soft tissue injury of the spine is an important cause of back pain but because of diagnostic difficulties, the size of the problem is uncertain. Back pain diagnoses which had favour in a previous generation, such as 'lumbago', 'fibrositis' or 'back strain', inferred a soft tissue pathology; but they have largely been discarded in favour of more easily identifiable disorders of the intervertebral disc and the spinal column. Nevertheless, disease of the musculoligamentous structures of the lumbar spine must be considered as a source of back pain.

Certain studies have given a better understanding of the soft tissue anatomy (Macintosh & Bogduk 1987) and the biomechanics (Myklebust et al 1986) of the spine, and there has been an improvement in diagnostic skills and better soft tissue imaging (Tracy et al 1989). These improvements may show that many acute episodes of back pain are the results of soft tissue injury which may precede disc and segmental disorders.

BIOMECHANICAL DEFINITION OF STRESS AND STRAIN

Stress is an internal force generated in a material in response to an external load. Strain is the change that develops in the material as a result of that stress; it may be an axial change in length, or a torsional or angular change. If the strain is within the elastic limit (Fig. 25.1) the material will return to the preformed state. The elastic limit in biological tissues varies with the speed of the applied stress, the duration of the load and its frequency. It is reached sooner if the force is

applied rapidly, and if the tissue is fatigued by repetitive loading (Fig. 25.2).

Plastic deformation occurs when the tissues are strained beyond the elastic limit. The tissue fails to return to the preformed state. Under further stress the tissues fail by disruption. This applies to all the soft tissues of the spine, muscles, tendons, fascia, ligaments, annulus, nerves, vessels, fat and skin. These tissues will be particularly vulnerable to strain beyond the elastic limit when fatigued by high frequency repetitive loading and then stressed by a fall, with the resulting failure of the protective reflexes.

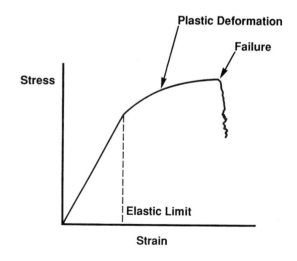

Fig. 25.1 A stress/strain graph showing how with increasing stress a material is deformed. It initially returns again to the predeformed state. When the elastic limit is reached plastic deformation occurs, and when the stress is reduced the material is permanently deformed. The material eventually fails with further stress.

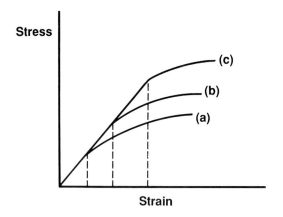

Fig. 25.2   In biological tissues when the stress is applied rapidly (**a**) the elastic limit is reached at a lesser stress than if it is applied more slowly (**b** and **c**). It is also reached at a lesser stress if that stress is applied frequently (**a**) rather than with less frequent repetition (**b**) and (**c**).

Clinical definition of 'strain'

A strain is an injury to muscle, tendon or fascia beyond the elastic limit (Baker 1984). It will produce plastic deformation with irreversible axial stretching and then, with increased stress, complete disruption of the tissues. The musculo-tendinous units repair by formation of fibrous tissue and, according to the amount of tissue damage, leave some reduction in function. Marked fibrosis of muscle can impair recovery from muscle injury (Lehto et al 1989). In practice, however, this reduced function is not apparent clinically; it reduces power, but does not significantly affect joint function.

Muscle rupture, disruption at a musculo-tendinous junction, or avulsion of ligamentous attachments is probably just as common in the spine as in the limbs, but because of the inaccessibility of the spinal structures, isolated muscle injury is less easily diagnosed. It may be suspected, however, in a young athlete or an individual suddenly experiencing unusually high stress, whose tenderness is localized away from the mid-line. Discomfort is experienced when the muscle involved is stretched, or when movement is resisted. Tenderness above the posterior iliac crest with pain extending into the buttock in a young footballer — whose pain is aggravated by spinal flexion and adduction of the hip, or resisted spinal extension or resisted abduction of the hip — probably results from musculo-tendinous injury rather than a mechanical disturbance of the lumbar spine.

Clinical definition of 'sprain'

A sprain is an injury to the ligaments of a joint; they are either stretched by plastic deformation or disrupted, perhaps both types of injury occurring in one ligament. By contrast to muscle injury, fibrous repair is a poor substitute for a ligament. The repaired ligament is an inefficient restrainer of the joint and, depending on the degree of the injury, a sprain carries a poor prognosis.

Isolated disruption of spinal ligaments is a difficult diagnosis to prove, except in the combined bony ligamentous injury of unstable fracture and fracture-dislocation of the spine (Nicoll 1949). Adams and Hutton (1982) suspected that interspinous ligament failure may be the precursor of the disc injury by permitting an unacceptable degree of segmental flexion, subsequently overloading the disc. Disruption of the interspinous and supraspinous ligaments may also precede degenerative spondylolisthesis (Newman 1963), but see page 36 (Hukins et al 1990).

DIAGNOSIS OF THE SOFT TISSUE INJURY OF THE SPINE

By definition a muscle strain or a ligamentous sprain is the result of injury. The history at the onset of pain is therefore important (Nicholas & Reilly 1985). Whilst the first symptoms of a disc protrusion may initially be mild and then steadily increase over a few hours or days, a muscle ligament or fascial injury will be most painful immediately, and gradually improve (Fig. 25.3). The events surrounding the onset of the pain are highly relevant. If the patient was hit by an object, or fell against a surface and contact was made with contusion, this is more likely to have caused muscle or fascial injury than ligamentous damage and therefore carries a good prognosis. An indirect injury, however — a slip, trip or fall — could produce ligamentous injury as well as a musculotendinous strain with less satisfactory recovery.

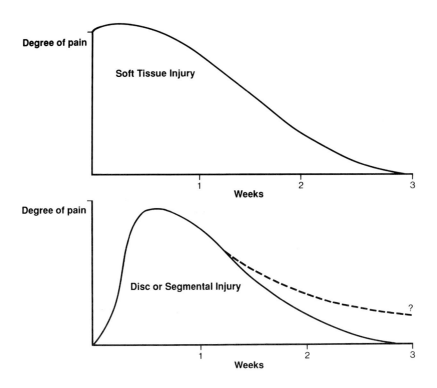

Fig. 25.3 (Top) Pain from a soft tissue injury is initially severe, and it slowly resolves over a few days or weeks. (Bottom) Pain from a disc or segmental injury can take several hours to develop. Most patients recover in a short period, but a few have persisting symptoms.

The mechanism of injury, therefore, has important medico-legal consequences. A blunt injury, though very painful initially, is less likely to result in ligamentous or disc damage than an indirect strain, and it carries a better prognosis.

The diagnosis of soft tissue injury is also a process of elimination. Soft tissue injury is excluded when pain below the knee in a root distribution suggests disc protrusion, root canal degeneration, spinal stenosis or vascular disturbance of the root. However, proximal pain in the lower limb can be referred from soft tissues in the back. Criteria of disc protrusion, even without leg pain — a list, pain aggravated by coughing, some reduction of straight leg raising, recurrent episodes of pain — would be unusual with soft tissue injury. Symptoms of inflammatory causes of back pain also have typical features: stiffness after rest, pain referred to one or other side alternately and variable in degree. The presence of a

spondylolysis or spondylolisthesis is no reason for excluding soft tissue injury. Such a defect occurs in 5% of the population and may be an incidental finding.

Abrasions or bruising of the back favours a diagnosis of soft tissue injury. Tenderness is more likely to be lateral to the midline, and sacral or sacroiliac tenderness is suggestive of contusion rather than segmental injury. Lateral flexion of the spine, which is usually well preserved in disc or segmental lesions, may be affected unilaterally with soft tissue injury. Resisted lateral flexion to the ipsilateral side is likely to be painful. Serious disruption of the interspinous ligament can be recognized by a palpable gap between the adjacent spinous processes.

Surgery provides a model of the natural history of musculotendinous injury to the spine. After discectomy many patients make a full recovery and within a few months have no troublesome symptoms in the back. A traditional operation, with fenestration, stripping muscle from the laminae and spinous processes, and fairly strong retraction on the sacrospinalis muscles, is compatible with a full functional recovery. We have yet to discover if more restricted surgery by microdiscectomy confers any long-term benefits to soft tissues, but in practice it seems that the spine can recover from moderate musculotendinous trauma. It is reasonable to assume that closed soft tissue injury to muscle, tendons and fascia, though painful initially, carries a good long-term prognosis. Symptoms which continue beyond 3 months must have another explanation.

Severe blunt contusion to the loin will produce not only bruising to the soft tissues, but frequently avulsion of the lumbar transverse processes through the attachment of the lumbar fascia and the quadratus lumborum. There are usually abrasions of the skin and deep bruising associated with severe pain. Radiographs show avulsion of one or more transverse processes on the side of injury. It is the possible association with visceral complications — kidney, liver, spleen or lung — that should concern the clinician.

Macroscopic or microscopic haematuria suggests the possibility of serious renal injury, and investigation is essential. Most patients with blunt renal trauma, no shock and only microscopic haematuria have contusion to the kidney alone. They should be admitted for observation but about 1% will have severe renal injury, such as a laceration, rupture or pedicle injury which would not be diagnosed without further investigation (Cass et al 1986). The renal area should first be examined by ultrasound, which will generally identify a rupture (Furtschegger et al 1988). Urography, however, probably remains the best method to exclude significant renal injury. Dynamic computerized tomography (CT) is useful to assess parenchymal injury, and angiography to identify renal artery damage (Lang et al 1985, Bretan et al 1986). Sometimes avascularity on early angiography can mimic a tumour (Weichen & Muller 1986).

The liver can be damaged by blunt trauma in the region of the twelfth thoracic and first lumbar vertebrae, and the spleen, with its lower border along the eleventh rib and its lower pole at the level of the first lumbar vertebra, is at risk from injury in the left loin. Injuries to the thoracolumbar region can rupture the diaphragm and contuse the lung. These more serious visceral complications usually declare themselves with abdominal and chest symptoms and signs. Though uncommon, the visceral complications of blunt trauma to the lumbar region must always be considered because they are life-threatening. The prognosis regarding the musculoskeletal injury, however, is excellent. Full function is generally restored whether or not the transverse processes unite. The patients benefit from the assurance of a full recovery and they should begin to mobilize after a few days.

Local haematomas usually resolve over 3 weeks with no continuing disability. The application of ice can hasten recovery time, probably by the vasoconstrictor effect and haemostasis from histamine release; oedema and microhaemorrhage are reduced.

Chronic expanding haematoma (cystic haematoma)

On rare occasions a haematoma will slowly expand, forming a pseudocapsule with a gradual collection of central serous fluid (Friedlander & Bump 1968, Sterling et al 1977, Vecchione 1977, Reid et al 1980) (Fig. 25.4). This can occur in any muscular compartment, including the paraspinal tissues. It may be difficult to exclude sarcoma, even with sonography and CT or magnetic resonance imaging. MRI may be necessary to ensure there is no solid tissue within the pseudocapsule. The capsule of the cystic haematoma is composed of dense fibrous tissue with haemosiderin deposits and iron-laden macrophages, with an inner lining of granulation tissue and fibrin with capillary ingrowth. The cause of the cystic formation is not well understood. Blood breakdown products can create an osmotic gradient causing fluid to be imbibed into the centre of the haematoma, a process enhanced by the inflammatory reaction (Labadie & Glover 1976). Animal experiments have shown that cystic formation is more likely, the larger the amount of blood injected. A cycle may develop in

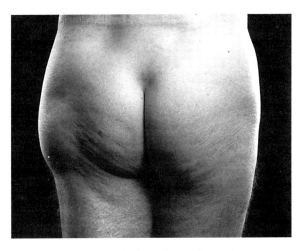

Fig. 25.4 A photograph of a patient with a cystic haematoma of the left buttock behind the greater trochanter.

which blood breakdown and liquefaction activate vasoactive substances and induce capsule formation, and continued inflammation produces effusion and new bleeding from damaged capillaries (Lewis & Johnson 1987).

If the diagnosis is not in doubt, the cystic haematoma can be left to resolve spontaneously. It may take many months but a conservative approach is preferable to surgical excision, which is often followed by a recurrence of the lesion.

Contusion and pathology within the vertebral canal

The contents of the vertebral canal are singularly well protected from the effects of contusion by the bony ligamentous anatomy and the protective cerebrospinal fluid in the envelope of the dura. There are records, however, of neurological concussion and neurapraxia from injury to the thoracolumbar region without vertebral damage. Predisposing factors are spinal stenosis or pre-existing segmental instability (Bigo & Johnson 1989). Extradural spinal haematomas are uncommon but can occur after injury in an individual with an underlying blood dyscrasia, and occasionally in the absence of coagulation disorders (Combelles et al 1983). Spinal haematoma can occur in patients with ankylosing spondylitis.

Chronic compartment syndrome in the erector spinae muscle

Spinal muscle compartment syndrome has been suggested as an occasional cause of low back pain (Carr et al 1984, Peck et al 1986, Bullock 1988). Criteria for suspecting this syndrome are paravertebral low back pain induced only by exercise, relieved by rest and with no lower limb neurological deficit. It might be expected to occur in athletic subjects. Of 12 patients with these criteria investigated by Styf and Lysell (1987), only one had raised intramuscular pressure which did not normalize with 20 min at rest. MRI will support the diagnosis (Difazio et al 1991). Fasciotomy normalized the pressure in this patient and relieved the exercise-induced pain. Though a genuine cause of low back pain, it is extremely uncommon.

Painful muscle 'spasm'

Spinal muscles may fail to relax voluntarily, and be in reflex 'spasm'. This is frequently observed in patients with lower lumbar disc protrusion. Asymmetrical spasm produces the deformity of a list, sometimes described as a 'wind-swept spine'. This characteristic distinguishes the list from a structural scoliosis. It is affected by gravity (Porter & Miller 1984). It is present only when the patient stands and is abolished by lying down or hanging from a bar. The list may be apparent only when the patient flexes forwards, and when the 'spasm' is symmetrical there may be a loss of lumbar lordosis.

Spasm associated with an osteoid osteoma and with spinal infection is not abolished by lying down. An osteoid osteoma will produce a painful scoliosis with marked spasm, as distinct from the painless idiopathic scoliosis. It is not known, however, whether the muscle spasm is painful of itself. If the underlying condition producing the spasm is the pain source, pharmaceuticals to relieve the spasm would not be appropriate.

Some believe that anxiety and fear can produce increased muscle tension with resultant ischaemia and a nociceptive stimulus from accumulation of metabolites, much like the muscular pain of intermittent claudication. Relaxation, biofeedback and the Alexander technique (Gelb 1981) which train for poise, posture and balance are recommended. There is, however, no good evidence that muscle tension is a cause of low back pain.

Fibrositis — fibromyalgia

This is a diagnosis without any objective evidence of pathological change. Smythe (1985) believed that the nociceptive source was neither in muscle nor fascia, but was a disturbance of pain modulation in the central nervous system. Patients complained of vague pain and tenderness in the muscles of the back which was said to be more common with sleep disturbance, and after sleep deprivation in healthy subjects. They had backache, muscle tenderness and stiffness, especially in the mornings, sometimes associated with headaches (Thould 1988, Yunus 1989). They complained of fatigue during the day, and symptoms were said to be affected by the weather. Symptoms may extend to other parts of the spine and limbs, and the condition is more common in tense, compulsive, energetic individuals (Cailliet 1988). Unfortunately there are no laboratory tests to confirm the organic nature of such a condition. Biopsies of tender tissue are negative. Those who believe in this condition recommend strategies: improving sleep patterns, applying heat or ice, massage, relaxation, biofeedback and a functional rehabilitation programme; in the absence of objective diagnostic criteria, however, the benefits of treatment are not easily assessed.

Polymyalgia rheumatica produces similar symptoms, but the erythrocyte sedimentation rate (ESR) is raised, usually above 50 mm/h. Acute infective polyneuritis (Guillain–Barré syndrome) may produce back pain with weakness and aching in the limbs, headaches and vomiting; the protein level in the cerebrospinal fluid is usually raised.

Tender soft tissue nodules are not uncommon in patients with back pain. They have attracted interest from clinicians over many years (Froriep 1943, Granham 1912, Steindler & Luck 1938, Travell 1942). They are circumscribed tender masses of connective tissue, sometimes infiltrated with lymphocytes. Pressure on these tissues can produce distal referred pain, and they are called 'trigger zones'. Spraying the overlying skin with coolant, stretching the tissue or injection with local anaesthetic and/or steroid is said to relieve the pain, though there are no adequate scientific studies.

Contusion to the buttock can cause ischaemia to the subcutaneous fat with atrophy and fibrosis and depression of the soft tissue contour. This is a cosmetic problem only (Fig. 25.5).

Piriformis syndrome

The piriformis muscle leaves the pelvis through the greater sciatic foramen. The sciatic nerve lies anterior to the muscle, and passes inferiorly between the muscle and the superior gemellus of the obturator internus muscle to lie posterior to obturator internus. Sciatic pain is said to result from entrapment of the nerve deep and inferior to the piriformis muscle. The piriformis muscle arises from the front of the sacrum, the margin of the greater sciatic notch, and from the upper part of the anterior surface of the sacrotuberous ligament. In 15% of individuals the sciatic nerve leaves the pelvis between two bellies of this muscle rather than below its inferior surface. Entrapment is believed to be more common in women, and is associated with dyspareunia. Pain and paraesthesia is felt in the buttock and posterior thigh. The lumbar spine has a full range of motion, straight leg raising is reduced, and

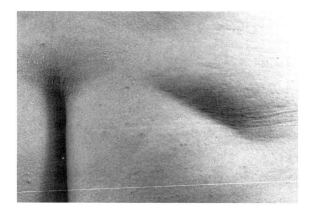

Fig. 25.5 A photograph of a patient with atrophy of the subcutaneous fat over the right sacroiliac region, following blunt trauma and fat necrosis.

internal rotation of the leg at the limit of straight leg raising is said to increase the pain in this syndrome. However, Brieg and Troup (1979) showed that this test is positive whenever straight leg raising is limited by increased root tension, and it would not appear to be specific to this syndrome. Piriformis, being an external rotator of the hip, is stretched by internally rotating the hip, especially the extended hip; resisting internal rotation should therefore increase the pain in this condition. The piriformis is also an abductor of the flexed hip; thus resisted abduction of the legs in the seated patient should be painful and reduced in power in this syndrome. Symptoms may follow a fall. Contrast-enhanced CT or MRI may show an enlarged piriformis muscle (Jankiewiez et al 1991). Relief of pain by injection of local anaesthetic into the piriformis is said to be diagnostic.

Soft tissue injury a precursor to instability

Although there is no universal agreement about the term spinal instability (Nachemson 1985), a segment is probably unstable if it moves beyond its normal bounds of restraint and returns again to its preformed position (Farfan & Gracovetsky 1984). Some unstable segments are not painful at all, and when an unstable segment is painful it is not easy to identify the source of pain.

Various methods have been used to measure normal and unnatural segmental movement by serial radiological images of the spine (Pearcy et al 1984, Seligman et al 1984, Ogston et al 1986, Stokes & Frymoyer 1987). Attention has been focused on the vertebrae and discs, with little interest in the soft tissues. There are, however, a number of features about the instability syndromes that suggest a study of the soft tissues would be rewarding. It is possible that soft tissue injury is the precursor to an unstable lumbar segment, and subsequently a degenerative disc.

Macnab (1971) described traction spurs arising a few millimetres from the adjacent margins of the vertebral bodies as a sign of instability. It is generally thought that disc degeneration produces unnatural segmental movement and that the anterior longitudinal ligament is strained at the vertebral attachment, causing small osteophytes to grow into the ligament. However, discs between vertebrae with traction spurs are not inevitably degenerate and may be well hydrated on MRI scan. An alternative hypothesis is that a soft tissue ligamentous injury is the primary pathology; the ligamentous structure no longer prevents the normal restraint on the segment. The disc is initially normal and instability, not disc degeneration, is responsible for the spurs. The very large claw spurs that develop on adjacent vertebrae may sometimes result from a soft tissue injury. These also can be compatible with a normal discogram.

The hormone relaxin, which increases in the last trimester of pregnancy, may increase not only the elasticity of the pelvic ligaments but also the laxity of spinal ligaments, and may be responsible for back pain which begins in pregnancy and then continues as a chronic instability problem. More patients with instability symptoms believe that pregnancy was responsible for the onset of their pain than do patients with other back pain syndromes (Porter & Jiang 1990).

Some patients may have primary disc degeneration with subsequent instability which stresses the ligaments, causing lengthening, disruption and fibrous repair. Others, however, may have primary ligamentous injury which causes an unstable segment, and insignificant disc pathology.

In the appendicular skeleton, ligamentous injury will produce an unstable joint. There is no reason why the axial skeleton should be the exception. If soft tissue injuries are suspected clinically, we now have new imaging techniques to help in diagnosis, and we may well find that these injuries have been seriously underestimated in the past.

REFERENCES

Adams M A, Hutton W C 1982 Prolapsed intervertebral disc — a hyperflexion injury. Spine 7: 184–191
Baker B E 1984 Current concepts in the diagnosis and treatment of musculo-tendinous injuries. Medical Sciences, Sports and Exercise 16: 323–327
Bigo M R, Johnson G E 1989 Clinical presentation of spinal cord concussion. Spine 14: 37–40
Bretan P N, McAninch J W, Federle, M P, Jeffrey R B 1986

Computerised tomographic staging of renal trauma: 85 consecutive cases. Journal of Urology 136: 561–565

Brieg A, Troup J D G 1979 Biomechanical considerations in the straight leg raising test. Spine 4: 242–250

Bullock N 1988 Idiopathic retroperitoneal fibrosis. British Medical Journal 297: 240–241

Cailliet R 1988 Soft tissue pain and disability, 2nd edn. FA Davis, Philadelphia, PA

Carr D, Frymoyer J W, Krag M H, Pope M H 1984 The lumbo-dorsal fascial compartment. Transamerican Orthopedic Research Society 9: 252

Cass A S, Luxenberg M, Gleich P, Smith C S 1986 Clinical indications for radiculographic evaluation of blunt renal trauma. Journal of Urology 136: 370–371

Combelles G, Blond S, Lesoin F, Bousquet C, Rousseax M, Christiaens J L 1983 Hematomes extraduraux rachidiens sans lesion osseuse traumatique. A propos de 9 cas. Neurochirurgie 29: 417–422

Difazio F A, Barth R A, Frymoyer J W 1991 Acute lumbar paraspinal compartment syndrome. Journal of Bone and Joint Surgery 73-A: 1101–1103

Farfan H F, Gracovetsky S 1984 The nature of instability. Spine 9: 714–719

Friedlander H L, Bump R G 1968 Chronic expanding haematoma of the calf. Journal of Bone and Joint Surgery 50A: 1237–1241

Froriep 1943 Ein Beitraq zur Pathologie and therapie des rheumatismus. Weimar, Germany

Furtschegger A, Egender G, Jakse G 1988 The value of sonography in the diagnosis and follow up of patients with blunt renal trauma. British Journal of Urology 62: 110–116

Gelb M 1981 Body learning — an introduction to the Alexander technique. Aurum Press, London

Granham M 1912 Uberdeen anatomeschon Bofience bel einem Fall von myositis Rheumatica. Doctoral dissertation, Cassel, Weber, Weidemeyer

Hukins D W L, Kirby M C, Sioryn T A, Aspden R M, Cox A J 1990 Comparison of structure, mechanical properties, and function of lumbar spinal ligaments. Spine 15: 787–795

Jankiewiez J J, Hennrikins W E, Hawkson J A 1991 The appearance of the piriformis muscle syndrome in computed tomography and magnetic resonance imaging. Clinical Orthopaedics 262: 205–209

Labadie E L, Glover D 1976 Physiopathogenesis of subdural haematomas: I. Histological and biochemical comparisons of subcutaneous haematoma in rats with subdural haematoma in man. Journal of Neurosurgery 45: 382–392

Lang E K, Sullivan J, Frentz G 1985 Renal trauma: radiological studies. Comparison of urography, computed tomography, angiography and radionuclide studies. Diagnostic Radiology 154: 1–6

Lehto M, Hurme M, Alaranta H, Einola S, Falak B, Jarvinen M, Kalimo H, Mattila M, Paljarvi L 1989 Connective tissue changes of the multifidus muscle in patients with lumbar disc herniation. Spine 14: 303–309

Lewis V L, Johnson P E 1987 Chronic expanding haematoma. Plastic and Reconstructive Surgery 79: 465–467

Macintosh J E, Bogduk N 1987 The morphology of the lumbar erector spinae. Spine 12: 658–668

Macnab I 1971 The traction spur. Journal of Bone and Joint Surgery 53A: 663–670

Myklebust J B, Pintar F, Yoganadan N, Cusik J F, Maiman D, Myers T J, Sances A 1986 Tensile strength of spinal ligaments. Spine 13: 526–531

Nachemson A 1985 Lumbar spine instability: a critical update and symposium summary. Spine 10: 290–291

Newman P H 1963 The etiology of spondylolisthesis. Journal of Bone and Joint Surgery 45B: 139–159

Nicholas J A, Reilly J P 1985 Orthopaedic problems in athletes. Comprehensive Therapy 11: 48–56

Nicoll E A 1949 Fractures of the dorso-lumbar spine. Journal of Bone and Joint Surgery 31B: 376–394

Ogston N G, King G J, Gertzbein S D, Tile M, Kapasouri A, Rubenstein J D 1986 Centrode patterns in the lumbar spine: baseline studies in normal subjects. Spine 11: 591–595

Pearcy M, Protek I, Shepherd J E 1984 Three dimensional x-ray analysis of normal movement in the lumbar spine. Spine 9: 294–297

Peck D, Nicholls P J, Beard C, Allen J R 1986 Are there compartment syndromes in some patients with idiopathic back pain? Spine 11: 468–475

Porter R W, Jiang B 1990 Pregnancy and chronic back pain. Presented to the International Society for the Study of the Lumbar Spine, Boston

Porter R W, Miller C 1984 Back pain and trunk list. Spine 11: 596–600

Reid J D, Kommareddi S, Lankerani M 1980 Chronic expanding haematomas, a clinicopathologic entity. Journal of the American Medical Association 224: 2441–2442

Seligman J V, Gertzbein S D, Tile M, Kapasouri A 1984 Computer analysis of spinal segment motion in degenerate disc disease with and without axial loading. Spine 9: 556–573

Smythe H A 1985 Fibrosis and the referred pain syndromes. Rheumatology Forum 3 (1)

Steindler A, Luck J V 1938 Differential diagnosis of pain in the low back. Journal of the American Medical Association 110: 106–113

Sterling A, Butterfield W C, Bonner R, Quikley W 1977 Post-traumatic cysts of soft tissue. Journal of Trauma 17: 392–396

Stokes I A F, Frymoyer J W 1987 Segmental motion and instability. Spine 12: 688–691

Styf J, Lysell E 1987 Chronic compartment syndrome in the erector spinae muscle. Spine 12: 580–582

Thould A K 1988 Any questions. What is fibromyalgia and how should it be treated? British Medical Journal 297: 1326

Tracy M F, Bibson M J, Szypryt E P, Rutherford A, Corlett E N 1989 The geometry of the muscles of the lumbar spine determined by magnetic resonance imaging. Spine 14: 186–193

Travell J 1942 Pain and disability of shoulder arm: treatment by intramuscular infiltration with procaine hydrochloride. Journal of the American Medical Association 121: 417

Vecchione T R 1977 Persistent post-traumatic pseudo-sheath formation secondary to a moveable organised blood clot. Journal of Traumatology 17: 481–482

Weichen P J, Muller W 1986 The contused kidney, an angiographic picture. Diagnostic Imaging in Clinical Medicine 55: 270–272

Yunus M B 1989 Fibromyalgia syndrome: new research on an old malady. British Medical Journal 298: 474–475

26. Conservative management

Low back pain is often a self-limiting disease which will settle spontaneously and it can usually be managed satisfactorily by non-operative methods. Although 400 000 patients are referred to British hospitals with back pain each year, only 7500 have surgery (Jayson 1981, Nelson 1982). A general practitioner will see approximately 200 patients each year with low back pain but on average, only one will require an operation (Drinkall et al 1984).

Patients with mechanical back pain are a heterogeneous population, and for conservative management as well as for surgery the first priority is to identify a back pain syndrome. Not only do these patients appreciate an attempt to identify the pain source, but unless the underlying syndrome is recognized, the clinician can only treat symptomatically. The first objective is therefore to make a diagnosis and communicate this to the patient.

DIAGNOSIS

The syndromes in which the diagnosis is not in doubt are those in which root pain extends below the knee. Pain is in a root distribution, and it is worse in the leg than in the back. However, greater controversy surrounds the diagnosis when there is only back pain or referred pain. The referred pain may be in the buttock, round the pelvis, or down to the knee (Kellgren 1977), but it is always worse in the back than in the legs. In these the diagnosis is difficult. If there are sufficient criteria to identify a back pain syndrome, the natural history and ways of resolving the problem can be explained and the patient may need no active treatment. Without a diagnosis

the patient may well get better, but we are working in the dark.

Lumbar disc herniation

This topic is covered in greater detail in Chapter 15. There are two symptoms and two signs which suggest a lumbar disc protrusion in the presence of root pain:

- Root pain aggravated by coughing, laughing or sneezing
- Difficulty putting on shoes and socks in the morning
- A trunk list
- Marked limitation of straight leg raising.

The patient may have signs of a neurological deficit (areflexia, motor weakness, wasting or sensory loss). These are signs of a pathological nerve root, but they are not specific for the cause of that pathology.

Most patients with a protrusion (as distinct from an extrusion or sequestration when the annulus is completely torn) will have recurrent episodes of pain which settle down with conservative management. If the pain is severe, then the patient has no choice but to rest in bed; they should, however, mobilize as soon as possible to avoid the deleterious effects of disuse. They need counselling about prognosis and rehabilitation, which may best be reinforced in the Back School. For most, the prognosis is good (Saal & Saal 1988).

When there are clear criteria of disc protrusion with straight leg raising less than 50°, enforced bed rest for as much as 2 weeks can allow a resolution in symptoms and signs.

Signs which carry a poor prognosis for conservative management are:

- A trunk list
- Cross-leg pain
- No diurnal change in straight leg raising (Porter & Trailescu 1990).

In these patients, especially when these three signs coexist (Khuffash & Porter 1989), early surgery may be appropriate. Discectomy, either by open or percutaneous operation, is reserved for those patients with a protrusion whose symptoms do not resolve. Those with a complete annular tear need open discectomy; otherwise, sequestrated nuclear disc material will compromise the vertebral canal indefinitely.

Bony entrapment of the nerve root

Root entrapment from lateral canal stenosis is the subject of Chapter 16. Patients with root pain due to bony compression by stenosis in the lateral recess or in the nerve root canal have pain in a similar distribution to those with disc protrusion, but with different features. They do not have a list, pain is not aggravated by coughing, the symptoms are not affected by diurnal changes, and they have no difficulty with socks in the morning. Sitting for long becomes painful and straight leg raising is not severely limited. They may or may not have signs of neurological deficit.

These patients are usually in an older age group, and there are radiological features of degenerative change. A myelogram is generally negative unless there is lateral encroachment from apophyseal joints at one segmental level. A CT scan will show bony and/or ligamentous encroachment into the lateral recess of the central canal or into the root canal. MRI studies are positive, with an absence of epidural fat. There may be rotational or sagittal vertebral displacement. Imaging is not necessary for the diagnosis; it is a clinical diagnosis, and CT or MRI is only useful to show the site of the degenerative pathology in those few patients who require surgery.

Treatment initially should be conservative, because most patients recover (Porter et al 1984). They require counselling about the mech-

anism of the pain and the prognosis. Some with severe pain benefit from an epidural injection and the support of the Pain Clinic. Surgical decompression is indicated when a short period of conservative management is unproductive, and when there is not a natural resolution of symptoms.

An isthmic spondylolisthesis, either bilateral or unilateral, can be associated with root entrapment syndrome when degenerative change compromises the adjacent nerve root (Porter & Park 1982, Porter & Hibbert 1984). Once established, the symptoms fail to settle down without surgical intervention. A fusion rather than decompression is generally sufficient to abolish the dynamic effects of instability and relieve root symptoms.

Neurogenic claudication

The problem of neurogenic claudication is discussed in Chapter 17. Patients with neurogenic claudication due to nerve root compression experience pain or discomfort in the legs above and below the knees, limiting the walking distance. This is relieved by a short period of rest, and if the spine is not too rigid (Dong & Porter 1989), by stooping forwards. There is always radiological evidence of spinal stenosis on myelogram, CT or MRI. There may be partial, subtotal or complete occlusion of the metrizamide column of the myelogram, often at several levels. The diagnosis cannot be made in the presence of a normal myelogram. The critical cross-sectional area of the cauda equina is 100 mm (Bolender et al 1985), though this is probably too generous and 75 mm may be more appropriate. This is further reduced by the dynamic changes of sagittal or rotational instability. There is usually a two-level compression, either two levels of central canal stenosis or central and root canal stenosis, causing a double nerve root block. In addition to the spinal pathology, there may be associated peripheral vascular disease (Johansson et al 1982).

Once established, the symptoms of neurogenic claudication rarely resolve, but there is no evidence that increasing deterioration occurs. Major neurological damage is unusual.

Many patients accept their disability after an explanation of the pathology and the likelihood that symptoms will not increase. They modify their life-style and avoid surgery. A course of calcitonin is worthwhile (Porter & Hibbert 1983, Porter & Miller 1988) — 100 units subcutaneously four times a week for 4 weeks. If there is no improvement at 4 weeks, then a response is unlikely. Some, however, will obtain a dramatic improvement in their walking distance and avoid surgery.

Painful unstable spondylolysis or spondylolisthesis

Chapter 19 deals with this problem in greater detail. It is not easy to be sure of the pain source for the patient with back pain alone. There is, however, less controversy about the diagnostic criteria for an unstable spondylolisthesis than for other causes of back pain. Isthmic spondylolisthesis occurs in approximately 5% of the Caucasian population, with a greater incidence in athletes and gymnasts (Roche & Rowe 1951, Kono et al 1975, Troup 1975, Jackson et al 1976, Murray Leslie et al 1977, Bird et al 1980, Hitoshi 1980, Hardcastle et al 1992). The pars defect is common and frequently symptomless. It is important to exclude other causes of back pain.

Pain from an unstable spondylolisthesis often radiates into the buttocks and round the pelvis, but unless a nerve root is affected, the pain is always worse in the back. It is aggravated by walking, shopping and driving, and partially relieved by lying down. There is sometimes a precipitating injury often many years before, and many women date their first symptoms to pregnancy (Porter & Hibbert 1984).

Although the results of fusion are good, not every patient with spondylolisthesis requires an operation. A slight increase in the displacement is possible over a few decades of adult life (Postacchini 1989) but this may not produce symptoms. Many patients have instability symptoms in early adult life with no discomfort thereafter, and some develop strong bony stability.

The young adolescent with spondylolisthesis and the first attack of back pain may have a stress fracture apparent on a scintiscan. Immobilization in a half-spica may allow the defect to unite. An acute episode of pain in adult life requires a lumbar corset, help in the Back School and dietary advice.

One can expect excellent results from a spinal fusion, but it is indicated only when acute severe symptoms are not resolving naturally, when chronic symptoms are unacceptable, and when the quality of working and sporting life is significantly curtailed by back pain.

Chronic low back pain

There is considerable disagreement about the causation and the pain source in chronic low back pain. Some look for certain criteria to incriminate an unstable intervertebral segment (Farfan & Gracovetsky 1984, Nachemson 1985); others describe facet joint pain (Rashbaum 1983, Helbig & Lee 1988). Some authorities attempt to make a specific soft tissue diagnosis such as sacroiliac, gluteus maximus or piriformis syndromes purely on clinical diagnosis (Kirkaldy-Willis 1988). It is not yet possible to establish the credibility of these syndromes when the symptoms have not been correlated with demonstrable pathology. If the pain is sufficiently disabling, and it is possible to identify the intervertebral segment responsible for the pain, then it is reasonable to hope that the prevention of movement at this level by surgical fusion will relieve the pain. Indications for fusion are more fully discussed in Chapter 24, but random fusion for low back pain is not very successful. This is probably because patients with chronic low back pain are a heterogeneous population with different pathologies.

If fusion is being considered for a patient with chronic low back pain, most would agree that it should be preceded by an adequate trial of conservative management. This includes counselling, attending the Back School, functional rehabilitation, and assessment for a behavioural disorder. Some would offer short-term tricyclic anti-depressant therapy (Ward 1986).

Once an attempt has been made to reach a diagnosis and to identify the source of the pain, only rarely is it necessary to progress directly to surgical treatment. There are a multitude of conservative approaches available, and the most commonly used will be discussed.

TREATMENT

Counselling

Patients with back pain have two main areas of concern: What is wrong? Can it be cured? They are often troubled most by the former. The clinician's role is to allay fears that there is serious underlying disease by explaining that it is not a crippling condition, that it will not result in paralysis or a spreading rheumatism, and that it is not a tumour. It is erroneous for surgeons to believe that patients with back pain consult them only for an operation.

It generally requires no more than an adequate history and examination supported by basic radiological investigation to decide that the pain is of mechanical origin and not due to an inflammatory disorder or more sinister pathology. There may be sufficient criteria to identify one of the specific back pain syndromes, allowing an explanation of the pathology and probable source of pain, which is a great relief to an anxious patient. Failure to receive an early and adequate explanation of the back pain problem is a major source of patient dissatisfaction (Deyo & Diehl 1986).

Half of the patients with an acute episode of back pain resolve within a week, 80% in 2 weeks, and only a minority are still in pain at the end of a month. Reassurance is therefore important at the start of an acute episode. For the patient whose pain is more persistent, counselling and advice on self-management can be as productive as active therapy. In the long term, many patients find that their back pain becomes less of a problem in later life and they need to know that age is kindly to the spine (Porter 1987a) (Fig. 27.2). It is not necessary to 'do something' for every patient; what is said may be more important.

Bed rest

There are times when the patient can do nothing other than rest in bed, but once the most acute symptoms have settled, mobilization should be encouraged. Recumbency has adverse effects on many systems including the spine. Whilst in bed it is immaterial whether the patient lies supine or on the side. A pillow beneath the knees can be helpful. Bed rest need not be total as personal hygiene may be more difficult to achieve in bed than out of it. Analgesics round the clock are necessary at first, but they should be reduced as soon as possible.

There is no good evidence that tranquillizers hasten recovery (Weber 1980). Anti-inflammatory drugs, however, do appear to be effective in relieving back pain if started within 2 days of the onset of an attack (Amlie et al 1987), and the early use of antispasmodic drugs also has benefit (Basmajian 1989).

In the presence of nerve root tension signs, 2 weeks of bed rest is useful (Weber 1983). With severe back pain only, 2 days of bed rest appears to produce results equivalent to 7 days of rest in bed (Deyo et al 1985), whilst an earlier study demonstrated that 10 days of bed rest produces a better recovery and a faster return to work than no rest (Wiesel et al 1980).

Too much rest is counter-productive. Not only does recumbency weaken the musculoskeletal system, delaying recovery (Van der Wiel et al 1991), but the anxious patient may become distressed by the fear of pain, and develop abnormal pain behaviour. Many a chronic disability could have been avoided by timely advice and early mobilization. Rest, though beneficial in the short term, should be kept to a minimum.

Spinal orthoses

Lumbar supports have been widely used for relief of back pain, but there is no documented evidence that they reduce the period of disability. Fidler and Plasmans (1983) showed that a canvas corset reduced the angular movement of the lumbar spine by one-third, but there are times when it will actually increase movement at the lumbosacral junction (Norton & Brown 1957, Lumsden & Morris 1968). A support within the corset gives better relief than the same canvas without support (Million et al 1981). Besides limiting lumbar mobility (Willner 1985), an orthosis can decrease intradiscal pressure

(Nachemson 1985) and provide relief, perhaps by local warmth and by stimulation of mechano-receptors; however, compliance is poor.

Back School

Starting in Scandinavia, the Back School concept has spread across the industrialized world (Zachrisson-Forsell 1972). It is a structured intervention programme for a group of individuals and provides patients with information about back pain of mechanical origin, about the types of stress that can injure the spine, how this knowledge can be applied in day-to-day activities, and how the spine can be strengthened by improving fitness. They are informed about self-management for the acute attack and how such attacks generally get better without active treatment, how to manage recurrent and chronic back pain, and how to reduce the incidence of attacks. Back School programmes have been shown to be a better use of resources and time than other unproven therapeutic methods (Berquhist-Ullman & Larson 1977, Williams 1977, Attix & Tate 1979, Aberg 1982, Fisk et al 1983, Moffett et al 1986, Berwick et al 1989). A tailor-made Back School programme can reduce absenteeism by at least 5 days per year per employee and is cost-effective to industry (Versloot et al 1992). The clinician can discuss the problem, the present management and prognosis during the first consultation, but he cannot spend 2 or 3 hours with the patient explaining and demonstrating the correct use of the spine. This is the role of the Back School (Andersson 1987), well reviewed by Klaber Moffett (1989).

Back Schools have no rigid structure, but each department offers instruction tailored to the needs of its own community (Pawlicki et al 1982), with variation in content, duration and class size. It is helpful to discuss first spinal anatomy and function, with appropriate demonstrations. Disc protrusion and degeneration are described, as well as the vulnerability of the nerve roots in middle life. If the probable cause of the patient's pain is known to the physiotherapist, they ask the patient if the pain mechanism explained by the doctor has been understood.

Relaxation is demonstrated and lifting techni-ques are practised. Advice is offered about posture and how everyday activities can be accomplished with minimal stress. Dialogue is encouraged. Some Back Schools incorporate exercises into their programme (White 1983). Exercises can be dynamic, with active contraction of a muscle group to bring about a change in length and cause articular movement, or static and isometric producing a voluntary contraction without change in length or joint movement. Certainly subjects with improved fitness and endurance are less prone to back problems (Mayer et al 1987), but dynamic exercises may increase the intradiscal pressure.

Back School education does seem to make good sense; it seems to meet the needs of many patients seeking medical help. Patients realize for the first time that management is in their own hands. It lowers the anxiety level of many bewildered patients who have suffered with back pain for a long time without an explanation of their problem.

Functional rehabilitation

Many patients fail to recover from an acute episode of back pain because they have been led to believe that they should treat their back with great caution. Any activity that produces back pain is noted and avoided, more because of anticipated pain and suffering rather than the actual experience of pain (Fordyce et al 1983, Linton 1985). It has been suggested, however, that avoidance behaviour is as unproductive in reducing pain as it is in reducing fear (Philips & Hunter 1981).

Not only does passive avoidance lead to psychological reinforcement of the invalidity status, but it also has adverse physical effects. Joints become stiff, soft tissues weak, and protective reflexes are impaired — the 'deconditioning syndrome'. This is further complicated by wearing corsets and jackets, and the injudicious use of analgesics. An acute episode of back pain which would be expected to resolve within a short period may therefore persist as chronic disability, with psychological disturbance and physical disuse phenomena.

Functional rehabilitation attempts to reverse this situation. It aims to improve physical fitness and influence low back pain by improving disc nutrition, assisting healing of connective tissues and increasing endorphins (Dale et al 1987). Mechanical forces have important effects on most tissues — musculoskeletal, skin, lung and blood vessels (Evans & Egan 1988). Several studies have shown a correlation between fitness and recovery from back pain (Cady et al 1979, Mellin 1986). Good isometric endurance of the back muscles may prevent the first-time occurrence of back pain (Biering Sorensen 1984), and hard work may protect against disc protrusion (Porter 1987b, Porter et al 1989a, Porter 1992). Coal miners are remarkably protected against disc protrusion (Porter 1991) but they are prone to a variety of degenerative spinal disorders.

The programmes of rehabilitation vary, but have a common content of increasing activity and restoration of function through vigorous physical exercise. Pain does not limit the activity; rather, the concept of activity being detrimental to chronic low back pain is challenged (Nachemson 1983a, Waddell 1987). Fear inhibits functional restoration (Kohles et al 1990). The activity programme is carefully monitored, sometimes with inclinometers and isokinetic or isometric strength measurement devices, to record strength, endurance, flexibility and co-ordination (Mayer et al 1985). Feedback is used to encourage the patient.

Patients with chronic back pain for whom surgery has no place and for whom traditional therapies have had little to offer, have frequently responded to a programme of functional rehabilitation, developing a new quality of life and many returning to work (Mayer et al 1987, Hazars et al 1989, Sachs et al 1990, Mitchell & Carmen 1990, Mayer 1992). Similarly, patients who have been off work for more than 8 weeks with an acute episode of back pain, and who are treated with a vigorous exercise regimen, not only return to work more quickly than an untreated control population, but they are also significantly better than the control group at 1 year (Lindstrom et al 1989).

Behaviour modification programme — 'School for Bravery'

Those patients whose chronic disability has a large non-organic component of abnormal pain behaviour respond well to a pain modification programme. Our own programme, designed by Mrs J Williams (Porter et al 1989b) is called 'School for Bravery'. Entry is possible for those with courage. It is similar to the functional rehabilitation programme, but those who respond change their behaviour so quickly that it cannot be attributed to improving fitness. It is a psychological approach, though psychology is never mentioned.

Patients joining the programme have many inappropriate symptoms and signs, and have had a full but unrewarding investigation for treatable pathology. They spend all day in the department, 5 days per week, wearing track-suit and trainers. Their disability is monitored on video, and their goals agreed. Pain is not discussed. They enter a demanding vigorous exercise programme. Improved performance is rewarded with praise, and illness behaviour ignored. Initially they have individual management, graduating into group activity with the encouragement of others who are further advanced.

Those who respond suddenly convert to wellness behaviour in a few days, much earlier than can be explained by improved physical fitness. They are initially unstable for a few days, until healthy function becomes established. A new video is taken, and most patients are surprised to see how gross was their original degree of disability. They are assured that by their own efforts, they have achieved a new quality of life, and they usually vow never to return to their previous state. The experience of pain may not be diminished when successful illness behaviour is abandoned.

Manipulation

The role of manipulative treatment for mechanical low back pain is uncertain and controversial, and a literature review provides only limited empirical support (Ottenbacher & Difabio 1985). Many different techniques are practised with little agreement about when it is indicated, what is being treated, what happens when it is effective, and what are the short- and long-term results.

An osteopath will identify the level of the lesion, and relax the muscles by careful stretching and manipulations of the part. The patient usually lies on the side with the trunk twisted so that some joints are believed to be locked and others free. Using lever techniques on the pelvis and other parts, a high velocity thrust is applied, often with audible cracks and clicks (Hadler et al 1987, MacDonald & Bell 1990). Manipulative treatment seems to be marginally and significantly better than heat, exercises and massage for patients with persistent back pain (Koes et al 1992).

The chiropractor will manipulate the individual vertebrae with a rapid but not very powerful thrust. He decides which type of thrust is appropriate, and applies it with precision. A randomized comparison of chiropractic and hospital outpatient treatment found chiropractic treatment slightly more effective in those patients with chronic or severe low back pain, with continued benefit at 2 years (Meade et al 1990). It is difficult to unravel the placebo response, but manual therapy and physiotherapy were both more effective in relieving complaints than no treatment at all (Koes et al 1992).

Some surgeons will manipulate a patient with chronic back pain under general anaesthesia, but the effects are generally less effective with time. The analgesic benefits from spinal manipulation do not appear to be mediated by increased endorphin production (Christian et al 1988).

Physiotherapists, though they may use different manipulative techniques, frequently practise the method described by Maitland. Oscillatory movements are applied to the spinous processes at the affected level, rotating away from the pain. A comparison of Maitland mobilization with placebo shows that:

— most episodes of back pain settle with or without treatment
— those likely to be helped with manipulation have only limited benefit with little long-term effect
— although some patients are immediately improved after manipulation, many other patients have similar improvement after a placebo session (Sims-Williams et al 1978).

The personal attention and interest of a physiotherapist probably plays a great part in hastening recovery (Jayson 1986).

Other techniques often accompany manipulation therapy (Burn & Paterson 1990). Cryotherapy with the application of ice, or ice and water with ice wrappings or compresses, aims to reduce oedema and pain, but except in spinal contusion it has not been demonstrated as efficacious. Nor have the benefits of the local application of superficial or deep heat, the use of diathermy, ultrasound, infra-red rays, warm fomentations, heating pads or hydrotherapy been shown to be effective. Deep or superficial massage of the soft tissues is useful in controlling pain, but it has not been supported in a controlled study. The elevation of endorphins in the central nervous system may explain some of the beneficial effects (Kosierlitz et al 1977, Terenius & Wahlstrom 1979).

Spinal traction — intermittent or continuous, manual or mechanical — has been widely used on the spine, but studies comparing different methods have not demonstrated their value (Weber et al 1985, Zylbergold & Piper 1985).

The McKenzie treatment

This is designed for patients with mechanical low back disturbance (McKenzie 1981). Three groups of patients are defined. Those with a 'postural syndrome' are young adults who have intermittent episodes of pain believed to be the result of prolonged stress on the soft tissues around the lumbar spine. They have no deformity and full movements, and they are treated by postural advice.

The second group have a 'dysfunctional syndrome'. They are older patients who are believed to have had trauma or a postural problem producing adaptive shortening of the soft tissues. Pain is triggered by over-use. Posture is poor, movements are restricted, and the pain is felt at the end of the range. They are given postural advice and gentle stretching exercises to the limit of a little pain.

The third group have a 'derangement syndrome' of the lumbar intervertebral disc, with a kyphotic deformity or a list when standing or stooping. Seven stages are described, and treatment is designed to move patients up to stage one, when they can manage themselves. After test movements the deformity is manually corrected, attempting to centralize the pain (Donelson et al 1990) and produce a situation whereby the patients can care for themselves with extension activity, maintain a lumbar lordosis, and subsequently perform flexion exercises to obtain a functional recovery.

The goal of the technique is to introduce the patient to a self-care programme, eventually avoiding the need for therapists or clinicians.

Posture

Frederick Matthias Alexander was born in Tasmania in 1869. He had a precarious acting career until he discovered how to improve his voice by correcting his posture. The teachers of the technique that bear his name (Gelb 1981) believe that poor posture can affect function and produce musculoskeletal pain; as a result of 'imbalance' some tissues suffer over-use and fatigue, and others disuse and atrophy. The Alexander technique is popular with musicians and athletes, who because of poor posture may under-perform and suffer pain. It is also suggested that inefficient use of the spine accounts for much backache.

The teachers of the technique seek to inhibit unnecessary tension and produce 'poise and harmony, balance and coordination'. They describe 'pause before action and stillness in activity'. Their approach is also holistic, believing that a distorted posture produces distorted perceptions, that poise affects personality. A good posture certainly is attractive and it makes sense. There are many followers of the technique, but it has yet to be assessed scientifically.

The Pain Clinic

The advent of pain treatment as a clinical speciality has provided a new method of management for patients with back pain. When surgery or further surgery is not indicated and when intractable pain is a problem, the Pain Clinic, which attempts to modify the patient's perception of pain, has much to offer. Most patients have received counselling and Back School advice; they have had manipulative therapy and

exercise programmes, and pain still remains. If they exhibit inappropriate symptoms and signs of abnormal pain behaviour, they are unlikely to respond to pain-relieving procedures in the Pain Clinic. Further invasive procedures will only be counter-productive and will reinforce illness behaviour. However, for patients with back or leg pain when the non-organic component is small, the Pain Clinic may be the only source of help.

Many patients with intractable pain suffer from the effects of excessive medication. The clinician in the Pain Clinic is probably best fitted to review the drug regimen and to evaluate and prescribe appropriate analgesics, anti-inflammatory drugs, antidepressants and hypnotics (Sullivan 1992). Paracetamol is the commonest non-narcotic prescribed for pain. It is probably not addictive, but in overdose can cause liver disease. It is often combined with weak narcotics, and an inadvertent overdose is possible.

Many patients attending a Pain Clinic are already taking narcotics and are often unaware of this potential for developing tolerance and addiction. There is no evidence that the prolonged use of narcotic drugs is beneficial for chronic benign pain, and their continued use is inadvisable.

Non-steroidal anti-inflammatory drugs (NSAIDs) are beneficial in the partial control of inflammatory conditions, and are helpful in acute episodic back pain (Orava 1986, Amlie et al 1987). Their use in chronic low back pain is equivocal, and because of significant gastrointestinal side-effects, especially in the elderly, they should be avoided. Antidepressant drugs can elevate mood and may increase pain tolerance in the depressed patient, reducing chronic low back pain (Ward 1986). Low-dose tricylic antidepressants may enhance the effect of transcutaneous nerve stimulation.

Antiepileptic drugs have been used for shooting, 'lancinating' pain (Swerdlaw & Cundill 1981), though with some side-effects in the elderly.

Sometimes the most important role of the clinician in the Pain Clinic is to re-evaluate the drug regimen. Too often drugs have lost their efficacy, have become addictive and are producing side-effects. Patients can be weaned from habit-forming drugs by prescribing a cocktail of increasing dilution.

Severe root entrapment pain from lateral canal stenosis or root canal stenosis can be helped by one or more epidural injections of 40 ml saline, with Marcaine and hydrocortisone. Although clinical trials to confirm its efficacy are still awaited, there is no doubt that many individual patients are supported through a stressful time with an occasional epidural injection. This regimen is sometimes proposed for the root pain of a disc protrusion, to economize on bed rest. If one believes that extradural scarring can produce pain after a discectomy or decompression, then an epidural injection may help by breaking down adhesions and reducing inflammatory change. It can be useful therapy when postoperative recovery is slow, but it has not been scientifically assessed. Some have suggested that the vehicle in which the steroids are dissolved may cause extradural scarring (Andersson & Mosdal 1987). The value of epidural injection is still controversial (Snoek et al 1977, Bourne 1984, Cuckler et al 1985, Bush & Hillier 1991, Power et al 1992).

Similarly, without clear evidence of efficacy, trigger points and fibrositic nodules are often injected with local anaesthetic and steroid, giving temporary relief. Superficial injection into a tender sacroiliac joint can be helpful, but in the absence of a controlled trial one cannot be sure that these procedures are successful only by their placebo effect. They will be counter-productive and should be avoided in the patient with abnormal pain behaviour.

The apophyseal joint may be an important pain source. It can be examined by percutaneous injection of local anaesthetic into the joint under radiographic control (Lippitt 1984). Relief of symptoms may convince the clinician that this is an important pain source, and the joint can then be denervated by radio-frequency block (Mehta & Sluijter 1979). The critics rightly remind us that it is difficult to place a needle accurately into a small joint, and local anaesthetic will diffuse widely into the root canal and epidural space, making interpretation of pain relief difficult (Fig. 26.1) (Moran et al 1988). Denervation can also produce a Charcot joint with subsequent problems. Marks and Thulbourne (1991) report encouraging results from injecting painful anomalous lumbosacral articulations with steroid and local anaesthetic. The facet joint syndrome, however, is still controversial (Jackson et al 1988).

Transcutaneous electrical nerve stimulation (Pike 1978, Melzack et al 1983, Ottosen & Lundeberg 1988, Deyo et al 1990) probably involves the endorphin system. The analgesic effect is blocked by naloxone. The peripheral nerves are stimulated by an electric current transmitted transcutaneously, and this can relieve low back pain in some patients. It has the advantage

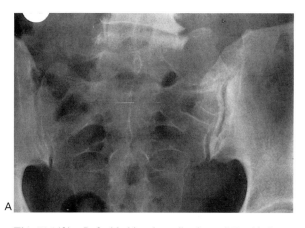
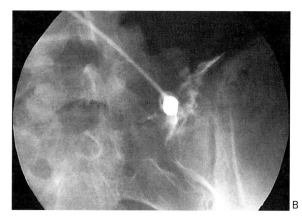

A   B

Fig. 26.1(A)   Left-sided hemisacralization at L5, with degenerative changes in the sacroiliac joint.
(B) Arthrography showing either wide extension of the hemisacralized joint, or extravasation of the radio-opaque fluid. It is difficult to interpret the significance of pain relief after instillation of local anaesthetic.

that the patient can position the electrodes on the back for best effect, and can regulate the intensity of the stimulus. In the short term, percutaneous dorsal column stimulators can also help patients with chronic back pain (Racz et al 1989). The long-term response to electrical nerve stimulation is poor in patients displaying abnormal illness behaviour.

Biofeedback (electromyography, EMG) transposes the physiological activity of the muscle response into a visual or auditory signal, enabling the patient to modify that response. It is designed to inhibit excessive or unbalanced muscle activity but, although sometimes used in patients with chronic back pain, there is no scientific study demonstrating its benefit.

Acupuncture can relieve low back pain for some patients, but it is not possible to predict success. It has proved difficult to design satisfactory trials in order to judge its value (Lewith & Machin 1983, Lewith 1984, Vincent & Richardson 1986). The counter-irritant effect of stimulating the skin in a noxious manner with subcutaneous acupuncture needles was found to be superior to placebo dummy surface electrodes on both subjective and objective assessment of back pain (MacDonald et al 1983, Deluze et al 1992). Though few individual trials favour acupuncture, a meta-analysis of randomized controlled trials seems to suggest some benefits (Patel et al 1989).

Not all the methods used in the Pain Clinic are of proven value, but many patients with severe pain for which no remedy has been found are grateful that someone is still prepared to try.

The aim of the Pain Clinic is to help the patient to manage their own pain, so that they can regain levels of function within the bounds of their spinal problem. In isolation the Clinic will fail, but with good co-operation from the referring spinal clinician, and with the therapist in the functional rehabilitation programme or behavioural modification programme, success rates can be high.

The management of patients with low back pain stretches clinical judgement as perhaps in no other field of medicine. Only a minority of the patients require surgery. Good results require judicial patient selection — which means understanding the back pain syndromes and their natural history, careful patient assessment, keeping up to date with the conservative options, and having the facilities available for the new methods of non-operative management.

REFERENCES

Aberg J 1982 Evaluation of an advanced back pain rehabilitation programme. Spine 7: 317–318

Amlie E, Weber H, Holme I 1987 Treatment of acute low back pain with Piroxicam: results of a double-blind placebo-controlled trial. Spine 12: 473–476

Andersson G B J 1987 Back Schools. In: Jayson M I V (ed) The lumbar spine and back pain, 3rd edn. Churchill Livingstone, Edinburgh, p 315–320

Andersson K H, Mosdal C 1987 Epidural application of cortico-steroids in low back pain and sciatica. Acta Neurochirurgica (Wein) 87: 52–53

Attix E A, Tate M A 1979 Low Back School: a conservative method for the treatment of low back pain. Mississippi State Medical Association 20: 4

Basmajian J V 1989 Acute back pain and spasm; a controlled multicentre trial of combined analgesic and anti-spasm agents. Spine 14: 438–439

Berquhist-Ullman M, Larson V 1977 Acute low back pain in industry. Acta Orthopedica Scandinavica Suppl 170

Berwick D M, Budman S, Feldstein M 1989 No clinical effect of back school in an HMO; a randomised prospective trial. Spine 14: 338–344

Biering Sorensen F 1984 Physical measurements as risk indicators for low back trouble over a one year period. Spine 9: 106–109

Bird H A, Eastmond C J, Hudson A, Wright V 1980 Is generalised joint laxity a factor in spondylolisthesis? Scandinavian Journal of Rheumatology 9: 203–205

Bolender N F, Schonstrom N S R, Spengler D N 1985 Role of myelography and computerised tomography in the diagnosis of central spinal stenosis. Journal of Bone and Joint Surgery 67A: 240–246

Bourne L H J 1984 Treatment of chronic back pain comparing corticosteroid lignocaine injections with lignocaine alone. Practitioner 228: 333–338

Burn L, Paterson J K 1990 Musculoskeletal medicine. The spine. Kluwer Academic Publisher, Dordrecht, p 204–227

Bush K, Hillier S 1991 A controlled study of caudal epidural injections of triamcinalone plus procaine for the management of intractable sciatica. Spine 16: 572–575

Cady L D, Bishoff M P H, O'Connell M S, Thomas B A, Allan J H 1979 Strength and fitness and subsequent back injuries in firefighters. Journal of Occupation Medicine 21: 269–272

Christian G F, Stanton G J, Sisson D, How H Y, Jamison J, Alder B, Fullerton M, Funder J W 1988 Immunoreactive ACTH, β-endorphin, and cortisol levels in plasma following spinal manipulative therapy. Spine 13: 1411–1417

Cuckler J M, Bernini P A, Wiesel S W et al 1985 The use of epidural steroids in the treatment of lumbar radicular pain. Journal of Bone and Joint Surgery. 67A: 63–66

Dale D, Fleetwood J A, Weddell A, Ellis R D, Sainsbury J R C 1987 Endorphin: a factor in 'fun run' collapse? British Medical Journal 294: 1004

Deluze C, Bosia L, Zirbs A, Chantraine A, Vischer T L 1992 Electroacupuncture in fibromyalgia: results of a controlled trial. British Medical Journal 305: 1249–1252

Deyo R A, Diehl A K 1986 Patient satisfaction with medical care for low back pain. Spine 11: 28–30

Deyo R A, Diehl A K, Rosenthal M 1985 How much bed rest for backache? A randomised clinical trial (abstract). Conference of the American Federation for Clinical Research, Dallas

Deyo R A, Walsh N E, Martin D C, Schoenfeld L S, Ramamnurthy S 1990 A controlled trial of TENS and exercise for chronic low back pain. New England Journal of Medicine 322: 1627–1634

Donelson R, Silva G, Murphy K 1990 Centralisation phenomenon: its usefulness in evaluating and treating referred pain. Spine 15: 211–213

Dong G X, Porter R W 1989 Cycling and walking tests in neurogenic and intermittent claudication. Spine 14(2): 201–203

Drinkall J N, Porter R W, Hibbert C S, Evans C 1984 The value of ultrasonic measurement of the spinal canal diameter in general practice. British Medical Journal 288P: 121–122

Evans G, Egan J M 1988 Catching up with the orthopods: mechanical forces matter in tissues other than bone. British Medical Journal 297–936

Farfan H F, Gracovetsky S 1984 The nature of instability. Spine 9: 714–719

Fidler M W, Plasmans C M T 1983 The effect of four types of support on the segmental mobility of the lumbo-sacral spine. Journal of Bone and Joint Surgery 65A: 943–947

Fisk J R, DiMonte P, Courington S McK 1983 Back schools: past, present and future. Clinical Orthopedics and Related Research 179: 18–23

Fordyce W E, Shelton J L, Dundore D E 1983 The modification of avoidance learning pain behaviour. Journal of Behavioural Medicine 4: 405–414

Gelb M 1981 Body learning — an introduction to the Alexander technique. Aurum Press, London

Hadler N M, Curtis P, Gillings D B, Stinnett S 1987 A benefit of spinal manipulation as adjunctive therapy for acute low back pain: a stratified controlled trial. Spine 12: 703–706

Hardcastle P, Annear P, Foster D H, Chakera T M, McCormick C, Khangure M, Burnett A 1992 Spinal abnormalities in young fast bowlers. Journal of Bone and Joint Surgery 74-B: 421–425

Hazars R G, Fenwick J W, Kalisch S M, Redmond J, Reeves V, Reid S, Frymoyer J W 1989 Functional restoration with behaviour support: a one year prospective study of patients with chronic low back pain. Spine 14: 157–161

Helbig T, Lee C K 1988 The lumbar facet syndrome. Spine 13: 61–64

Hitoshi H 1980 Spondylolysis in athletes. Physical Sports Medicine 8: 75–79

Jackson D W, Wiltse L L, Cirincone R J 1976 Spondylolysis in the female gymnast. Clinical Orthopaedics 117: 68–73

Jackson R P, Jacobs R R, Montesano P X 1988 Facet joint injection in low back pain; a prospective statistical study.

Spine 13: 966–971

Jayson M I V 1981 Back pain: the facts. Oxford University Press, New York

Jayson M I V 1986 A limited role for manipulation. British Medical Journal 293: 1454–1455

Johansson J E, Barrington T W, Ameli M 1982 Combined vascular and neurogenic claudication. Spine 7: 150–158

Kellgren J H 1977 The anatomical source of back pain. Rheumatology and Rehabilitation 16: 3–12

Khuffash B, Porter R W 1989 Cross leg pain and trunk list. Spine 14: 602–603

Kirkaldy-Willis W H 1988 The site and nature of the lesion. In: Kirkaldy-Willis W H (ed) Managing low back pain, 2nd edn. Churchill Livingstone, Edinburgh, pp 135–154

Klaber Moffett J A 1989 Back Schools. In: Roland M O, Jenner J R (eds) Back pain. New approaches to rehabilitation and education. Manchester University Press, Manchester

Koes B W, Boulter L M, van Mameren H, Essers A H M, Verstegen G M J R, Hofhnizen D M, Houben J P, Knipschild P G 1992 The effectiveness of manual therapy and physiotherapy and treatment by the general practitioner for non specific back and neck complaints. Spine 17: 28–35

Kohles S, Barnes D, Gatchel R J, Mayer T G 1990 Improved physical performance outcome after functional restoration treatment in patients with chronic low back pain: early versus recent training results. Spine 15: 1321–1324

Kono S, Hayashi N, Kashahara G, Akimoto T, Keneko F, Suguira Y, Harada A 1975 A study on the aetiology of spondylolysis with reference to athletic activities. Journal of the Japanese Orthopaedic Association 49: 125–131

Kosierlitz H W, Hughes J, Law J H, Waterfield J A 1977 Encephalins, endorphines and opiate receptors. Neurosciences Symposium vol 2, Society for Neuroscience, p 291–307

Lewith G T 1984 Can we assess the effects of acupuncture? British Medical Journal 288: 1475–1476

Lewith G T, Machin D 1983 The evaluation of the clinical effects of acupuncture. Pain 16: 111–127

Lindstrom L, Ohlund C, Eek C, Peterson L E, Nachemson A 1989 Work return and LBP disability. Presented to the Society for the Study of the Lumbar Spine, Kyoto, Japan

Linton S J 1985 The relationship between activity and chronic back pain. Pain 21: 289–294

Lippitt A B 1984 The facet joint and its role in spine pain: management with facet joint injections. Spine 9: 746–750

Lumsden R M, Morris J M 1968 An in vivo study of axial rotation and immobilisation at the lumbo sacral joint. Journal of Bone and Joint Surgery 50A: 1591–1602

MacDonald A J R, Macrae K D, Master B R, Rubin A P 1983 Superficial acupuncture in the relief of chronic low back pain. Annals of the Royal College of Surgeons of England 65: 44–46

MacDonald R S, Bell C M J 1990 An open controlled assessment of orthopaedic manipulation in non-specific low back pain. Spine 15: 364–370

McKenzie R 1981 Spinal Publications Ltd PO Box 2, Waikanae, New Zealand

Marks R C, Thulbourne T 1991 Infiltration of anomalous lumbosacral articulations with steroid and anaesthetic injections in 10 back-pain patients. Acta Orthopedica Scandinavica 62: 139–141

Mayer T G 1992 Spine functional restoration. In: Rothman, Simeone (eds) The spine. W.B. Saunders, p 1929–1944

Mayer T, Gatchel R J, Kishino N, Keeley J, Capra P, Mayer H, Barnet J, Mooney V 1985 Objective assessment of spine function following industrial injury. Spine 6: 482–493

Mayer T G, Gatchel R J, Mayer H, Kishino N D, Keeley J, Mooney V 1987 A prospective two year study of functional restoration in industrial low back injury. Journal of the American Medical Association 258: 1763–1767

Meade T W, Dyer S, Browne W, Townsend J, Frank A O 1990 Low back pain of mechanical origin: randomised comparison of chiropractic and hospital outpatient treatment. British Medical Journal 300: 1431–1437

Mehta M, Sluijter M E 1979 The treatment of chronic pain. A preliminary survey of the effect of radio frequency denervation of the posterior vertebral joints. Anaesthesia 23: 768

Mellin G 1986 Chronic low back pain in men 54–63 years of age. Correlations of physical measurements with degree of trouble and progress after treatment. Spine 11: 421–426

Melzack R, Vetere P, Finch L 1983 Transcutaneous electrical nerve stimulation for low back pain; a comparison of TENS and massage for pain and range of motion. Physical Therapy 63: 489–493

Million R, Nilsen K H, Jayson M I V, Baker R D 1981 Evaluation of low back pain and assessment of lumbar corsets with and without back supports. Annals of the Rheumatic Diseases 40: 449–454

Mitchell R I, Carmen G M 1990 Results of a multi-centre trial using an intensive active exercise programme for the treatment of acute soft tissue and back injuries. Spine 15: 514–521

Moffett J A K, Chase S M, Portek I, Ennis J R 1986 A controlled prospective study to evaluate the effectiveness of a back school in the relief of chronic low back pain. Spine 11: 120–122

Moran R, O'Connell D, Walsh M G 1988 The diagnostic value of facet joint injections. Spine 13: 1407–1410

Murray Leslie C F, Lintott D J, Wright V 1977 The spine in sport and veteran military parachutists. Annals of the Rheumatic Diseases 36: 332–342

Nachemson A 1983a Work for all. Clinical Orthopaedics and Related Research 179: 77–85

Nachemson A 1983b Work for all, for those with back pain as well. Clinical Orthopaedics 179: 177–182

Nachemson A 1985 Lumbar spine instability; a critical update and symposium summary. Spine 10: 290–291

Nelson M 1982 Orthopaedic Surgery. Proceedings of International Symposium of the Low Back Pain Association, London

Norton P L, Brown T 1957 The immobilising efficiency of back braces. Their effect on the posture and motion of the lumbosacral spine. Journal of Bone and Joint Surgery 39A: 111–138

Orava S 1986 Medical treatment of low back pain. Diflunisal compared with indomethacin in acute lumbago. International Journal on Clinical Pharmacology and Research 6: 45–51

Ottenbacher K, Difabio R P 1985 Efficacy of spinal manipulation/mobilisation therapy. Spine 10: 833–837

Ottosen D, Lundeberg T 1988 Pain treatment by T.E.N.S. Springer Verlag, Berlin

Patel M, Gutswiller F, Paccard F, Marrazi A 1989 A meta-analysis of acupuncture for chronic pain. International Journal of Epidemiology 18: 900–906

Pawlicki R E, Gil K, Jopling C A, Bettinger R, Stevenson J M 1982 The low back school: a new palliative approach to low back pain. West Virginia Medical Journal 78: 249–251

Philips H C, Hunter M 1981 Pain behaviour in headache sufferers. Behaviour Analysis and Modification 4(10): 256–266

Pike P M H 1978 Transcutaneous electrical nerve stimulation. Anaesthesia 33: 165–171

Porter R W 1987a Should one operate on the elderly spine? In: Hukins, Nelson M (eds) The ageing spine. Manchester University Press, Manchester, p 79–83

Porter R W 1987b Does hard work prevent disc protrusion? Clinical Biomechanics 2: 196–198

Porter R W 1991 Is hardwork good for the back? The relationship between hard work and low back pain. International Journal of Industrial Ergonomics 9: 157–160

Porter R W 1992 Is hard work good for the back? International Journal of Industrial Ergonomics 9: 157–160

Porter R W, Hibbert C 1983 Calcitonin treatment for neurogenic claudication. Spine 8: 585–592

Porter R W, Hibbert C 1984 Symptoms associated with lysis of the pars interarticularis. Spine 9: 755–758

Porter R W, Miller C G 1988 Neurogenic claudication and root claudication treated with calcitonin: a double blind trial. Spine 13: 1061–1064

Porter R W, Park W 1982 Unilateral spondylolysis. Journal of Bone and Joint Surgery 64B: 344–348

Porter R W, Trailescu F 1990 Diurnal changes in straight leg raising. Spine 15: 103–106

Porter R W, Hibbert C, Evans C 1984 The natural history of root entrapment syndrome. Spine 9: 418–421

Porter R W, Adams M A, Hutton W C 1989a Physical activity and the strength of the spine. Spine 14: 201–203

Porter R W, Ellingworth C, Hughes T, Trailescu F 1989b Assessment of a 'school for bravery' — modification of abnormal pain behaviour. In: Roland M, Jenner J R (eds) Back pain. Manchester University Press, Manchester, p 157–165

Postacchini F 1989 Progression of spondylolysis in spondylolisthesis in adulthood. Presented to the International Society for the Study of the Lumbar Spine, Kyoto, Japan

Power R A, Taylor G J, Fyfe I S 1992 Lumbar epidural injection of steroid in acute prolapsed intervertebral discs: a prospective study. Spine 17: 453–455

Racz G B, McCarron R F, Talboys P 1989 Percutaneous dorsal column stimulator for chronic pain control. Spine 14: 1–4

Rashbaum R F 1983 Radio frequency facet denervation: a treatment alternative in refractory low back pain with or without leg pain. Orthopedic Clinics of North America 14: 569–575

Roche M B, Rowe G G 1951 The incidence of separated neural arch and coincident bone variation. A survey of 4200 skeletons. Anatomical Records 109: 233–252

Saal J A, Saal J S 1988 Nonoperative treatment of herniated lumbar intervertebral disc with radiculopathy; an outcome study. Spine 13: 431–437

Sachs B L, David J F, Olimpio D, Scala A D, Lacroix M 1990 Spinal rehabilitation by work tolerance based on objective physical capacity assessment of dysfunction: a prospective study with control subjects and twelve months review. Spine 15: 1325–1332

Sims-Williams H, Jayson M I V, Young S M S, Baddeley H, Colins E 1978 Controlled trial of mobilisation and manipulation for patients with low back pain in general practice. British Medical Journal 2: 1338–1340

Snoek W, Weber H, Jorgensen B 1977 Double blind evaluation of extradural methyl prednisolone for herniated lumbar discs. Acta Orthopedica Scandinavica 48: 635–641

Sullivan J B G 1992 Chronic pain management. In: Rothman, Simeone (eds) The spine. W.B. Saunders, p 1945–1961

Swerdlaw M, Cundill J G 1981 Anticonvulsant drugs used in the treatment of lancinating pain. A comparison. Anaesthesia 36: 1129–1132

Terenius L, Wahlstrom A 1979 Endorphines and clinical pain: an overview. Advances in Experimental Medicine and Biology 116: 261–277

Troup J D G 1975 Classical factors in spondylolisthesis and spondylolysis. Clinical Orthopedics and Related Research 117: 59–67

Van der Wiel H E, Lips P, Nauta J, Netelenbos J C, Hazenberg G J 1991 Biochemical parameters of bone turnover during ten days of bed rest and subsequent mobilisation. Bone Mineralization 13: 123–129

Versloot J M, Rozeman A, van Son A M, van Akkerveeckan P F 1992 The cost-effectiveness of a back school programme in industry. Spine 17: 22–27

Vincent C A, Richardson P H 1986 The evaluation of therapeutic acupuncture. Concepts and methods. Pain 24: 1–14

Waddell G 1987 A new clinical model for the treatment of low back pain. Spine 7: 632–644

Ward N G 1986 Tricyclic antidepressants for chronic low back pain: mechanisms of action and predictors of response. Spine 11: 661–665

Weber H 1980 Comparison of the effect of diazepam and levomepromazine on pain in patients with acute lumbago–sciatica. Journal of Oslo City Hospital 30: 65–68

Weber H 1983 Lumbar disc herniation: a controlled prospective study with ten years of observation. Spine 8: 131–140

Weber H, Ljunggren A R E, Walker L 1985 Traction therapy in patients with herniated lumbar intervertebral discs. Journal of Oslo City Hospital 34: 61–70

White A H 1983 Back school and other conservative approaches to low back pain. CV Mosby, St Louis

Wiesel S W, Cucker J M, Deluca F et al 1980 Acute low back pain: an objective analysis of conservative therapy. Spine 5: 324–330

Williams S J 1977 Back school. Physiotherapy 63: 90

Willner S 1985 Effects of a rigid brace on back pain. Acta Orthopedica Scandinavica 56: 40–42

Zachrisson-Forsell M 1972 Low back pain school. Danderyds Hospital, Sweden

Zylbergold R W, Piper M C 1985 Cervical spine disorders: a comparison of three types of traction. Spine 10: 867–871

27. The elderly spine

Back pain does not spare the elderly. Its victims are claimed from every decade of life and the old are no exception. All the medical disciplines are reassessing their role in the treatment of the elderly, because they represent an increasingly large and important proportion of the population. In 1901 only 5% of the UK population was over 65 years of age, but by 1951 this had increased to 11%; it was 13% in 1981 (Hodkinson 1981) and 17% by 1991. How do we manage the elderly patient with back pain, and what is the role of surgery? Is surgery necessary, and is it appropriate?

IS SURGERY NECESSARY IN THE ELDERLY SPINE?

The prevalence of surgery for four back pain syndromes declines in later years (Fig. 27.1), and one might conclude that spinal surgery is generally unnecessary for the older patient.

One of the reasons for less spinal surgery in the elderly is a falling age-related hospital consultation rate for back pain. The age distribution of patients attending hospital back pain clinics also shows individual syndrome characteristics (Fig. 27.2). Patients with symptomatic lower lumbar disc lesions have a peak prevalence in the fourth decade, instability has the greatest prevalence in the fifth decade, and root entrapment in the sixth. There is a steady decline in attendance for each of these syndromes thereafter. This is still true when the numbers are corrected for the attendance per 100 000 in the population at that age (Fig. 27.3). There are relatively few elderly patients attending with these syndromes. By contrast, neurogenic claudication has its greatest prevalence in the sixth

decade, and does not decline significantly in later life.

General practitioner attendance for all conditions tends to increase steadily with the years, but with back pain there is a declining attendance

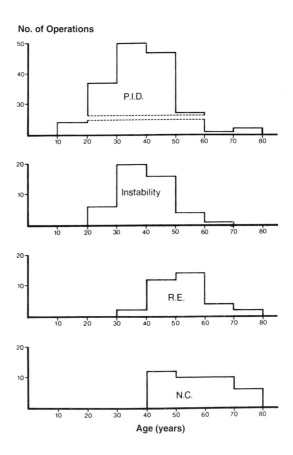

Fig. 27.1 The number of patients requiring surgery in one spinal unit during each decade of life for: disc protrusion (PID), instability, root entrapment for lateral stenosis (RE) and neurogenic claudication (NC).

307

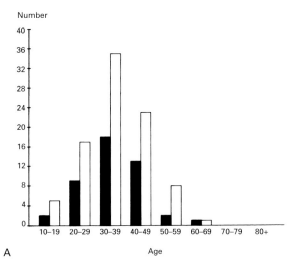

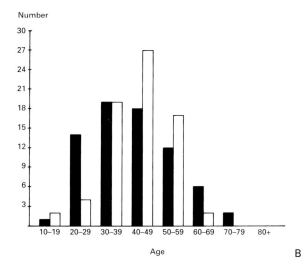

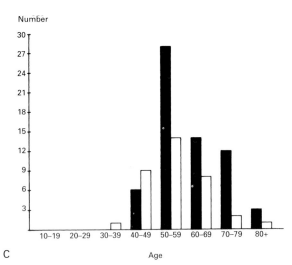

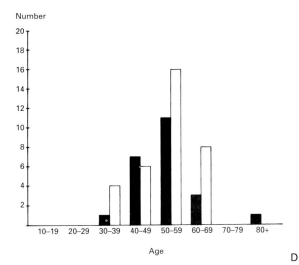

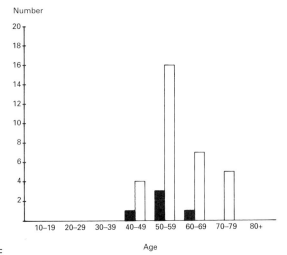

Fig. 27.2 Numbers of patients attending a spinal unit in each decade of life with (**A**) disc protrusion (**B**) instability symptoms, (**C**) degenerative spondylolisthesis, (**D**) root entrapment from lateral canal stenosis, and (**E**) neurogenic claudication. (Black bar = females, white bar = males.)

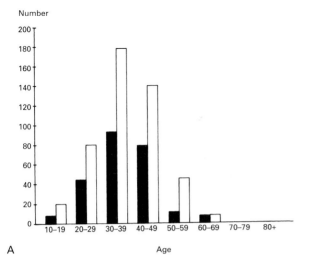

A

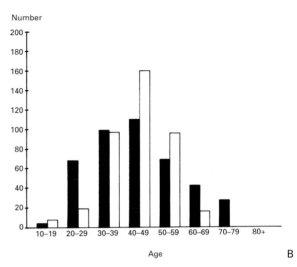

B

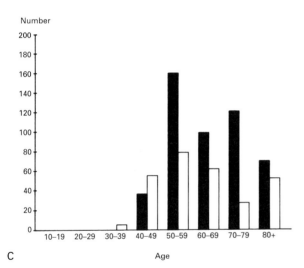

C

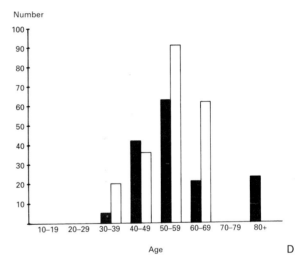

D

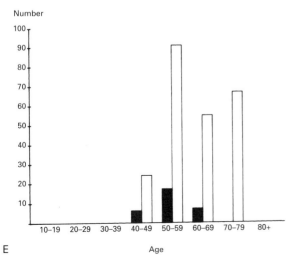

E

Fig. 27.3 Prevalence of attendance at a spinal unit, normalized per 100 000 population for each decade, for patients with (**A**) disc protrusion, (**B**) instability symptoms, (**C**) degenerative spondylolisthesis, (**D**) root entrapment from lateral canal stenosis, and (**E**) neurogenic claudication. (Black bar = females, White bar = males.)

in later life (Badley 1987). In a mechanistic age, we are conditioned to compare the human organism with a machine. Orthopaedic surgeons and bioengineers in particular can be excused for likening the jointed locomotor system to a machine. We then express surprise when human joints and motor car engines respond differently to age. The motor car deteriorates at a linear or even logarithmic rate, with ever-increasing garage repair bills, but the spinal locomotor system follows another course (Fig. 27.4). In the middle years of life it is prone to failure and needs surgical help, but built into the system is a repair and compensation mechanism that protects the elderly from the spinal surgeon. What is this mechanism?

The recovery we observe from each episode of back pain suggests that there is a mechanism of repair, though we do not understand it. We know little of the potential for repair of the annulus. An extruded nucleus can organize with fibrosis. An irritated nerve root in root entrapment syndrome can thicken with perineural fibrosis. Weber has shown that patients who make only a limited recovery after conservative treatment for disc protrusion have surprisingly good function 10 years later (1983). And the natural history for many patients with root entrapment syndromes is for the symptoms to reduce with time (Porter et al 1984). In addition to repair, there is the long-term compensation that assists the elderly.

Reduced demands

A lower prevalence of back pain in later life may in part be due to the reduced demands of the spine. Isometric strength tests suggest that a man without back pain has peak spinal strength between 30 and 40 years of age, declining by 20% at 65 years of age. An elderly spine will have to bear lesser loads and may cope with this when it would have been symptomatic in earlier life. A fusion may therefore be essential for an unstable spondylolisthesis in order to keep a young man at work, but quite unnecessary for a man in retirement.

Reduced expectations

Many elderly patients probably suffer from neurogenic claudication but fail to consult their doctor, accepting a reduced walking distance as the inevitable consequence of advancing years. Even when the diagnosis is confirmed, many refuse to consider surgery and prefer walking restrictions to an operation.

Expectations are also reduced when multiple pathology afflicts the elderly. A young man in good health will rightly expect a discectomy to relieve his root pain and restore function, whilst the elderly with root entrapment may consider this a lesser problem to angina and prostatism.

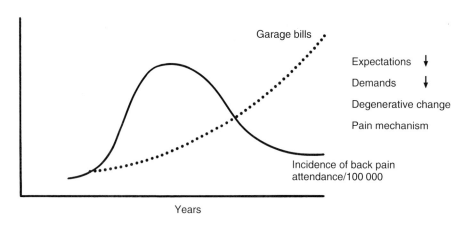

Fig. 27.4 Diagram comparing the requirements for failure of a motor car with those for back pain. Improvement is probably due to decreased expectations, decreased demands, the benefits of degenerative change and repair, and altered pain mechanism in the elderly.

Altered pain mechanism

Diagnosis in the elderly is sometimes made difficult by an altered pain mechanism. According to William Wordsworth, 'He is by nature led to peace so perfect that the young behold with envy, what the Old Man hardly feels'. It might lead to serious consequences in the silent myocardial infarction, the painless perforated duodenal ulcer and unrecognized urinary retention, but in non-life-threatening spinal pathology it can be a bonus.

Reduced spinal motion

The range of lumbar motion in general is reduced by approximately 30% between 20 and 70 years of age (Loebl 1967, Moll & Wright 1971, Fitzgerald et al 1983). This is an advantage in those syndromes where there is a significant dynamic component.

Degenerative change

Traction spurs developing in the vertebral ligaments are a sign of an unstable segment (MacNab 1971), but are equally a feature of attempted repair. For non-degenerative discs the position and length of the centrode during segmental motion is fairly uniform and small but with mild degeneration there is erratic movement of the centrode, and an increase in its length. This is more marked in the mildly degenerate spine, however, than with gross degeneration when the spine regains some stability (Seligman et al 1984). A middle-aged woman may require fusion for an unstable mildly degenerate segment, but given time some natural stabilization can occur with increasing degenerative change (Fig. 27.5).

Changes in the physical–biochemical properties of the disc

The behaviour of the disc is governed to a large extent by the composition and organization of its major macromolecules, collagen and proteoglycan. These change with age. There is a reduction in the proteoglycan concentration, and a corresponding reduction in water content from 90 to 70% which alters the diurnal fluid exchange in

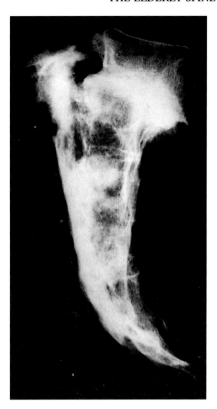

Fig. 27.5 A radiograph of an archaeological spondylolisthesis spontaneously fused at L5/S1.

the disc, its porosity and disc nutrition (Urban 1987). The effect of these changes in disc protrusion is not known, but as the symptoms of herniation are uncommon in the elderly, it can be assumed that they are not disadvantageous. This is good news for the young patient with episodic disc symptoms; because of repair, age-related changes and compensations, many back problems improve with time, and spinal surgery is frequently unnecessary in the elderly spine.

IS SURGERY APPROPRIATE FOR THE ELDERLY SPINE?

Some aspects of spinal assessment are unique for the elderly patient. One is more alert to the possibility of other lesions coexisting with a minor mechanical problem, which may be the main cause of disability (Paget's disease, metastasis, multiple myelomatosis, blood dyscrasia, tuberculosis); non-spinal pathology that causes back pain (aortic aneurysm, carcinoma of the pancreas); and pathology that disturbs walking (cervical stenosis, subacute combined degeneration of the cord, disseminated sclerosis, and arthritis of the hips). Difficulties of communication also increase the risk of making the wrong diagnosis.

With correct diagnosis, however, and exclusion of other pathologies, the spinal surgeon has an advantage when operating on the older patient; with rapid postoperative mobilization that is possible after spinal surgery, the complications are few and the results rewarding.

Root pain

An older patient with root pain is occasionally sufficiently disabled to warrant surgical decompression of the root canal. The symptoms and signs need to be appropriate, degenerative pathology must be identified on CT scan or MR, and perhaps electromyography should show abnormal nerve function. The root is decompressed by hemilaminectomy, following the root into the root canal and undercutting the superior facet. The root may be affected under the cranial lip of the lamina (Crock 1981). Irreversible root damage can be the price of delay. Disc herniation, though unusual, can occur in the elderly (Harada & Nakahara 1989). An elderly patient may present with signs of root entrapment from degenerative change with full straight leg raising, and a buttonholed disc extrusion is a surprise finding.

Sister N, a Catholic nun, was 72 years of age and had suffered intractable root pain in the left buttock, thigh and calf for 2 years. There were no abnormal neurological signs, but a CT scan showed some root canal stenosis, and also pelvic Paget's disease. The root canal was decompressed, and anterior to the root was a button-hole disc extrusion which was excised; 5 years later she still has some root pain, but writes to express her gratitude.

Sometimes the fragment of disc material causing root symptoms in the elderly is composed of avulsed cartilage end-plate in addition to the annulus fibrosus (Harada & Nakahara 1989).

Neurogenic claudication

This is the most common indication for spinal surgery in the elderly. Ami Hood and Weigl (1983) reported pain relief and an improved quality of life in 20 out of 21 central canal decompressions for elderly patients with spinal stenosis. This is a relatively simple procedure with short anaesthesia and few complications.

LT, a peer of the realm and 76 years of age, had back pain and claudication. He had difficulty walking from the upper chamber to his car. The myelogram showed partial occlusion at L4/5. Frustrated with his limitations he had a spinal decompression at L4 and L5 with hemifacetectomy. Not entirely free of pain, but with an improved walking distance, he was delighted to be able to fulfil his role as University Chancellor at the next graduation ceremony.

There are, however, a few pitfalls. Decompression and facetectomy for the osteoporotic patient with a minor compression fracture can have disastrous consequences, with the development of gross kyphosis and paraplegia (Natelson 1986). Epstein et al (1983) recommended decompression for stenotic symptoms in patients with degenerative spondylolisthesis and they were prepared to remove the facet unilaterally, but unless there is already a degree of natural spondylotic interbody fusion, further displacement can occur with subsequent root symptoms. An associated lateral fusion is therefore wise.

Instability

When segmental movement is judged to be causing pain, age is no contraindication to fusion provided the disability is sufficiently great. It is rarely indicated, however, after the seventh decade. Even in the elderly it is worth ensuring that the segment proximal to the proposed fusion is neither pathological nor stenotic.

Mrs AM at 65 years of age had had 10 years of increasing back pain, and eventually found relief lying on the floor. A degenerate unstable L4/5 segment was fused with L5/S1, with almost complete relief of back pain. She was able to lead a very active life for 13 years. She then developed right thigh pain, and at 79 years of age was admitted with reduced right knee reflex and positive femoral stretch test. She had a degenerative retrolisthesis at the segment proximal to the fusion, with encroachment into the right root canal (Fig. 27.6). After 6 weeks rest, the root pain resolved but the reflex did not recover.

Some patients with vertebral metastasis will benefit from surgical stabilization (Galasco 1991).

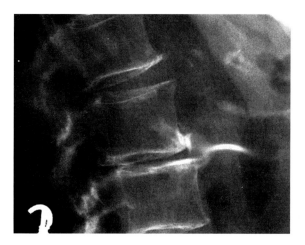

Fig. 27.6 Lateral radiograph of retrolisthesis at L3/4 above an Attenborough fusion. This 79-year-old lady had anterior thigh pain which settled with 6 weeks' rest. The reduced knee reflex failed to recover.

Good results are to be expected from anterior surgery, when vertebral body metastasis has caused wedging and neural deficit. Less successful is posterior decompressive surgery (Onimus et al 1986).

Osteomyelitis

Osteomyelitis may be missed in elderly patients with back pain when they already have degenerative spinal disease. Pyogenic vertebral osteomyelitis is now more common than tuberculous lesions in white people but it is still uncommon, with an incidence of one in 250 000 a year in the UK (Digby & Kersley 1979). Whilst osteomyelitis of the vertebrae in the young is generally due to staphylococci, it is the gram-negative organisms that affect the elderly spine (Silverhorn & Gillespie 1986, Thomson et al 1988). Most proved bacteraemias in elderly patients are caused by gram-negative bacteria, the source being the urinary tract, so the preponderance of these organisms in spinal infection is not surprising. Unfortunately, the diagnosis is commonly delayed, and when vertebral collapse occurs it is often misdiagnosed as carcinoma. If suspected, a needle biopsy is mandatory; the choice of antibiotics depends on culture, and should continue for at least 6 weeks. Prolonged bed rest and immobilization in a cast should be avoided in the elderly. Surgical intervention is necessary with incipient paraplegia in the presence of large abscesses, and when there is a failure of response to antibiotics (Thomson et al 1988).

Osteoporosis

Surgery does little to help the lady with the osteoporotic spine unless it is a bone biopsy because the cause of demineralization is in doubt. On rare occasions, however, impingement of the twelfth rib on the iliac crest can be a troublesome source of back pain. It is difficult to palpate between the rib and the pelvis in the seated patient. The offending rib is tender, and its excision can produce welcome relief (Nordin 1983).

Mrs CJ was 74 years of age and attended with severe left-sided low back pain under the left costal margin, aggravated by movement. She was grossly osteoporotic with a kyphotic lower thoracic spine. The lower ribs impinged on the iliac crest. After the lower left rib had been excised, she asked if the pain had been discovered, and if it had been removed. She was told it had and she remains satisfied.

The indications for spinal surgery in the elderly are relatively few, but with a correct diagnosis and sufficient disability it can give encouraging results and restore an acceptable quality of life.

REFERENCES

Ami Hood S, Weigl K 1983 Lumbar spinal stenosis: surgical intervention for the older person. Israel Journal of Medical Sciences 19: 169–171

Badley E M 1987 Epidemiological aspects of the ageing spine. In: Hukins D W L, Nelson M A (eds) The ageing spine. Manchester University Press, p 13

Crock H V 1981 Normal and pathological anatomy of the lumbar spinal nerve root canals. Journal of Bone and Joint Surgery 63-B: 487–490

Digby J M, Kersley J B 1979 Pyogenic non-tuberculous spinal infection. Journal of Bone and Joint Surgery 61-B: 47–58

Epstein N E, Epstein J A, Caras R, Lavine L S 1983 Degenerative spondylolisthesis with an intact neural arch; a review of 61 cases with analysis of clinical findings and the development of surgical management. Neurosurgery 13: 555–561

Fitzgerald G K, Wynveen K G, Rhealt W, Rothchild B 1983 Objective assessment with establishment of normal values for lumbar spinal range of motion. Physical Therapy 63: 1776–1781

Galasco C S B 1991 Spinal instability secondary to metastatic cancer. Journal of Bone and Joint Surgery 73-B: 104–108

Harada Y, Nakahara S 1989 A pathologic study of lumbar disc herniation in the elderly. Spine 14: 1020–1024

Hodkinson H M 1981 An outline of geriatrics. Academic Press, London

Loebl W Y 1967 Measurement of spinal posture and range of spinal movement. Annals of Physical Medicine 9: 103–110

Macnab I 1971 The traction spur. Journal of Bone and Joint Surgery 53-A: 663–670

Moll J M H, Wright V 1971 Normal range of spinal mobility: an objective clinical study. Annals of Rheumatology 30: 381–386

Natelson S E 1986 The injudicious laminectomy. Spine 11: 966–969

Nordin B E C 1983 Osteoporosis. In: Wright V (ed) Bone and joint disease in the elderly. Churchill Livingstone, Edinburgh, p 167–180

Onimus M, Schraub S, Bertin D, Bosset J F, Guidet M 1986 Surgical treatment of vertebral metastasis. Spine 11: 883–891

Porter R W, Hibbert C, Evans C 1984 The natural history of root entrapment syndrome. Spine 9: 418–421

Seligman J V, Gertzbein S D, Tile M, Kapasouri A 1984 Computer analysis of spinal segment motion in degenerate disc disease with and without axial loading. Spine 9: 566–573

Silverhorn K G, Gillespie W J 1986 Pyogenic osteomyelitis: a review of 61 cases. New Zealand Medical Journal 99: 62–65

Thomson D, Bannister P, Murphy P 1988 Vertebral osteomyelitis in the elderly. British Medical Journal 296: 1309–1311

Urban J P G 1987 Physical chemistry of the disc. In: Hukins D W L, Nelson M A (eds) The Ageing Spine. Manchester University Press, p 135–143

Weber H 1983 Lumbar disc herniation: a controlled prospective study with ten years of observation. Spine 8: 131–140

The 'problem back' patient

28. Repeat spinal surgery

The failures of previous spinal surgery are amongst the most disabled of back sufferers (O'Brien 1983). Our natural response is to consider helping them with a further operation, but if the results of spinal surgery are uncertain, repeat surgery is much more unpredictable. The most recalcitrant pain problem is that associated with the multiply operated back. Further surgery should be approached with caution, not because the surgery is technically difficult. Our problems are with patient selection. When we are approached by a patient asking about the value of a further spinal operation, there are several possibilities to consider:

1. Was the first operation a failure because of a wrong diagnosis?
2. Was the first operation a failure because the diagnosis was correct but the operation was wrong?
3. Was the first operation a failure because, even though the diagnosis of the organic problem and the operation were correct, the patient assessment was inadequate?
4. Was the operation successful, but secondary pathology has developed producing a new genuine organic problem for which a new surgical remedy is worth considering?
5. Was the operation successful, but a new largely non-organic element has developed causing considerable distress to the patient?

In order to resolve the problem, the patient needs a great deal of our time. The correct decisions are most likely to be made by a multidisciplinary team approach. Where do we start? An accurate past history is essential, relying not upon the patient's memory alone, but upon all the available records from previous hospitals and from general practitioner notes. The memory can be clouded by grievances about litigation. The history prior to an accident is forgotten and previous operative failure confuses the record. Waddell et al (1979) showed that compensation has a significant negative influence on the results of surgery for lumbar disc disease. In a study of Philadelphia firemen having surgery for a herniated lumbar disc, only one in 13 had returned to work after 1 year (Menkowitz & Wittaker 1975).

An estimate of the severity of the present problem is measured not only by listening to the patient but by interviewing the spouse and talking to the general practitioner. An objective measure of the abnormal signs may need to be documented longitudinally. Hospital admission makes this possible, when the patient's activity and behaviour can be assessed by the physiotherapist, and drug requirements monitored by the nurses.

The length of the pain-free interval after the previous surgery is significant (Boden & Wiesel 1992). For example, if the preoperative leg pain was still present after surgery, then it is likely that the root was not decompressed. If, on the other hand, there was a 6-month pain-free interval, then there may be a disc recurrence at the same or a different level. A gradual recurrence within 6 months might suggest epidural fibrosis.

A detailed psychological assessment is essential. An abnormal profile on the Minnesota Multiphasic Personality Inventory (MMPI) does not mean that repeat surgery will fail, but it directs the surgeon to factors other than the spine that may be responsible for back pain. There is no clear evidence that the MMPI low back scale will differentiate between patients who will have a poor, fair or good outcome from spinal fusion (Wilfling et al 1973). Neither does it appear to help to differentiate the non-organic from the organic back pain patients (Tsushima & Towne 1979). Patients with a high hypochondriasis score generally have a poor outcome to treatment, but this is only one of many factors to be considered when contemplating repeat surgery.

Few surgeons relish re-exploration without hard clinical and radiological evidence of treatable symptomatic pathology. No investigation should be ignored that might help to determine the pain source and repeat radiculography, discography, MR or CT scan will be necessary. There is no place for an exploratory operation.

CT and MR provide unique evidence about the extent of previous surgery and demonstrate the shape and size of the vertebral canal. Epidural fibrosis is seen in 75% of postoperative studies (Teplick & Haskin 1983), but without gadolinium enhancement it is not easy to differentiate this condition from overlooked previous disc material. In distinguishing recurrent disc herniation from epidural scar, MRI has a 100% sensitivity, 71% specificity and 89% accuracy (Bundschul et al 1988, Hueftle et al 1988). However X-rays are not very good to identify whether a fusion is sound (Brodsky et al 1991). The place for fusion in the multiply operated back patient is based more on personal judgement than upon objective criteria.

Only when all the available evidence is assembled will a conference between the many disciplines produce the best decision. In practice, this time-consuming, laborious approach to repeat surgery is rarely followed outside a few centres of excellence, but the failures that accompany hastily conceived operations, the time involved in attempting to repair the results of failures and the distress caused to the patient, should make us pause before we recommend repeat spinal surgery. After two operations the patient is more likely to be made worse than better by further surgery. Rather than operate in desperation, we do well to recall the inverted proverb 'if at first you don't succeed, give up'.

CAUSES OF FAILED SURGERY

Wrong diagnosis

Case report — a tumour
Mrs JM, a 53-year-old housewife, had severe constant burning pain in the left leg from the buttock into the posterior thigh, behind the knee to the calf and ankle. It kept her awake at night and drove her husband and the local doctor to despair. She had treatment for a root entrapment syndrome, first with epidural injections and eventually a decompression of the left L5 root canal, where degenerative change had been encroaching from the apophyseal joints. The operation had relieved symptoms for a short time. Whilst in the hospital, the nurses had observed that she was fairly comfortable until her husband arrived to visit her, and then she requested analgesics. She was referred to a pain clinic, and several pain-relieving techniques were offered to her, but she was no better. On reviewing the details of the first operation, she had only had a CT scan at L4 and L5. Further imaging demonstrated a large neurofibroma at the level of L3. It was removed and she lost her pain.

Wrong operation

Surgery may fail because the diagnosis is right but the operation incorrect. Imaging may have identified a disc protrusion but the wrong level was approached. At times the wrong side is explored when a preoperative skin mark would have prevented the mistake.

A disc protrusion may have been correctly diagnosed in the older patient and excised with poor results because stenosis and/or instability were not recognized as associated factors.

Case report — unrecognized stenosis
Mr JK, a 47-year-old lorry driver, attended with pain in his back and root pain down to the left foot. Three years ago he had a disc removed without much success. The previous hospital notes suggested that he had had surgery for pain in the back and left thigh. Straight leg raising had been 80/80 and there were no abnormal neurological signs. The lateral view of a radiculogram had shown a disc protrusion at L4/5 but there was not cut-off of the nerve root dural sheath. The disc protrusion had been excised, but with no relief of symptoms. Once on his feet, his pain recurred.

A new radiograph showed further narrowing at the L4/5 disc space. Posterior indentation of the dural column remained on the radiculogram much as three years before, and a CT scan identified a very shallow vertebral canal at L5 with overhanging facets. Originally he had certainly had symptoms related to a disc protrusion but with associated lateral canal stenosis. We would not expect such a combination of factors to be helped by removing the disc protrusion alone. A lateral canal decompression would have had more chance of success, possibly without incising the annulus of the disc.

Operative risk demands informed consent, so that the patient understands that even in the best hands there is a risk to nerve root and dura, and possible infection. Damage to a major vessel is a failure of technique.

Inadequate patient assessment

Inadequate patient assessment combined with over-diagnosis and over-confidence will inevitably lead to failed surgery (Dhar & Porter 1992).

Case report — symptoms mainly due to distress
Mr PT said he first hurt his back lifting at work, quickly developed pain down the right leg, and was admitted for bed rest. He failed to respond and was given a jacket, which he found uncomfortable. The surgeon was reluctant to operate because although the symptoms remained, there were some signs of exaggeration. A neurologist confirmed the opinion that the symptoms were not all related to an organic problem, but the patient found his way to another surgeon who performed a CT scan. It demonstrated a small disc protrusion at the L4/5 level. This was removed through a fenestration, but the patient was no better. He says he is in constant pain; he walks with a stick and is seeking recompense for a disabling industrial accident.

Recurrence of back pain after successful surgery

Iatrogenic

Case report — iatrogenic disc degeneration and root entrapment
Mrs FW had an L4/5 disc sequestration removed through a fenestration at 32 years of age and had 12 good years without any back symptoms. She then presented with left L5 root pain from the buttock and thigh to the calf, with pins and needles in the big toe. It was fairly constant, worse when sitting for long and walking far. Straight leg raising was 90/80 and there were no abnormal neurological signs. She had some reduction of the L4/5 disc space with osteophyte formation of the vertebral margins. She was given two epidural injections which provided only temporary relief, and because of continuing pain over an 18-

month period she requested further surgery. A CT scan confirmed a shallow central canal at L5, trefoil in shape with lateral canal stenosis. At operation, there was a posterior vertebral bar on the lower border of L4 and upper border of L5 with a tough ridged annulus, to which the thickened L5 root was closely apposed. Half the laminae of L5 and L4 were removed, undercutting the superior facet at L5 and decompressing the shallow trefoil canal, following the L5 root well into the root canal. There was a slow improvement with reduction in the degree of root pain over 12 months, but she still admits to some intermittent root pain.

A further disc fragment

Case report — a further disc fragment
Mrs GE at 34 years of age had several pieces of disc material removed which had extruded deep to the posterior longitudinal ligament at L5/S1 on the left. The surgery had relieved L5 root symptoms, straight leg raising had been 70/40 and she had quickly returned to a normal active pain-free life. Two years later she developed pain in the opposite thigh which spread to the calf. It varied in severity, sometimes putting her to bed for days at a time. Two epidural injections gave temporary relief but she began taking large doses of analgesics and tranquillizers. She listed to the left, was a little tender at L5, had straight leg raising of 70/90, and a CT scan showed an overhanging superior facet at S1 on the right with probable disc material anterior to the L5 root (Fig. 28.1). The root was decompressed surgically by undercutting the facet and after incising the annulus anterior to the root, a large sequestrated piece of disc material was removed. This was either symptomless from the first operation or was 'fresh herniation' of nucleus.

The recurrence of disc herniation after initial successful disc surgery varies from 3 to 15% (White 1984, Hanley & Shapiro 1989), and the sciatica is not uncommonly on the other side. Further surgery for these patients is usually successful (Frymoyer et al 1978).

Postoperative arachnoiditis

The cause of failed spinal surgery when a patient has continuing back pain and discomfort in the legs for no apparent cause is often attributed to 'arachnoiditis' — an inflammatory subdural process leading to fibrosis, which binds together the roots of the cauda equina. It is probably over-diagnosed. A repeat MR, CT or myelogram may show concentric narrowing of the terminal theca

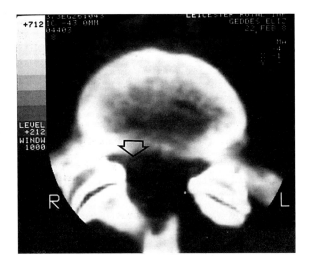

Fig. 28.1 CT scan showing a large right-sided disc protrusion, with an overhanging superior facet compromising the L5 root.

with occlusion of the root sheaths and tapering of the metrizamide column (Fig. 28.2), and the term 'arachnoiditis' becomes a convenient diagnosis. It can be generalized or localized to one root (Wilkinson 1979). Repeat imaging on symptomless postoperative patients shows that these radiological appearances are often the inevitable consequence of surgery for many healthy patients, and generally they are the result of extradural scarring and not subdural arachnoiditis.

The appearance of arachnoiditis at operation, however, is not in question. The dura appears white instead of blue, it is opaque rather than translucent, and its contents firm and resistant to pressure. A small incision into the dura will fail to produce a bead of cerebrospinal fluid, but rather the dura and underlying arachnoid are adherent in a mass of fibrous tissue. A subdural fibrinous exudate has formed similar to the fibrous adhesions which develop in the peritoneum. It covers the nerve roots. Proliferating fibrocytes then form dense collagen adhesions.

Arachnoiditis produces aching and burning pain in the lower back, buttocks and perineum. Pain in a root distribution, although it may co-exist, is probably from other causes. Extradural scarring often accompanies arachnoiditis, which will limit the normal excursion of the nerve roots. Associated bony or soft tissue encroachment into

the root canal adds to the problem and produces root symptoms. MR is the imaging of choice, showing peripheral, eccentric or damaged roots (Delmarter et al 1990).

Historically, a major cause of arachnoiditis was oil-based myelography, and the material was often aspirated after injection to prevent this complication. Current causes are surgical trauma, infection (bacteriological, viral or fungal), foreign material, intrathecal haemorrhage, intrathecal steroid or anaesthetic agents (Burton 1978, Quiles et al 1978).

Postoperative extradural fibrosis

Fibrosis can densely surround or indent the dura, sometimes extending to the exit foramen. It can be distinguished from extruded disc material by gadolinium-enhanced CT or MR. Altered tissue density by gadolinium enhancement will also distinguish extradural scarring, with its stenosing effects on the roots, from arachnoiditis, in which the roots are dispersed in intradural fibrosis.

Such scarring can result from organized postoperative haematoma, from infection, from swab debris or from an iatrogenic leak of cerebrospinal

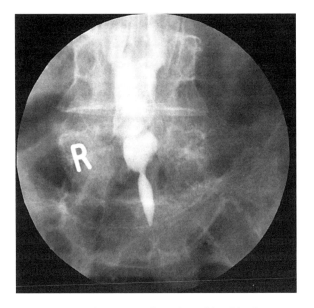

Fig. 28.2 A radiculogram of a patient with epidural scarring. There is some oil-based metrizamide from a previous myelogram, and probably some arachnoiditis.

fluid, especially if there was a postoperative fistula (Kitchel et al 1989). Fibrinolysis will generally prevent the deposition of extradural scar tissue, but the mechanism can vary in efficiency and may at times be defective (Poutain et al 1987, Zebonni et al 1990). Disc protrusion may be a cause of some perineural scarring, but surgeons do not encounter dense extradural scarring in a virgin spine; it is usually the result of some invasive procedure. Physical activity increases fibrinolytic activity (Deoijoward et al 1990), but when activity-induced fibrinolytic activity has a half-life of only about 5 min, the therapeutic benefits of exercise can be questioned.

Extradural fibrosis can be reduced by the application of a fat graft over the dura at the time of operation. This is probably unnecessary if only a small area of dura is exposed, such as when removing a disc protrusion through a fenestration, but with a larger area of decompression it is worth applying a prophylactic fat graft. The graft can be obtained from the subcutaneous tissues at the site of incision in women, but a separate buttock incision may be necessary for donor fat in the less obese male.

The principles of skin grafting apply to fat grafts. Vascularization depends on peripheral ingrowth of vessels and firm apposition to the recipient bed. A large volume of fat with small surface area is less likely to survive than a smaller volume with larger surface area. Thin postage stamp-size grafts of 5 mm thickness are probably ideal. If the graft is floating in haematoma it is less likely to vascularize than a graft seated between the dry dura and paraspinal muscles. A loose deep muscle suture helps to reduce the dead space, and good haemostasis and vacuum drainage reduce the possibility of haematoma. Several patients have developed a cauda equina syndrome from the compressive effect of a fat graft and it should not be inserted within the proximal vertebral canal (Stromqvist et al 1991).

Extradural scarring should not preclude further operation when attempting to treat the post-laminectomy back pain, but excision of scar should be combined with other procedures. If restriction of space within the vertebral canal is an associated factor, then good results can be expected from decompression if it is sufficiently radical (Parke et al 1981). If, however, the symptoms are related to instability, decompression can only compound the problem. O'Brien (1983) has some success from combined anterior and posterior fusion for selected post-laminectomy back pain patients, suggesting that for some, instability is a significant factor.

Late distress

Case report — claudication or distress?
Mr HW, now 62 years of age, can walk only 200 yards before he stops with tired legs. Twenty years ago he had a disc removed, and worked consistently at a light job until 5 years ago. He became unemployed and his legs started to ache at that time. Does he have neurogenic claudication requiring canal decompression?

He complains not only of the legs and back, but of the thoracic spine and anginal pain. Previous depressive illness has made him seek psychiatric help. He exhibits several inappropriate clinical signs, has good peripheral pulses, and a CT, although suggesting some epidural scarring, confirms an adequate canal above L5. There is so much evidence of distress that, although there may well be an organic element to his back symptoms, further spinal surgery is likely only to add to them.

Repeat spinal surgery can be rewarding, but should be approached with great care. There are too many patients who have followed a disastrous trail — first a disc operation, then dissection of adhesions, a spinal fusion, followed by further rhizolysis or correction of a failed fusion, and then a decompression, even rhizotomy, or spinothalamic tractotomy. Before embarking on any spinal operation, we would do well to consider whether every reasonable conservative approach has been tried. Unsatisfactory surgical procedures produce far greater degrees of disability than does the unoperated lumbar spine.

REFERENCES

Boden S D, Wiesel S W 1992 The multiple operated low back patient. In: Rothman, Simeone (eds) The spine. WB Saunders, p 1899–1905

Brodsky A E, Kovalsky E S, Khalil M A 1991 Correlation of radiologic assessment of lumbar spine fusions with surgical exploration. Spine 16: 261–265

Bundschul C V, Modic M T, Ross J S 1988 Epidural fibrosis and recurrent disc herniations in the lumbar spine: MR imaging assessment. American Journal of Radiology 150: 923–932

Burton C V 1978 Lumbosacral arachnoiditis. Spine 3: 24–30

Delmarter R B, Ross J S, Marsaryk T J, Modic M T, Bohlman H H 1990 Diagnosis of lumbar arachnoiditis by magnetic resonance imaging. Spine 15: 304–310

Deoijoward G, de Boer A, Turion P N C, Kluft C, Cohen A F, Breimer D D 1990 Physical exercise induces enhancement of plasma U-PA. Fibrinolysis 4 (Suppl 3): 131

Dhar S, Porter R W 1992 Failed lumbar spinal surgery. International Orthopedics 16: 152–156

Frymoyer J W, Matter R W, Hanley E N, Kuhlmann D, Howe J 1978 Failed lumbar disc surgery requiring second operation: a long term follow-up study. Spine 3: 7–11

Hanley E N, Shapiro D E 1989 The development of low-back pain after excision of a lumbar disc. Journal of Bone and Joint Surgery 71-A: 719–721

Hueftle M G, Modic M J, Ross J S 1988 Lumbar spine: post operative MR imaging with Gd-DTPA. Radiology 167: 817–824

Kitchel S H, Eismont F J, Green B A 1989 Closed subarachnoid drainage for management of cerebrospinal fluid leakage after an operation on the spine. Journal of Bone and Joint Surgery 71-A: 984–987

Menkowitz E, Wittaker R 1975 Spine 2: 503

O'Brien J P 1983 The role of fusion for chronic low back pain. Orthopaedic Clinics of North America 14: 639–647

Parke W W, Gammell K, Rothman R H 1981 Arterial vascularisation of the cauda equina. Journal of Bone and Joint Surgery 63-A: 53–61

Poutain G D, Keegan A L, Jayson M I V 1987 Impaired fibrinolytic activity in defined chronic back pain syndromes. Spine 12: 83–86

Quiles M, Marchisella P T, Tsairis P 1978 Lumbar adhesive arachnoiditis: etiologic and pathologic aspects. Spine 3: 45–50

Stromqvist B, Jonsson B, Annertz M, Holtar S 1991 Cauda equina syndrome caused by migration of fat grafts after lumbar spinal decompression. Spine 16: 100–101

Teplick J G, Haskin M E 1983 CT of the post-operative lumbar spine. Radiological Clinics of North America 21: 395–420

Tsushima W T, Towne W S 1979 Clinical limitations of the low back scale. Journal of Clinical Psychology 35: 306–308

Waddell G, Kummel E G, Lotto W N, Graham J D, Hall H, McCulloch J A 1979 Failed lumbar disc surgery and repeat surgery following industrial injuries. Journal of Bone and Joint Surgery 61-A: 201–207

White A A 1984 Overview of and clinical perspective on low back pain syndrome. In: Gonant H K (ed) Spine update. Radiology Research and Education Foundation, San Francisco, p 127–130

Wilfling F J, Klonoff H, Kokan P 1973 Psychological, demographic and orthopaedic factors associated with prediction of outcome of spinal fusion. Clinical Orthopaedics and Related Research 90: 153–160

Wilkinson H A, Schuman N 1979 Results of surgical lysis of lumbar adhesive arachnoiditis. Neurosurgery 4: 401–409

Zebonni L M P, Heillwell P S, Davies A, Wright V 1990 Defective fibrinolytic activity in chronic low back pain: causal effect. British Journal of Rheumatology 24 (Suppl 2): 68

29. Back pain — an exhibition of distress

We have previously discussed ways of recognizing patients whose behaviour appears to be disproportionate to the organic spinal problem (page 96). The clinician begins to recognize these patients intuitively though Waddell and colleagues (1980, 1984) have encouraged a more systematic documentation of those spinal symptoms and signs that suggest exaggeration.

AETIOLOGY

For the majority of patients, exaggeration is an unconscious response to one of several motivating causes. Fear of cancer, fear of a crippling illness, or fear of paralysis may initiate a psychoneurological process that results in exaggeration. The same process may develop from a desire to gain, whether it be financially by litigation, socially by not having to continue in an unpleasant occupation, or domestically by receiving the sympathy of family and friends. Other emotions may trigger the same response. Aggression and a desire for vengeance on the employer, the medical profession, or the spouse may stimulate the same exaggeration.

There is some evidence that this exaggerated reaction to a relatively less significant organic spinal problem is constitutionally or environmentally predetermined from an early age, though a life-changing event may be the precipitating cause of symptoms (Leavitt et al 1979, Higgs 1984). Early work on the tourniquet test suggested that people differ in terms of their pain threshold. Letham and associates (1983) have shown that individuals in early adult life tend to react in a consistent way to any external pain source, some making much of it and others little. Psychological studies of patients with chronic back pain show that some subjects with low extraversion, high neuroticism and high somatization suffer greatly (Hanvik 1966, Sternback et al 1973, Maruta et al 1976). This suggests that personality may influence the way in which a patient will respond to a mechanical disturbance of the spine. How much of this is genetically determined, and how much related to environment has yet to be resolved.

Patients attending a general practitioner with back pain are no more likely to have psychological or psychiatric problems than other patients (Gilchrist 1983), but when assessing the relatively few patients with chronic back pain, there does seem to be a high proportion with psychological and psychiatric disturbance (Lloyd et al 1979). Psychosocial problems can prolong the course of physical illness and lead to chronic invalidism. Alcohol abuse can be a hidden problem, its onset generally preceding the chronic back pain (Atkinson et al 1991).

The clinician who is first consulted about back pain bears a great responsibility for the subsequent behaviour of the patient. If he fails to recognize the potential for abnormal pain behaviour, he may unwittingly enhance fears by over-investigation, unnecessary treatment and advising prolonged rest, when confident encouragement to graduated increasing activity may be in the patient's interest.

We are still appallingly ignorant about abnormal illness behaviour. We can recognize it, and postulate about causative mechanisms, but still do not understand the neurological and physiological factors responsible. It is not surprising that our attempts to modify it usually fail (McCreary et al 1979).

RECOGNITION OF DISTRESS

One of the benefits of clinical maturity is a growing ability to recognize the patient whose distress outweighs the recognizable organic pathology. One is constantly alert for mistakes and the possibility of overlooking a treatable lesion, but intuitively it becomes possible to recognize those patients with an exaggerated response (Fig. 29.1). Their facial expression and the adjectives they use for pain suggest distress.

We recognize psychological disturbances in the unco-operative, noisy, weepy, agitated patient, but these are often hidden in the quiet and uncomplaining (Nabarro 1984). Ransford et al (1976) have popularized the use of 'pain drawings'

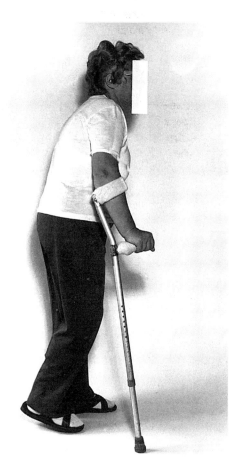

Fig. 29.1 A patient complaining of back pain, walking with two elbow crutches. She either has a serious neurological problem or is exhibiting signs of distress.

which can be assessed at a glance, avoiding the need for a complicated scoring system. A disability score can be obtained at the initial consultation and used to measure the effects of rehabilitation (Deyo & Diehl 1983, Fairbank et al 1980, Lehmann 1983, Roland & Morris 1983, Saunders 1985, Pynsent & Fairbank 1989, Greenough & Fraser 1992). Pain drawings provide a baseline for comparison with time, but in practice do not help distinguish the organic component of disability from that perceived by the patient. This distinction must be made on clinical grounds. Main and colleagues (1992) suggest a structured screening assessment for use as a first-stage procedure in a problem back clinic.

Clinical signs which are suggestive of abnormal pain behaviour are:

- Use of a stick, crutches, wheelchair
- Wearing of a collar and a corset
- Slow movements
- Staggering movements, though never falling
- Needing help to dress and undress
- Grasping movements
- Keeping the eyes closed during physical examination
- Low back pain to axial loading
- Low back pain to simulated rotation
- Excessive tenderness of the skin
- Tenderness over the sacrum, sacroiliac joints and coccyx
- Resisted straight leg raising
- Non-dermatomal sensory loss
- Inappropriate motor weakness

A few of these signs are quite compatible with a normal response to pain, but when many are present, the patient is exhibiting abnormal behaviour. It is not the recognition of abnormal behaviour, but its modification which is difficult.

WHAT IDENTIFIES THE MALINGERER?

Exaggeration may, of course, be a deliberate attempt to deceive, but this probably represents only a small proportion of exaggerating patients. How can we identify the patient who complains of back pain and disability, but is consciously deceiving us? It is naive to suggest these patients do not exist. The monetary gain provided by government to compensate for illness and injury is too tempting for some in society. The bonus of avoiding unpleasant work and difficult social interactions with workmates, plus financial gain, may at times result in a conscious decision to deceive. Such a malingerer may appear outwardly to be the same as the psychologically disturbed distressed patient. They both have sticks or crutches, request help getting dressed and undressed, move slowly, overreact, and have inappropriate physical signs.

Consistency of behaviour is important. It is not an absolute criteria, but when a patient can be shown to be inconsistent in behaviour, this is strongly suggestive of malingering. By contrast, the patient with consistent inappropriate signs is probably not aware of any attempt to deceive.

Mrs JR was a club hostess, and slipped at work twisting her ankle. She took to her bed a week later with pain in her back, and has not worked now for 2 years. If she could prove that her back pain prevents her from working, and that the fall was responsible, she would still receive her old salary and need never work again.

She preferred to stand in the consulting room and would not sit down. She needed help getting undressed. She had no active movement of the spine. There were many inappropriate physical signs.

Some weeks later an investigator provided video evidence that she hurried out to her car, drove to the supermarket and returned to unload several bags of shopping from the boot of the car, without any apparent disability. In court she needed assistance to reach the witness box. The inconsistency of behaviour in the consulting room, in the street and in court was proof of conscious deception.

Marked inconsistency during one examination, between examinations, or between examiners suggests deceit, provided the measurements are outside the accepted range of intra- and inter-observer error, and provided the changing signs are not matched by changing symptoms. Inconsistency of isometric and dynamic muscle testing is objective evidence in support of deceit. A dynamometer can provide objective evidence of poor co-operation and amplification of symptoms. There are inconsistencies between isometric and dynamic tests, between trials of the same test, and between the torque in the primary and secondary axes (Spengler 1992).

If malingering is suspected, one should not necessarily exclude a patient from a rehabilitation programme such as the 'School for Bravery'. This can provide a respectable escape route for a confused patient, when fresh discussion about financial gain and the benefits of work by an impartial therapist can be productive.

The doctor providing an opinion for litigation may have to express a view about conscious deceit or unconscious psychological disturbance. For the therapist, however, it matters little whether or not the apparent distress is consciously motivated. Some patients may begin their illness behaviour with conscious deceit, and play-act so long that they truly believe they are ill. The therapist need not be concerned with the question of malingering, and can attempt behavioural modification for these patients whatever their motivation.

MANAGEMENT

We are singularly unsuccessful with invasive approaches to help the patient with abnormal illness behaviour. It is a source of disappointment that we are least able to help those chronically disabled patients with the most intense suffering. We cannot detect much organic pathology (though it does not mean that it is not there), and generally our therapeutic efforts fail to reduce the level of distress. If we try to identify a motivating cause such as fear, attempts to reassure are often unrewarding. It is sometimes suggested that when litigation has been settled and the gainful motive is no longer necessary, symptoms will resolve, but this is rarely true. Although it is essential to be sure that there is no treatable organic problem that has caused exaggerated pain behaviour, negative invasive investigations sometimes actually increase the morbidity (Herkowitz et al 1983). All too often imaging shows no pathology or irrelevant pathology and the procedure increases the anxiety level of the patient. This must be weighed against ignoring a possible spinal tumour.

Some patients with back pain benefit from a team approach (Bartorelli 1983), and probably none more than the distressed patient. A psychiatric and psychological assessment is time-consuming but helpful. It often explains the distress, though cannot change it.

BEHAVIOUR MODIFICATION

For these patients the general medical approach has failed, and the 'Back School' only reminds them of their disability. A pain modification programme, however, does hold out a promise of a cure (Main & Parker 1989). We have had some success using the methods of Bonica and Fordyce (1974) and Roberts and Reinhardt (1980) with the more modern cognitive behavioural approaches (Turk et al 1983). We attempt to modify behaviour in a programme called 'School for Bravery'. When a patient shows gross signs of exaggeration, provided there is no significant organic problem that requires treatment and no psychiatric disorder, they are offered this programme of non-reward for abnormal behaviour. Patients are not excluded if they are seeking compensation. But to enter they must accept the objectives and methods of the programme.

The patient and spouse attend a multidisciplinary conference with their general practitioner, orthopaedic surgeon, pain specialist, psychologist, physiotherapist and pharmacist. This is helpful in excluding any previously unrecognized treatable pathology. If accepted for the programme, they are asked to agree to identify defined objectives, such as withdrawing from all analgesic drugs, removing walking aids, correcting abnormal posture, performing household chores, gardening, improving social contacts, developing hobbies and recreations, even returning to work. The relief or reduction of pain is not included in the objectives. Any financial benefits of illness are frankly discussed, and they are asked to decide on priorities. Is disability and financial support a better bargain than less disability and no financial benefit? Without exception the patient opts for good health.

On the first day the patient lies on the floor, and a video (Begg et al 1990) monitors their struggle to stand upright, their awkward posture and hesitant gait. Over a 3-week period the patient is seen daily as an out-patient in the physiotherapy department. Abnormal behaviour is actively discouraged, and acceptable behaviour com-

mended. The patient is commended for walking without aids and for correct posture, but reprimanded for unacceptable behaviour. Behavioural techniques are employed specifically to eliminate undesirable pain behaviour, and to re-establish more acceptable behaviour relevant to the patient's life. The spouse is asked to take the same attitude at home, being unsympathetic to any pain responses, and a diary for the patient and spouse helps to confirm compliance (Petty & Mastria 1983). The general practitioner likewise refrains from an attitude supporting pain. A cocktail of the patient's analgesic drugs is administered with decreasing concentration until there are no active ingredients at all.

Increasing activity in spite of pain may in fact reduce the level of suffering. β-endorphins and meta-encephalins are released with treadmill exercise (Howlett et al 1984), and by encouraging a more energetic life-style we may increase the release of these endogenous opioid peptides.

After 3 weeks some patients surprise themselves by their achievements, discarding their therapeutic and walking aids and living more purposeful lives (Delargy et al 1986). They review the first video with incredulity (Fig. 29.2). However, not all are successful.

Many behaviour modification programmes have been established in the past two decades (Pither 1989). Most include mobility and fitness training as well as some type of behaviour modification. Some are outpatient and others inpatient programmes. Recently a more psychological focus has become apparent in many behaviour modification programmes. Our own 'School for Bravery' begins as psychological behaviour therapy, to be followed after conversion by a programme of fitness.

WARNING

Inappropriate symptoms and signs are an attempt by the patient to communicate their distress. The organic component of lumbar spine disability may be small or non-existent, and illness behaviour more a failure to cope with the pressures of life and a cry for help. However, the same inappropriate symptoms and signs may be a cry for attention from the patient with serious organic

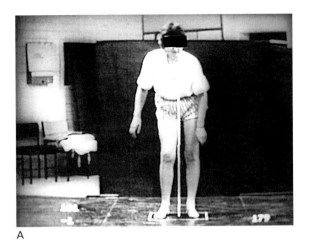
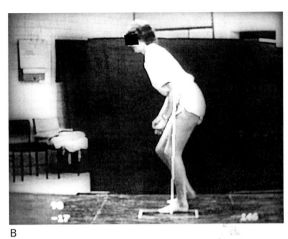
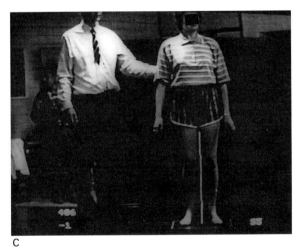
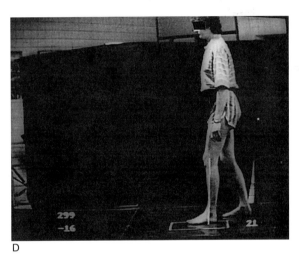

Fig. 29.2   A print from a video of a patient who first had a discectomy, then a fusion and finally an exploration of the fusion. Before the first operation she could not stand upright, and now 4 years later she has the same stooped posture. When viewed on the Aberdeen Video-Vector (Begg et al 1990) from the front (**A**) and from the side (**B**), she had flexed hips and knees. One month after completing a 3-week course in a 'School for Bravery' she maintains an erect posture (**C** and **D**). She stands symmetrically and is developing a normal gait.

pathology in the lumbar spine which he feels is being neglected by disinterested clinicians.

JP was a 41-year-old housewife who was referred to the outpatient clinic by her general practitioner. She had had 5 years of intermittent back pain after a fall down stairs. The whole of the right leg had been numb for 2 weeks. She was distressed and described her symptoms with bizarre adjectives. She had hesitancy passing urine. SLR was 40/60. There were no abnormal motor signs, and reflexes were normal. Axial loading and simulated rotation of the spine were painful. She had pins and needles in both arms. She was thought to have a large non-organic component to her back pain problem, but because of her urinary symptoms and the widespread numbness, she was

admitted. A myelogram showed a complete block at L5/S1 (Fig. 29.3) and a massive sequestrated fragment of disc was excised surgically with complete and dramatic relief of symptoms.

FAM was a labourer, and when 37 years of age he was lifting a sheet of metal and hurt his back. He could not work again, and attended 4 years later for a medical report to support a compensation claim. He had many inappropriate signs. He held himself very stiffly and walked with an awkward gait. He was tender over a wide area of the spine including the sacrum. Straight leg raising was resisted, and he had non-dermatomal sensory loss over various parts of the lower limbs. He was described to the solicitors as having had a mechanical strain to his back, but his disability could

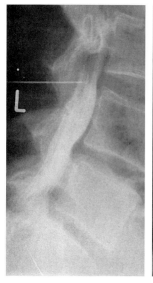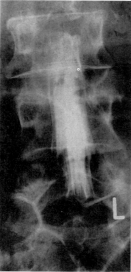

Fig. 29.3 Myelogram showing complete block of the metrizamide column at L5/S1 from a massive disc protrusion. This was excised with good results.

not now be explained in terms of continuing organic pathology. Subsequent reading of the general practitioner's records showed that he had attended with intermittent pain and stiffness in his back for a number of years before his accident, and there was a previous blood test recording an ESR of 44. He was asked to re-attend, and it was noted that his chest expansion was limited. A further ESR was raised, and an X-ray now showed signs of ankylosing spondylitis.

WR, a 65-year-old man, fell 6 feet when some steps on which he was standing gave way. He was shaken but after a rest continued working for 10 days. He slowly developed pains in the neck and the middle of his back. He came off work, and claimed compensation. He attended walking with a stick, and said his legs became stiff after walking only short distances. He was taking a lot of analgesics. He wore a corset. Simulated rotation of the spine gave him discomfort. SLR was a little restricted and seemed to be resisted voluntarily. There was stocking–glove sensory loss below the left knee, but no other abnormal neurological signs. There were marked degenerative changes of the lumbar spine, and a provisional diagnosis was made of neurogenic claudication with a litigation problem and a large non-organic component. He was not

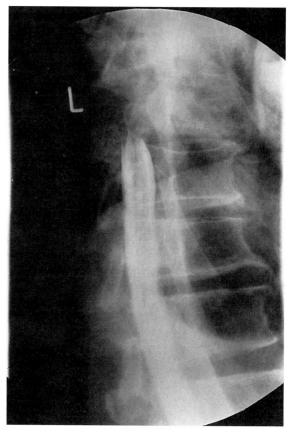

Fig. 29.4 Myelogram showing complete block of metrizamide at D10. Chronic back pain had been associated with degenerative change, but the new lesion was a secondary deposit from a prostatic carcinoma.

investigated further, but returned a month later in a wheelchair. A myelogram showed a block of the metrizamide column at D10 from what proved to be a prostatic metastatic vertebral deposit (Fig. 29.4).

These genuine histories make the clinician constantly afraid of neglecting organic pathology that might be hidden beneath bizarre symptoms and signs. Too much investigation will only perpetuate abnormal pain behaviour, but neglect can sometimes be costly. The reasons for distress may be grounded in serious organic pathology, and good clinical judgement is essential.

REFERENCES

Atkinson J H, Slater M A, Grant I 1991 Prevalence, onset, and risk of psychiatric disorders in men with chronic low back pain: a controlled study. Pain 45: 111–121

Bartorelli D 1983 Low back pain: a team approach. Journal of Neurosurgery 15: 41–44

Begg R K, Wytch R, Major R E 1990 A microcomputer based video-vector system for clinical gait analysis. Journal of Biomedical Engineering 12: 383–388

Bonica J J, Fordyce W E 1974 Operant conditioning for chronic pain. In: Bonica J J et al (eds) Recent advances in pain: pathophysiology and clinical aspects. C C Thomas, Springfield, Illinois

Delargy M A, Peakfield R C, Burk A A 1986 Successful rehabilitation in conversion paralysis. British Medical Journal 292: 1730–1731

Deyo R A, Diehl A K 1983 Measuring physical and psychosocial function in patients with low back pain. Spine 8: 635–642

Fairbank J C T, Davies J, Couper J, O'Brien J P 1980 Oswestry disability questionnaire. Physiotherapy 66: 271–273

Gilchrist J C 1983 Psychological aspects of acute low back pain in general practice. Journal of the Royal College of General Practitioners 33: 417–419

Greenough C G, Fraser R D 1992 Assessment of outcome in patients with low-back pain. Spine 17: 36–41

Hanvik L J 1966 MMPI profiles in patients with low back pain. In: Welsh G S, Dahlstrom W G (eds) Basic readings on the MMPI in psychology and medicine. University of Minnesota Press, Minneapolis

Herkowitz H N, Romeyn R L, Rothman R H 1983 The indications for metrizamide myelography. Journal of Bone and Joint Surgery 65-A: 1144–1149

Higgs R 1984 Life changes. British Medical Journal 288: 1556–1557

Howlett T A, Tomlin S, Nghafoong L, Rees L H, Bullen B A, Skrinar G S, McArthur J W 1984 Release of β endorphin and met-enkephalin during exercise in normal women: response to training. British Medical Journal 288: 1950–1952

Leavitt F, Garron D C, D'Angelo C M and McNeill T W 1979 Low back pain in patients with and without demonstrable organic disease. Pain 6: 191–200

Lehmann T R 1983 A low back rating scale. Spine 8: 308–315

Letham J, Slade, P D, Troup J D G, Bentley G 1983 Outline of a fear–avoidance model of exaggerated pain perception. Behaviour Research Therapy 21: 401–408

Lloyd G G, Wolkin S N, Greenwood R, Harris D J 1979 A psychiatric study of patients with persistent low back pain. Rheumatology and Rehabilitation 18: 30–34

McCreary C, Turner J, Dawson E 1979 The MMPI as a predictor of response to conservative treatment for low back pain. Journal of Clinical Psychology 35: 278–284

Main C J, Parker H 1989 The evaluation and outcome of pain management programmes for chronic low back pain. In: Roland M O, Jenner J R (eds) Back pain: new approaches to rehabilitation and education. Manchester University Press, p 129–156

Main C J, Wood P L R, Hollis S, Sponwich C C, Waddell G 1992 The distress and risk assessment indices. A simple patient classification to identify distress and evaluate the risk of poor outcome. Spine 17: 42–52

Maruta T, Swanson D W, Swenson W M 1976 Pain as a psychiatric symptom: comparison between low back pain and depression. Psychosomatic 17: 123–127

Nabarro J 1984 Unrecognised psychiatric illness in medical patients. British Medical Journal 289: 635–636

Petty N E, Mastria M A 1983 Management of compliance to progressive relaxation and orthopaedic exercises in treatment of chronic back pain. Psychological Reports 52: 35–38

Pither C E 1989 Treatment of persistent pain. British Medical Journal 299: 1239

Pynsent P B, Fairbank J C T 1989 Computer interview system for patients with back pain. Journal of Biomedical Engineering 11: 25–29

Ransford A O, Carins D, Mooney V 1976 The pain drawing as an aid to the psychogenic evaluation of patients with low back pain. Spine 1: 127–134

Roberts A H, Reinhardt L 1980 The behavioral management of chronic pain: long term follow up with comparison groups. Pain 8: 151–162

Roland M O, Morris R 1983 A study of the natural history of back pain. 1. Development of a reliable and sensitive measure of disability in low back pain. Spine 8: 141–144

Saunders S H 1985 Cross validation of the back pain classification scale with chronic intractable pain patients. Pain 22: 271–277

Spengler D M 1992 Newer assessment approaches for the patient with low back pain. In: Rothman, Simeone (eds) The Spine. WB Saunders, Philadelphia, p 1921–1928

Sternback R A, Wolf S R, Murphy R W 1973 Aspects of chronic low back pain. Psychosomatic 18: 52–56

Turk D C, Meichenbaum D, Genes K M 1983 Pain and behavioural medicine: a cognitive behavioural perspective. The Guildford Press, New York

Waddell G, McCulloch J A, Kummell E, Venner R M 1980 Nonorganic physical signs in low back pain. Spine 5: 117–125

Waddell G, Main C T, DiPaola M, Gray I C M 1984 Chronic low back pain, psychological distress and illness behaviour. Spine 9: 209–213

Prevention

30. Prevention of back pain

WHY PREVENTION?

There is no lack of enthusiasm for treating patients with back pain. General practitioners, therapists, rheumatologists and surgeons receive great respect as they diagnose, lay on hands and wield the knife. Only a handful of epidemiologists and basic scientists with limited funds are left to look for the source of the problem, and some of them do not expect to find an answer.

The direction of our research, therapeutic or preventative, will be affected by our concept of the spine's design (Ch. 1). If, for instance, we believe that there is an inherent defect in the design, with vestigial structures being a handicap to the upright posture, we shall reluctantly have to accept a faulty spine as a problem common to the human race. But what if we consider that the design of the spine is good, that its form matches its function? Then back pain is not a consequence of poor adaption to the upright posture and impossible to modify, but it is related more to the life-style of modern man. Prevention then becomes a possibility. There is a source to find and rectify. How can it be done? The following are aspects of prevention of back pain:

- Changing the environment — ergonomics
- Changing the individual — morphology
- Changing attitudes — education
- Deployment of individuals at risk — screening

ERGONOMICS

Ergonomics attempts to match the demands of the work to the ability of the worker by modifying the working environment. Employers, if they would consider it (Nordin et al 1991), and employees, if they knew it, have equal opportunity to ensure a safe working environment. There is broad agreement about what is unsafe for a spine. Posture is important. Lifting is often the final insult with its three variables: the weight of the object, how it is lifted and how often. Avoidance of accidents comes a close third, and vibration is unhealthy for the disc.

Posture

Unacceptably high static spinal loads can develop when standing or sitting for long in the stooped posture, which probably affects disc nutrition and produces spinal muscle fatigue. At such a time the disc is vulnerable to injury from inadvisable lifting or accident. Modification of the working environment to provide a more acceptable working posture should reduce the incidence of back pain.

Attempts have been made to evaluate certain working activities, postures and spinal strength by measuring intradiscal pressure (Nachemson & Elfstrom 1970); intra-abdominal pressure; electromyography (Schultz et al 1982); time spent in the flexed posture by using inclinometers (Burton et al 1989); and computerized models (Fothergill & Grieve 1991). These techniques need further assessment and comparison before they can be meaningfully used in the working environment to measure spinal stress. Changing from the supine to the erect stooped posture increases the intradiscal pressure sixfold (Nachemson & Elfstrom 1970), and patterns of lifting correlate with intra-abdominal pressure (Davis & Stubbs 1976, 1977). By looking critically at working activities and postures that produce these high pressures, these can be modified to generate more acceptable spinal loads.

Lifting

There is obviously a limit to the weight that can be safely lifted, but it is arbitrary. We probably have a built-in warning mechanism about weights that are too heavy, and trouble arises when a load is not properly assessed, and when it is lifted without preparation. The working environment should allow for unacceptable loads to be lifted with assistance from colleagues or by mechanical aids, hoists, barrows and trolleys.

The manner of lifting is important, and if loads must be lifted at a distance from the body either they should be reduced proportionally, or the method of lifting altered (Davis & Stubbs 1977). Lifting can be made acceptable by altering the height and location of the working surface. Wearing suitable clothes for the job is important for the man afraid of getting his clean trousers dirty, or the nurse limited by stooping in a tight skirt. Safety training in industry has for many years emphasized the presumed advantage of lifting with the trunk erect, using the lower limb muscles to reduce the compressive load on the lumbar spine (Troup 1977). There is no doubt that this requires a greater expenditure of energy because there is a vertical displacement of a greater proportion of the body weight when lifting with bent knees. It is, however, thought to be less stressful on the lumbar spine. Leskinen and colleagues (1983) have shown that the benefits of the leg lift are only superior to the back lift provided the weight is kept close to the body, and this is not always possible if the knees are bent. Advocates of kinetic lifting believe there is less spinal stress if the load is first pulled horizontally towards the body before being swung upwards (the load kinetic lift), or if the hips are first moved vertically before the load is lifted from the floor (the trunk kinetic lift), but this has yet to be proved. Perhaps the best advice to protect the lumbar spine is to lift from the bent knee position, having the load as close to the body's centre of gravity as possible, stoop slightly forwards with a lordotic spine and do most of the work with the legs. The initial major work is accomplished by the hip extensors. Watching a weight lifter can be informative (Fig. 30.1).

There is no doubt that a man with a healthy back can do more work and expend less energy by using a back lift with extended legs, but this is not a position to recommend if the spine is weak.

Spinal structures are more subject to injury when fatigued, and the frequency of lifting must be considered in any job. Periods of rest can be productive.

Injury

It is not possible to estimate the importance of 'accidents' at work, because of the tendency to associate a causative episode to the experience of pain. As many as a third of back pain episodes at work are recorded as truly accidental injuries

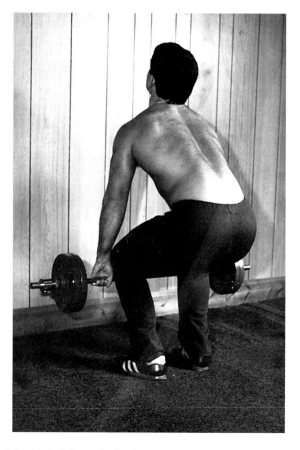

Fig. 30.1 The professional weight-lifter lifts without flexing the lumbar spine.

(Troup 1981). Many patients blame some injury like slipping, stumbling, falling or having something fall on them with subsequent back pain, but the avoidance of accidents should be as much the responsibility of the employee as the employer. Although falls are not the major cause of accidental back pain, they do have a poor prognosis (Manning & Shannon 1979, Troup 1981). Fatigued muscles are less able to protect the spine against potential injury (Parnianpour et al 1988). Respect for the regulations, clean floor surfaces and care in performing the job are as important as adequate lighting, plenty of space and safe machinery. Anticipation is an essential part of avoiding back injury.

Vibration

Epidemiological studies have shown that men working in occupations exposed to vibrations, such as drivers of trucks, tractors and cranes, are at greater risk of back pain complaints than men in other occupations (Weinstein et al 1988). This has been examined in the laboratory, when a disc exposed to vibrations at 5 Hz for 25 min becomes significantly dehydrated. Vibration may cause spasm in the vessels of the vertebral end-plate, affecting disc nutrition (Pope et al 1991). Vibration can be reduced by seat design, which might have some effect in reducing work-related back pain.

Job satisfaction

The Boeing study demonstrated that the strongest predictors for low back pain were job satisfaction and good relationships (Battie et al 1989). Those who most enjoyed their work had lowest reported back pain. When considering absenteeism with back pain, psychosocial factors are more important than load (Magnusson et al 1990).

Some employers concerned about the incidence of back pain amongst their staff are prepared to seek the help of ergonomists. They can identify the areas of high and low incidence of back pain by documentation of every back injury and absenteeism due to back pain, and then study the working activities in the area of high risk. Sophis-

ticated measuring apparatus may help (Otun et al 1984), but this is not always necessary in order to recommend modifications. Advice about working postures, seat design, work surfaces, material handling, design of containers, design of the workplace and reduction of vibration can all help to reduce work-related back pain (Chaffin et al 1991).

There are, however, limitations to the application of ergonomic principles in real life. The mining industry is an example of excellent mechanization on the surface, where in the stock yard, tons of equipment are moved with little or no manual handling. Underground, however, although the backbreaking pick and shovel belong to another era, there are times when heavy machinery must be manipulated into a confined coal face, or repaired when it fails. The fluid nature of the underground strata means constant damage to supports and machinery, which can only be corrected by physical spinal effort (Fig. 30.2).

The nurse is faced with the same dilemma (Scholey 1983). Areas of high and low risk have been identified in hospitals. Orthopaedic and geriatric wards are more hazardous for the nurse's back than surgical wards and outpatient departments (Lloyd et al 1979). The relationship between back pain and patient handling and nurse status is conflicting (Stubbs et al 1983). Nursing administrators aware of the risks are obliged to provide lifting hoists for patients in hospital and at home. The height of beds and nurses uniforms are planned with spinal safety in mind. But in spite of every care and effort to improve the environment, the unexpected can happen; a heavy patient moves awkwardly, the nurse slips, and an injury occurs.

MORPHOLOGY

Changing spinal morphology is at present but a dream, but there are four areas that demand our attention. The disc is the first culprit (Ch. 4), with a quest for environmental factors that affect its nutrition. The pain mechanism is the second (Ch. 5), and here our understanding is still in its infancy. The vertebral canal is the third (Ch. 6), reduced in size largely by early growth disturbance.

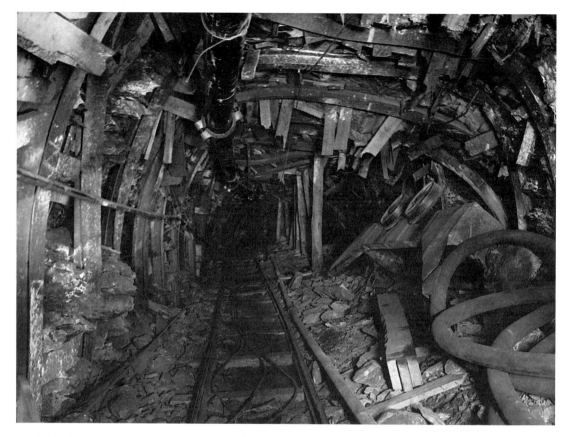

Fig. 30.2   Photograph showing the fluid nature of the geological conditions of a coal mine. Without constant repair, the roadways are crushed.

And fourth is the neuromuscular control of the spine (Ch. 7), partly affected by poor development, and partly by lack of fitness. All of these areas are potentially amenable to prevention, as we seek a healthy spine.

EDUCATION

Education of the young

Every patient with a degenerate spine would choose to turn the clock back and start again, with a knowledge about the limitations of the spine's anatomy and physiology. But it is too late. They regret the abuse of earlier years, and wish someone had told them that there was a correct way to lift, and that the spine has limited strength.

We can only speculate at present whether there would be less back pain if the sufferers had been better informed. We can argue that if a disc is inherently weak, it will prolapse under normal stresses and that education is ineffective. Even if it were of value, information may be quickly forgotten by those for whom back pain is not part of their experience. 'What I hear I forget, what I see I remember, what I do I know.' Education may even be counter-productive. Furthermore, to concentrate on spinal pain in a neurotic society, of which back pain is but one symptom, may only fuel back pain disability.

Others would suggest that all knowledge is valuable, and that with something as important as the human spine it is unreasonable to withhold information about its structure and limited strength. Health education shares knowledge of diet, sex and addiction. Why should a healthy spine be excluded? If it is accepted that knowledge important to our well-being should be shared, then the young deserve 'back education':

1. Teachers of biology have an opportunity to teach spinal structure, function and limitations in their syllabus. The lumbar spine is a prime example of the wedding between structure and function, but compared with other human systems it receives a disproportionately smaller share of study. A healthy theoretical understanding of the spine, reinforced by its rightful place in an examination, may be remembered with benefit in later years (Fig. 30.3).

2. Teachers of physics already teach principles of levers, arches, stress and strain, pressures and osmosis. An application of these to the function of the spine would not only reinforce the physics, but focus on the importance of the spine (Fig. 30.4).

3. We do not truly learn until we apply what we have been taught. As practice produces the musician or sportsman, so only applied instruction can be expected to produce skilled handling and lifting techniques. Teachers of physical education are in a unique position to

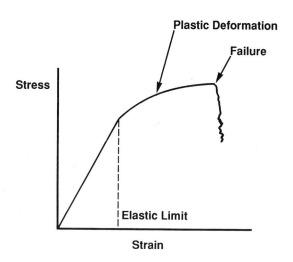

Fig. 30.4 A stress/strain curve demonstrating the pattern of tissue failure.

show and train the young as week by week they reinforce what has been learnt in the classroom, demonstrating and correcting as the children lift and move apparatus about the gymnasium. They can instill a pride of achievement in their charges, that instead of being 'weak' if they cannot move a heavy weight, they are skilled when they learn how to lift.

4. Spinal strength and spinal fitness are part of the health education programme we have so far failed to communicate. Living tissues respond physiologically to stress by increasing their strength, whilst too much stress produces degeneration and injury.

Young spines benefit from mechanical stresses within the physiological range, and provided injury is avoided, sporting activity and supervised weight training must be good for the spine.

At a local level it is possible to arouse enthusiasm amongst teachers for this multidisciplinary approach to back education with seminars for teachers of biology, physics and physical education. There is no evidence that this will affect the incidence of back pain, but it is not unreasonable, and it may offer a way forward to reduce a major sickness problem in our society.

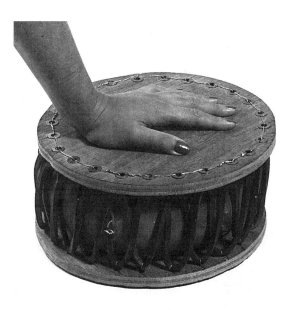

Fig. 30.3 A model of an intervertebral disc constructed from a football bladder laced with rubber strands.

Educating the recruit

The heavy manual worker is 50% more likely to recollect a history of back pain than the sedentary worker, 100% more likely to visit his general practitioner with back pain, and 200% more likely to be off work with back pain. It would seem sensible to offer some teaching programme to recruits entering heavy manual industries, in the hope that they may take reasonable care with their backs. Many industries now give instruction in safe handling techniques, with talks, films and demonstrations reinforced by in-service training. The value of such training programmes is still dubious, and opinions vary about their effects. Probably recruits who have no experience of back pain themselves remember only for a short period information gathered at a 'Back School'. It is the established worker with a personal knowledge of back pain who will continue to apply the principles he has learnt.

Educating the back pain sufferer — the Back School

How can he avoid the next attack? How can he keep at work without repeated periods of absenteeism? It may be done if the patient is fully informed about the types of stress that injure the spine, and is prepared to apply this in day-to-day activities. The hospital-based 'Back School' is a good place for this education.

How to prevent the next attack is the most important advice we can offer. This present attack will generally settle in spite of us, but the next episode depends very much on whether we can generate new attitudes. For this reason clinicians are tending to offer a 'Back School' programme rather than using resources and time on dubious therapeutic methods (Berquist-Ullman & Larson 1977, Williams 1977, Attix & Tate 1979, Fisk et al 1983).

What are the results? Versloot and colleagues (1992) showed that a tailor-made back school was cost-effective, reducing absenteeism by at least 5 days per year per employee. Our own attempts comparing patients who attended the 'Back School' with defaulters, showed in fact that the non-attenders were just as satisfied. They returned to work as quickly and had as little trouble over the subsequent year as the attenders. 'Back School' education, however, does seem to make good sense; it seems to meet the needs of many patients seeking medical help, and it does lower the anxiety level of many bewildered patients who have suffered with back pain for a long time with no-one attempting to explain the problem to them.

Rehabilitation

The natural history of most episodes of back pain encourages physicians to be more active in advocating a patient's return to work. Patients should be convinced that strict bed rest is usually necessary for only a few days after an acute episode, and then a gradual increase in activity helps a functional recovery. Outpatient functional rehabilitation can hasten the return to work after acute pain and restore the confidence of the chronic sufferer (Lindstrom et al 1989, Hazard et al 1989) (Ch. 26). A few patients benefit from residential rehabilitation in their progress to return to work, with the psychological and physical stimulus of competitive group therapy. They should be helped to return to work gradually and gently, preferably to an environment that is kind to the back. Such concepts need the support of social workers, employers and politicians (Nachemson 1983). Alternatively, a long period of enforced rest, with no hope of work ultimately, is counter-productive to restoring a healthy back.

Education of the chronic sufferer

Self-help groups have developed over recent years to support patients and their families with many different medical problems (Gunn 1984). Self-help groups are usually originated by people with some common problem where existing services and facilities are seen as unsatisfactory (Williamson & Danaker 1978), and this is certainly true for some chronic back pain sufferers. There are many such groups now in the United Kingdom with common objectives:

- To provide a venue for back pain sufferers and their families to meet together and improve their understanding of back pain and its management. The meetings are regular, friendly and informal, with a strong medical support but a lay organization. Those who appreciate such a group are often the middle-aged who at least have found others who understand their predicament. Many distressed patients find support from such a group when traditional management has failed. Perhaps they have met for the first time someone else like themselves. Talking out the problem and sharing experiences does not necessarily reduce the pain, but it can reduce the anxiety. One in 10 back pain sufferers offered a self-help group may actually attend (Webb 1982), and two-thirds of the group admit to benefit.

- To promote an understanding of back pain prevention in the local community. The drive of a well organized lay group can alert the community to its responsibility in back care, in industry, education and the wider society. Health education and preventive policies cannot be imposed on a community but they become effective by a one to one contact (Williams 1984). Who better to make that contact at a local level than the informed patient, backed by doctors, physiotherapists and health workers.
- To raise funds for local and national research. The appeal of back pain is less emotive than cancer, the illnesses of children, the elderly and the crippled. Self-help groups recognize the dearth of back pain research.

DEPLOYMENT OF THE INDIVIDUAL AT RISK

Some individuals working in the same environment and subjecting their backs to identical stresses are at greater risk than others of sustaining a back injury. Of coal miners, 20% can work underground lifting excessive loads in unacceptable positions and never experience back pain (Dales et al 1986), yet a colleague may leave the industry after only a few years and become a 'back cripple' for life. What is the difference? There are probably many factors:

The shape and size of the vertebral canal

Our own studies using ultrasound suggest that individuals with small sagittal diameters of the central lumbar vertebral canal are prone to develop low back pain. They are more likely to attend hospital (Porter et al 1980), to be admitted and to have spinal surgery than subjects with deeper canals. The small canal with a trefoil shape is a particularly sinister combination if that canal is compromised by a disc protrusion, by osteophytic degenerative change or by segmental instability. It is necessary to have a relatively inexpensive and non-invasive method of identifying the canal's size and shape, and ultrasound does appear to have the potential needed for screening. Vertebral canal measurement alone, however, is an inefficient method of screening, because so many other factors are related to back pain disability.

Pre-employment strength testing

Chaffin has found a correlation between the ability of a man's back to stand up to the demands of his work, and his strength for the task (Chaffin & Park 1973, Chaffin et al 1978). He has designed apparatus to record dynamic strength testing with initial optimism for pre-employment screening (Troup 1979, Biering-Sorensen 1984). However, men with a pre-existing history of back pain will have reduced muscle strength and will be prone to further back pain; unless recognized in any prospective series, they will invalidate the results. A prospective study of nurses using a Cybex machine showed that strength was a poor predictor of subsequent low back pain (Mostardi et al 1992).

Previous history

The best predictor of back pain is a previous history (Roland et al 1983, Lloyd & Troup 1983, Drinkall et al 1984). A man is at high risk entering a heavy labouring industry with a previous history of back pain, but this is an insensitive measure for young recruits.

The presence of abnormal signs

Lloyd and Troup (1983) recorded that subjects with reduced straight leg raising were more likely to have subsequent absenteeism due to back pain. This reflects a pre-existing spinal pathology, and although a useful observation when recruiting older subjects, it is not particularly helpful when recruiting the young.

Anthropometry

Lawrence (1955) suggested that taller miners were prone to develop back pain, and Kelsey (1975) noted that taller women who had multiple full-term pregnancies were at risk. Merriam et al (1983), in a careful anthropometric study, concluded that the pelvic height was significantly related to the incidence of back pain. A small skull and small biacromial diameter are related to a small vertebral canal (Porter et al 1980). Perhaps these and other body measurements may become useful predictors, but the subject requires further study when other epidemiological data suggest that neither height nor weight are associated risk factors for back pain (Buckle 1983).

The family history

There is circumstantial evidence that the family history is important. There are many families in which each member suffers from disabling back pain, often requiring similar surgical procedures. Twin studies have shown that the high familial relationship of disc pathology is affected more by environmental than genetic factors. It would not be unreasonable to expect inheritance to affect the morphology of the vertebral canal, the resilience of the disc and the tendency to develop degenerative change, but apart from ankylosing spondylitis, there is no proven genetic association with back pain.

Our own studies suggest a strong familial relationship in 50 patients who had disc excision, 48 of their first-degree relatives having significant low back pain. There were only 18 first-degree back-suffering relatives of 50 matched non-back pain control subjects (Porter & Oakshott 1988).

The tendency to develop abnormal pain behaviour

It is possible to identify patients exhibiting abnormal pain behaviour, and these attend their general practitioner with various conditions many times above the average attendance rate. They find their way to many hospital departments. The women visit gynaecologists for a hysterectomy, frequent the dieticians and complain of back pain. They have tomes of medical notes and bulging packets of radiographs. They describe inappropriate symptoms, exhibit inappropriate signs and are resistant to treatment. Their rate of absenteeism from work is high, from all conditions as well as back pain. They feel pain and who can contradict them.

It would be helpful if such individuals could be identified in early adult life to protect themselves from injuries of heavy manual work, their employers from absenteeism and their doctors from offering them harmful investigations and treatment. The imprinting of abnormal pain behaviour will be present in early life (Melzack 1973, Letham et al 1983), but can it be recognized? One may speculate that a good history, a record of school absenteeism and a suitable psychological questionnaire would help.

We are at present only at the earliest stages of identifying risk factors, but we may soon be able to combine several factors and suggest the probability of a young adult eventually suffering from back pain. The ethics of screening are complex, but we accept that a certain acuity of vision is necessary for a pilot, and that a coal face worker requires good hearing. A strong spine is requisite for the manual worker in a stressful environment, to protect him, his family and his employer from the complex physical and social distress of back pain. Where the environment cannot be changed and where education has its limitations, the back pain problem will be reduced if the man is matched to the job. The size of the back pain problem, and our limitations in effectively treating it, make prevention a high priority.

REFERENCES

Attix E A, Tate M A 1979 Low back school: a conservative method for the treatment of low back pain. Journal of the Mississippi State Medical Association 20: 4

Battie M C, Bigos S J, Fisher L D et al 1989 A prospective study of the role of cardiovascular risk factors and fitness in industrial back pain complaints. Spine 14: 141–147

Berquist-Ullman M, Larson U 1977 Acute low back pain in industry: a controlled prospective study with special reference to therapy and compounding factors. Acta Orthopaedica Scandinavica Suppl 170

Biering-Sorensen F 1984 Physical measurements as risk indicators for low back trouble over one year period. Spine 9: 106–119

Buckle P 1983 A multi-disciplinary investigation of factors associated with low back pain. PhD thesis, Cranfield Institute of Technology, Bedfordshire

Burton A K, Tillotson K M, Troup J D G 1989 Variation in lumbar sagittal mobility with low-back trouble. Spine 14: 584–590

Chaffin D B, Park K S 1973 A longitudinal study of low back pain as associated with occupation weight lifting factors. American Industrial Hygiene Association Journal 34: 513–525

Chaffin D B, Herrin G D, Keyserling W M 1978 Pre-employment strength testing: an updated position. Journal of Occupational Medicine 20: 403

Chaffin D B, Pope M A, Andersson G B J 1991 In: Pope M A, Andersson G B J, Frymoyer J W, Chaffin D B (eds) Occupational low back pain. Mosby Year Book, St Louis, p 251

Dales J L, MacDonald E B, Porter R W 1986 Back pain; the risk factors and its prediction in work people. Clinical Biomechanics 1: 216–221

Davis P R, Stubbs D A 1976 A method of establishing safe handling forces in working situations. Symposium on safety in manual materials handling at Suny, Buffalo, organised by National Institute of Occupational Safety and Health

Davis P R, Stubbs D 1977 Radio pills: their use in monitoring back stress. Journal of Medical Engineering and Technology 1: 209–212

Drinkall J N, Porter R W, Hibbert C S, Evans C 1984 The value of ultrasonic measurement of the spinal canal diameter in general practice. British Medical Journal 288: 121–122

Fisk J R, DiMonte P, Courington S McK 1983 Back schools: past, present and future. Clinical Orthopaedics and Related Research 179: 18–23

Fothergill D M, Grieve W D 1991 Human strength capabilities during one-handed maximum voluntary exertions in the fore and aft planes. Ergonomics 34: 563–573

Gunn A D G 1984 Self help. British Medical Journal 288: 1024–1025

Hazard R G, Fenwick J W, Kalisch S M, Redmond J, Reeves V, Reid S, Frymoyer J W 1989 Functional restoration with behavioral support: a one-year prospective study of patients with chronic low-back pain. Spine 14: 157–161

Kelsey J L 1975 An epidemiological study of acute herniated lumbar intervertebral discs. Rheumatology and Rehabilitation 14: 144–159

Lawrence J S 1955 Rheumatism in coal miners. British Journal of Industrial Medicine 12: 249–261

Leskinen T P J, Stalhammar H R, Kuorinka I A A 1983 A dynamic analysis of spinal compression with different lifting techniques. Ergonomics 26: 595–604

Letham J, Slade P D, Troup J D G, Bentley G 1983 Outline of a fear-avoidance model of exaggerated pain perception. Behaviour Research Therapy 21: 401–408

Lindstrom L, Ohlund C, Eele C, Peterson L E, Nachemson A 1989 Work return and low back pain disability. International Society for the Study of the Lumbar Spine, Kyoto, Japan

Lloyd D C E F, Troup J D C 1983 Recurrent back pain and its prediction. Journal of Society of Occupation Medicine 33: 66–74

Lloyd P, Allan M C, Haggerty A, Lee M E, Scrivenger M, Peake S 1979 Avoiding low back injury among nurses. Report of Royal College of Nursing of the United Kingdom

Magnusson N, Granqvist M, Jonson R 1990 The loads on the lumbar spine during work at an assembly line. The risk for fatigue injuries of vertebral bodies. Spine 15: 774–779

Manning D P, Shannon H S 1979 Injuries of the lumbosacral region in a gear box factory. Journal of Society of Occupational Medicine 29: 144–148

Melzack R 1973 The puzzle of pain. Penguin Books, Middlesex, England

Merriam W F, Burwell R G, Mulholland R C, Pearson J C G, Webb J K 1983 A study revealing a tall pelvis in subjects with low back pain. Journal of Bone and Joint Surgery 65-B: 153–156

Mostardi R A, Noe D A, Kovacik M W, Porterfield J A 1992 Isokinetic lifting strength and occupational injury. A prospective study. Spine 17: 189–193

Nachemson A 1983 Work for all. Clinical Orthopaedics and Related Research 179: 77–85

Nachemson A, Elfstrom G 1970 Intravital dynamic pressure measurements in lumbar discs: a study of common movements, manoeuvres and exercises. Almqvist and Wilksell, Stockholm

Nordin M, Crites-Battie M, Pope M H 1991 Education and training. In: Pope M H, Andersson G B J, Frymoyer J W, Chaffin D B (eds) Occupational low back pain. Mosby Year Book, St Louis, p 271

Otun E O, Henrich I, Anderson J A D, Crooks J 1984 'Padas' an ambulatory electronic system to monitor and evaluate factors relating to back pain at work. Journal of Ergonomics 27: 268–271

Parnianpour, Nordin M, Kahanovitz N, Frankel V 1988 The triaxial coupling of torque generation of trunk muscles during isometric exertions and the effect of fatiguing isoinertial movements of the motor output and movement pattern. Spine 13: 982–992

Pope M H 1990 Impact and vibration and their effects on the lumbar spine. Department of Orthopaedics and Rehabilitation, University of Vermont, Burlington, USA

Pope M H, Jayson M I V, Blau A D, Kaigle A M, Weinstein J N, Wilder D J 1991 The effect of vibration on serum levels of von Willebrand's factor. Presented to the International Society for the Study of the Lumbar Spine, Heidelberg, May 1991

Porter R W 1978 Measurement of the lumbar spinal canal by diagnostic ultrasound. MD thesis, University of Edinburgh

Porter R W, Oakshott G H L 1988 Familial aspects of disc protrusion. Journal of Orthopaedic Rheumatology 1: 173–178

Porter R W, Hibbert C, Wellman P, Langton C 1980 The shape and the size of the lumbar spinal canal. Spine

Roland M O, Morrell D C, Morris R W 1983 Can general practitioners predict the outcome of episodes of back pain? British Medical Journal 286: 523–525

Scholey M 1983 Back stress: the effects of training nurses to lift patients in a clinical situation. International Journal of Nursing Studies 20: 11–13

Schultz A B, Andersson G B J, Haderspeck K, Ortengren R, Nordin M, Bjork R 1982 Analysis and measurement of lumbar trunk loads in tasks involving bends and twists. Journal of Biomechanics 15: 669–675

Stubbs D A, Buckle P W, Hudson M P, Rivers P M, Worringham R J 1983 Back pain in the nursing profession, part 1. Epidemiology and pilot methodology. Ergonomics 26: 8: 755–765

Troup J D G 1977 Dynamic factors in the analysis of the stoop and crouch lifting matters. Orthopaedic Clinics of North America 8: 201–209

Troup J D G 1979 Biomechanics of the vertebral column. Physiotherapy 65: 238–244

Troup J D G 1981 Back pain in industry: a prospective survey. Spine 6: 61–69

Versloot J M, Rozeman A, van Son M A, van Akkerveeken M D 1992 The cost effectiveness of a back school. Spine 17: 22–27

Webb P 1982 Back to self care? Physiotherapy 68: 295–297

Weinstein J, Pope M, Schmidt R, Seroussi R 1988 Neuropharmacologic effects of vibration on the dorsal root ganglion. Spine 13: 521–525

Williams B T 1984 Are public health education campaigns worthwhile? British Medical Journal 288: 170–171

Williams S J 1977 Back School. Physiotherapy 63: 90

Williamson, Danaker 1978 Self care in health. Croom Helm, London

Index